Gluten-Free, Hassle Free

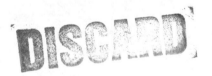

Gluten-Free, Hassle Free

A SIMPLE, SANE, DIETITIAN-APPROVED PROGRAM FOR EATING YOUR WAY BACK TO HEALTH

Marlisa Brown, RD, CDE

Illustrations by Kenneth Brown and William Cypser
Cartoon content by Marlisa Brown, RD, CDE

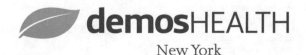

demosHEALTH

New York

Library of Congress Cataloging-in-Publication Data

Brown, Marlisa.
   Gluten-free, hassle free : a simple, sane, dietitian-approved program for eating your way back to health / Marlisa Brown ; illustrations by Kenneth Brown and William Cypser ; cartoon content by Marlisa Brown.
       p. cm.
   Includes index.
   ISBN 978-1-932603-79-8 (pbk.)
   1. Celiac disease—Diet therapy.   2. Gluten-free diet.   3. Gluten-free food.   I. Title.
   RC862.C44B76 2010
   616.3'990654—dc22

                                                    2009041763

TO MY PARENTS,
ANN AND STUART BROWN,
AND TO MY HUSBAND, RUSSELL SCHIMMENTI

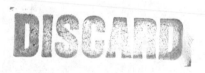

Contents

Foreword

In August 2006, when I started Allergicgirl.com, my blog about eating out in New York City with serious food allergies and dairy and wheat intolerances, I thought, *I'm alone*. But I was wrong. I quickly discovered a growing community of allergic girls and guys, celiac chicks and dudes, gluten-free men and women who were all trying to do the same thing: eat safely with joy.

I made it my personal mission to help others like me find that joy.

A licensed social worker since 2000, I established my food-allergy coaching practice, Allergic Girl Resources, Inc., in 2007 to work one-on-one with clients with dietary restrictions who want to overcome fear and anxiety and find a way back to loving and enjoying food. And in 2008, I launched my Worry-Free Dinners program to bridge the gap between restaurants that want to serve the food-restricted community and food-restricted diners who want to reclaim positive and enjoyable dining-out experiences.

But how do you regain the intoxicating mix of food and joy after the doctor tells you that you can no longer eat certain foods lest you suffer dire consequences?

You may feel waves of sadness, frustration, confusion, denial, anxiety, depression, and anger. Yet you may feel some relief that symptoms that have gone unchecked or unexplained now have a name, a diagnosis. Whether it is a food allergy, food intolerance, celiac disease, or non-celiac gluten sensitivity, a diagnosis will help you regain some sense of control over your health. However, one of the hallmarks of a diagnosis of a dietary restriction is that you can't eat certain things—ever.

But what *can* you eat? And where do you find reliable information about how to create quick, easy daily meals and snacks that will make you feel better, not worse?

A crucial path back to loving food again after you're diagnosed is to see a registered dietitian, especially one who is knowledgeable about your dietary restriction diagnosis and needs. I met Marlisa Brown—a compassionate registered dietitian with thirty years of experience and a chef with her own set of dietary restrictions—in 2007 at the International Foodservice and Restaurant Show. She was giving a talk about food allergies and food service, using her mango allergy as an example. She had yet to discover what she now knows: that she had an undiagnosed lifelong non-celiac gluten sensitivity.

Marlisa has written a book to help herself, her mother (who has celiac disease), and you get back on that path to loving food again. With easy-to-create menu ideas and suggestions, tons of gluten-free recipes, smart grain substitutions, safe gluten-free resources, and a massive list of naturally gluten-free foods, you'll be surprised how much food there is to choose from.

With Marlisa as your guide, enjoy all of the delicious gluten-free meals ahead!

Sloane Miller, MFA MSW LMSW
President, Allergic Girl Resources, Inc.
allergicgirl@gmail.com
http://allergicgirl.blogspot.com/
http://worryfreedinners.blogspot.com/
http://allergicgirlresources.com/
http://twitter.com/allergicgirl

Introduction

It's Much Easier
Than You Think

You're probably reading this book because you or someone you know may have celiac disease or a non-celiac gluten sensitivity. If so, you've taken the all-important first step to making gluten-free living easy and uncomplicated.

Gluten is often the hidden culprit at the root of many health problems. However, eating your way back to health doesn't have to be painful or difficult. Know that you are not alone. Millions of people of all ages and backgrounds share the challenges of living gluten-free. This book contains a wealth of information, including tips, strategies, and shortcuts to make your journey easier.

When people first learn (or suspect) that they can't eat gluten, they often feel scared, angry, frustrated, and confused—and with good reason. They have health problems that they don't understand, and they suddenly have to make huge, unexpected changes in what and how they eat. To most people, the whole prospect can seem overwhelming.

The transition can seem complicated, even to a dietitian. When I first began investigating gluten-free diets some years ago, I discovered layer upon layer of confusing (and sometimes contradictory) information on the subject. It took me some time to sort through it all and learn what was true, what was speculation, and what was somebody's best guess. My training made it easier for me to make sense of it all, but I saw how the details and contradictions could leave many people feeling lost. I also discovered that there was a great deal that science still didn't yet understand about the subject.

Even so, living without gluten doesn't have to be difficult or complex for you.

Part of my job as a registered dietitian and nutrition consultant is to make things simple and understandable for ordinary people. Over the past 15 years, many hundreds of people have come to me with gluten-related health problems, including my own mother. I still remember her reaction when she first found out about her condition. "I just want to be healthy!" she shouted at me over the phone. "Is that too much to ask? Can't you just tell me what I can and can't eat? The more I read about it all, the more complicated it gets. You're a dietitian, for heaven's sake! Can't you make it simple for me?"

I've also faced the same situation even more personally. For years I suffered from recurring stomach problems, but tests for celiac disease and other digestive ailments always came back negative. I was eventually given a diagnosis of irritable bowel syndrome. But after my mother tested positive for celiac, I decided that celiac disease might also be my problem, since it tends to run in families. I needed to find a solution, so as an experiment. I tried a gluten-free diet. Within a few days, my stomach pains began to disappear. What do you know!

I've been a foodie from birth. I was a chef before I became a dietitian. I love everything about food—cooking it, growing it, tasting it, and reading about it. So I knew I had to find ways to make the necessary dietary changes while still being able to enjoy the arts of cooking and eating.

In short, I know how you feel, and I am with you 100 percent. This book is an uncomplicated, easy-to-follow way to make gluten-free eating work for anyone who likes to eat: for you, me, other chefs, other foodies, and my mother.

Right now you're probably feeling stressed out, because you have to relearn how to shop, how to cook, and how to eat in restaurants. You also have to deal with your family, coworkers, friends, and acquaintances. They may not understand your diet, and they may not want to understand it—they may even think you're weird, neurotic, or just being difficult. This book will help you set them straight.

Maybe you've already looked at some of the other books on gluten-free cooking, eating, and living that have been so loaded with technical and scientific detail that you feel even more confused. You shouldn't need a PhD in nutrition in order to make the changes that will help you get and stay healthy. Gluten-free *can* be hassle-free.

As a registered dietitian and president of Total Wellness, Inc., a New York–based health consulting company, I have found that when people come to me for help, they don't want a long lecture or a longer list of things that they can't and shouldn't do. Instead, they want to know what they *can* do. They want someone who can lay things out for them and give them a step-by-step plan that lets them live their lives the way they're used to living them.

Everything about *Gluten-Free, Hassle-Free* is designed to make gluten-free living as simple, doable, worry-free, and easy to understand as possible. From "Safe Supermarket Shopping" to "Gluten-Free at the Deli Counter and in Fast Food Restaurants" to "Making Social Events Easier for Everyone" to "Stocking a Gluten-Free Kitchen," each section of this book is practical, down to earth, and easy to follow. You can quickly find what you need, immediately put it into practice, and instantly begin improving your life. You'll also find a wealth of shortcuts, tips, and special tools—each of which can save you time, trouble, headaches, and heartache.

Over the past 15 years, I've helped thousands of people dramatically improve their health through an easy step-by-step process. Many of these people have celiac disease or non-celiac gluten sensitivity. They come to my office looking for simple solutions; they leave not only with those solutions, but also with relief and hope.

I'm glad you're here. Your healthier, happier life begins right now.

Marlisa Brown

Acknowledgments

There are so many people who made this book possible that I would like to thank: my husband Russell for endless gluten-free tastings, my family for their support, my brother Kenneth Brown for his creative Dee cartoon character, and my agent Stephany Evans for her encouragement from the beginning of this project. In addition, special thanks go to Catherine Brittan for her hard work on all aspects of this book, and to Sloane Miller for her contributions. I would also like to thank my sisters-in-law (Rosemarie Kass, Barbara Schimmenti, and Eileen Ciaccio) for experimenting with gluten-free holiday meals. To my soul sister Constance Brown-Riggs for her continued encouragement during the development of this book. I also received a great deal of support from the nutrition department at CW Post, especially Sandy Sarcona and the following dietetic interns and students: Alessandra Pacino, Alision Gerber, Anne Dyling, Ariella, Joanne Johnson, Atsuko Shiraishi, Madeline Orland, Michelle Serpas, Ryan Whitcomb, and Nicole Cousins. Finally, I would also like to thank Shelley Case and Carol Fenster for their work with celiac disease and gluten-free cooking and for their creative feedback on this project.

Special thanks to:
- Catherine Brittan, MS, RD, LD
- Jodi Wright, MS, RD, CDN
- Yvonne Mullman, RD, CDN
- Randy Yaskal at the Center for International Studies and Foreign Languages, for her help with some of the more complex translations. Translatethisdocument.com.

Gluten-Free, Hassle Free

PART I: MAKING THE CHANGE

Is Your Diet Putting Your Health at Risk?

Finding Out Whether You Are Gluten-Intolerant

Are You at Risk?

When it comes to our own health, most of us feel that we are doing the best we can, and we accept our daily aches and pains as something which is normal for us. We tend to distance ourselves from the thought that our health could decline until it does, and then we are forced to deal with it.

None of us can predict the health challenges we'll encounter in our lifetime, but your body often does give clues, if you learn to listen and know what to look for. In the case of celiac disease, the symptoms show up in hundreds of different ways.

What Is Celiac Disease?

Celiac disease is thought to have been around for thousands of years, and may have started back when human kind switched to a diet that included wheat. Even though celiac disease has been around for so long, science has just begun to understand how to diagnosis and treat it as well as the risks associated with it. Only 10 years ago, celiac disease was considered a rare European disease. Recent research has discovered that celiac disease can affect as many as 1 in 133 Americans— approximately 2 million people. Celiac disease affects about 1 percent of the population in the world, including in North Africa, Asia, and South America. And yet about 97 percent of people living with celiac disease go undiagnosed.

Celiac disease is caused by a reaction to the gluten (pronounced glOO-ten) found in certain foods. Gluten is mostly found in wheat, rye, and barley, so when you eat these starches, or when they are added to your food, you are consuming gluten. It is the protein part of wheat, rye, and barley that contains gluten. Gluten is actually a mix of proteins, specifically gliadin and glutenin. When people suffer from food allergies or sensitivities, they are reacting to the proteins in those foods, which therefore should be avoided. Celiac disease is not considered an allergy, but rather a sensitivity to the gluten found in food. This sensitivity will cause an autoimmune response any time the protein gluten is ingested. Therefore gluten must be avoided at all times. Depending on whom you speak to, celiac disease may be referred to as a sensitivity or as a gluten intolerance, but no matter how you say it, if the diagnosis is celiac disease, gluten can never be consumed. In addition to being found naturally in grains, gluten is also added to many foods. You may ask why add gluten to food? Well, gluten is the "glue" that holds the ingredients together, giving breads and other foods the texture we are all used to.

Since celiac disease is activated by the foods we eat, it primarily affects the digestive system, but when left untreated it can affect the entire body. Celiac usually presents itself in the small intestine, a 22-foot-long organ covered with tiny hairlike things called villi. It is through the villi that our bodies absorb nutrients. Celiac disease flattens the villi, making it difficult for our gastrointestinal tract to function correctly. Although 50 percent of those with celiac suffer from gastrointestinal disturbances, many people who are affected often have no notable symptoms at all. It is often difficult to diagnose celiac disease, because the symptoms vary from person to person—and the villi get flattened in patchy segments. If not enough villi samples are taken, the flattened villi may not be identified, and the disease can easily be missed.

Celiac disease can affect every person differently; one may have stomach pains or be depressed and tired all the time, but another may feel sick only once in a while, and still another may feel just fine. And the disease can develop at any age, from infancy to old age, so it's hard to know when to look out for it. And because it can show up in many ways, your doctor may attempt to treat you for other ailments, such as Crohn's disease, chronic fatigue, irritable bowel syndrome, thyroid disorder, osteoporosis, diverticulitis, or rheumatoid arthritis—anything and everything but the celiac disease. Because there are no "typical" symptoms of celiac disease, it is not the first thing doctors think of. It's no wonder that so many who have celiac disease remain undiagnosed. It has been shown that most people with celiac disease will spend an average of about 11 years going to doctors and specialists before they figure out what the cause of their problems is.[1] Numerous studies have shown that many people diagnosed with other diseases, such as irritable bowel syndrome, are actually are suffering with undiagnosed celiac disease.

How do we get celiac disease? We don't know how, but we now know that it runs in families (90 percent of people with celiac disease have genetic markers) and involves the immune system, the part of our body that fights off infections. If you have a first-degree relative (sibling or parent) with celiac disease, you have a much higher chance of also having celiac disease. That is why if someone in your family has celiac disease, it is important that you be tested for it as well.

The following checklists will help you evaluate your risk and focus on prevention. If you have already been diagnosed with celiac disease or suffer from a non-celiac gluten sensitivity, proceed directly to "Learning the Basics" in Chapter 2.

Recognizing Symptoms of Celiac Disease

Section A

Put a check next to any of the health problems below that you have or think you may have experienced at one time or another:

———— Anemia
———— Behavioral changes
———— Bloating, gas, or abdominal pain
———— Bones that break easily
———— Bone or joint pain
———— Bruising
———— Chronic fatigue

---

[1] Fasano A., Berti I., Gerarduzzi, et al. A multicenter study on the sero-prevalence of celiac disease in the United States among both at risk and not at risk groups. *Arch Int Med* 2003; 163:268–292.

————— Delayed growth as a child
————— Dental enamel problems
————— Depression or irritability
————— Diarrhea or constipation
————— Discolored teeth or enamel problems
————— Canker sores
————— Dry eyes
————— Edema (swelling, especially found in hands and feet)
————— Epstein–Barr
————— Failure to thrive (in children)
————— Fatigue
————— Frequent bowel movements
————— Frequent infections
————— Frequent illness
————— Hard-to-flush stools
————— Inability to lose weight
————— Indigestion
————— Infertility
————— Irritability
————— Joint pain
————— Lactose intolerance
————— Learning difficulties
————— Memory problems
————— Menstrual problems
————— Migraines
————— Mouth sores and ulcers (canker sores)
————— Nutritional deficiencies (iron, calcium, vitamins A, D, E, and K)
————— Reflux (heartburn)
————— Seizures
————— Short stature
————— Skin problems and rashes
————— Tingling or numbness in hands and feet
————— Unexplained weight loss
————— Unexplained weight gain

Count how many items you have checked in Section A: _____.

If you have checked 2 or more of the items in this section, you should be screened for celiac disease.

Not everyone who has celiac disease will have symptoms!

Section B

Some diseases are sometimes attributed to celiac disease. Please check any of the following health problems with which you have been diagnosed:

———— Addison's disease

———— Alopecia areata

———— Anemia

———— Autoimmune disorders

———— Autism

———— ADHD

———— Central and peripheral nervous system disorders

———— Dermatitis herpetiformis

———— Down syndrome

———— Family history of celiac disease (any relative with celiac disease)

———— Gastro-intestinal malignancies

———— IBS (irritable bowel syndrome)

———— Inflammatory bowel disease (ulcerative colitis, Crohn's disease)

———— Intestinal lymphomas

———— Hepatitis

———— IgA deficiency

———— Infertility

———— Intestinal cancer

———— Juvenile idiopathic arthritis

———— Lymphoma

———— Myasthenia Gravis

———— Non-Hodgkin's lymphoma

———— Osteoporosis

———— Pancreatic insufficiency

———— Peripheral neuropathy

———— Primary biliary cirrhosis

———— Psoriasis

———— Recurrent aphthous ulcerations

———— Rheumatoid arthritis

———— Sarcoidosis

———— Scleroderma

———— Selective IgA deficiency

———— Sjögren's disease

———— Systemic lupus erythematosus

———— Thyroid disease

———— Turner syndrome

———— Type 1 diabetes (DM1) (in you or any of your first-degree relatives)

———— Williams syndrome

Count how many items have you checked in section B: _____.

If you have checked 1 or more of the items in this section, you should be screened for celiac disease.

You think, "These lists are so long—they can't all be linked to celiac disease, can they?" But celiac disease affects your immune system as well as your gastrointestinal system. Many problems begin when gluten is digested. It may trigger the autoimmune system in your body, which could lead to illness and the development of disease states. How you are affected depends on your body's weak spots, which will influence where your immune system decides to attack. For instance, it has long been known that there is a relationship between type 1 diabetes and celiac disease. This is why the American Diabetes Association recommends that all first-degree relatives of those who have type 1 diabetes be screened for celiac disease. More recently, scientists have been looking at the chromosomal abnormalities that are similar among those with type 1 diabetes and those with celiac disease. There is some speculation suggesting that gluten may even be the trigger for the autoimmune process that causes type 1 diabetes, but at this time it is only speculation. You can determine your potential risk by identifying the specific diseases that are most commonly associated with celiac disease, and by evaluating your symptoms and your family history.

Useful and Not-So-Useful Medical Tests

It is estimated that 1 in 100 people worldwide suffers from celiac disease. The easiest way to screen for celiac disease is with blood tests. Unfortunately none of the tests alone are 100 percent accurate, nor can they be used to rule out celiac or to diagnose you. But they can help indicate a potential risk.

When Screening for Celiac Disease, These Blood Tests Should be Used:

1. **IgA and IgG anti-tissue transglutaminase antibody (anti-tTG):** If this test is positive, it is very likely that you have celiac disease, but false positives are possible in people with type 1 diabetes and auto-immune hepatitis, and possibly in other autoimmune diseases.

2. **IgA and IgG anti-gliadin antibodies (AGA):** These tests have a low level of accuracy and are not used as much any more except with young children. In children, the EMA and anti-tTG is not as accurate due to the children's immature immune systems.

3. **IgA anti-endomysial antibodies (EMA):** This test has mostly been replaced by the anti-tTG test but is not reliable in children younger than 2. This test is highly specific but is not as sensitive as anti-tTG. Also, this test requires human analysis, which leaves room for human error if the slides are not read correctly.

4. **IgA and IgG anti-deaminated gliadin peptide antibodies (anti-DGP):** This test is a new version of the older AGA tests, and its accuracy is higher than that of the original tests. Although anti-tTG is still considered the best test for adults, in cases in which someone also has an IgA deficiency (see note below), the DGP may be more accurate than either of the anti-tTG antibody tests.

* Please note that when being screened for celiac disease it is also important to have a total serum IgA test, which is used to identify an IgA deficiency. Many of the screenings rely on the IgA to identify celiac disease; if you have an IgA deficiency, the results of celiac screening may not be accurate. Deficiencies in general are rare, but they are slightly more common in those who have celiac disease.

Genetic Tests

About 95 percent of patients with celiac disease have the genes HLA-DQ2 and HLA-DQ8. Thus, if an individual comes back negative on the above blood tests but has symptoms of celiac disease and are positive on the DQ2 and DQ8 tests, they most likely have celiac disease. If they do not have these genes it is unlikely that they have celiac disease.

* Please note DNA testing is available from Kimball Genetics: 101 University Blvd., Suite #350, Denver CO 80206; 1 (800) 320-1807; www.kimballgenetics.com.

Interpreting the Results

- If you are positive on any one of the blood tests, go directly to the diagnostic tests.

- If you are negative on all the blood screening tests but have checked several items in section A or B, and no other cause of your illness has been found, talk to your doctor about being tested further for celiac disease.

- If you are negative on all the blood screening tests but have checked off anything in section A or B, and have a relative who is suffering from celiac disease, talk to your doctor about further celiac testing.

- If you are either positive or negative on the blood tests and do not want to go for diagnostic tests right away, you can do a simple DNA test, as noted above. This test—which is sometimes covered by insurance—will isolate whether or not you have the gene or DNA that is found in 95 percent of those who develop celiac disease. If you do not have the DNA, it is very unlikely that you could have celiac disease. If this test is positive, you should go for diagnostic tests (see our resource section for more information on testing).

Diagnostic Tests

If you are positive on any of the blood tests, make sure you follow up by having an endoscopy of the small intestine (duodenum or jejunum). Blood tests are a good screening tool, but they cannot currently be used alone to diagnose celiac disease. The endoscopic procedure is done to identify flattened villi in the small intestine which are found in someone who has celiac disease. Villi are a fingerlike covering on the lining of your intestines and are responsible for nutrient absorption. An endoscopy, along with a biopsy, is the only way to get a conclusive diagnosis for celiac disease. You will need to have an endoscopy with multiple samples taken in a maize pattern, since celiac disease can be patchy and can easily be missed during testing. Taking a number of samples from various locations will give you a better chance of being properly diagnosed. The endoscopic procedure is a relatively quick, painless procedure that will be done while you are under anesthesia. Try to find a specialist or gastroenterologist who works often with patients who have celiac disease. A gastroenterologist is a doctor who specializes in treatment and diagnosis of gastrointestinal problems. Some doctors work more extensively with celiac patients than others and are more likely to give an accurate diagnosis. Often when a diagnosis of celiac disease is missed, it is due to either an insufficient number of samples taken or a misinterpretation of the test results. If a diagnoses of celiac is not found, it is important to have a full range of gastrointestinal tests done to rule out any other illness. If nothing is found, consider being retested for celiac disease.

 WHEN WORKING WITH YOUR DOCTOR

You have the right . . .
- to be heard.
- to have all your questions answered.
- to be retested if you do not have any diagnosis that explains your symptoms.
- to a second opinion.
- to see a specialist (such as a gastroenterologist that specializes in celiac disease).
- to be taken seriously. Just because they haven't found the root of your illness doesn't mean it is all in your head.
- to see a registered dietitian who specializes in celiac disease.

It is possible to pass screening and diagnostic tests and still be at risk, but if you do not have symptoms, the risk is minimal. If you do have symptoms, consider being retested. If you have symptoms and do not wish to have repeat testing, and no other medical explanation is found, consider experimenting with a test diet (by trying the quick-start meal plan found in Chapter 2) to see whether your symptoms improve. There is no cure for celiac disease; the only treatment is to follow a gluten-free diet. People with celiac disease begin to have some improvement in symptoms within a few days of initiating a gluten-free diet.

Although it's understandable that anyone would want to start feeling better right away, it's generally not recommended to start the gluten-free diet if you are still being tested for celiac disease, as it may interfere with your diagnosis, since your villi will begin to heal. And if you start the diet without being diagnosed, you may not be as committed to following the diet.

> **TIP**
> Prior to starting a gluten-free diet, it is important to first undergo needed medical tests to rule out the possibility of any serious health problems.

Another Sign of Celiac Disease

A skin disorder called **dermatitis herpetiformis (DH)**, a prickly, itchy skin rash usually found on elbows and knees, is closely associated with celiac disease. If a person has dermatitis herpetiformis and it has been sampled and shown to be positive for celiac disease, no further testing is needed to confirm the diagnosis of celiac.

If You Have Celiac Disease

Following a gluten-free diet works by allowing those villi covering your small intestine to heal and return to normal so that you can once again absorb all the nutrients from food. This, in turn, allows your immune system to improve. Many people who start the diet after discovering that they have celiac disease will begin to feel better within 48 hours. Younger people may completely heal in several months, but it can sometimes take two to three years for an adult's villi to heal entirely.

Now that so many people are being diagnosed with celiac disease, more research is being done that is helping provide us with new information. Scientists are looking for different ways to treat celiac disease. One approach is to develop medications to help the body handle the gluten protein so that gluten can be consumed safely; there is ongoing research in this area.

Presently, however, there is no magic bullet. If you are diagnosed with celiac disease, following a gluten-free diet must be taken seriously. It is a lifelong commitment that takes dedication. You may have already spent years feeling terrible and frustrated because you have been going to doctor after doctor, feeling like no one is helping. Initially, you may feel overwhelmed when you realize all the changes you will need to make to follow a gluten-free lifestyle. In Chapter 2, you will find an easy quick-start plan to begin following a gluten-free diet. It is also important to find a registered dietitian who specializes in celiac disease to answer any questions and to help you identify problem-solving issues. There is a listing of some dietitians specializing in celiac disease in the resource section of this book.

If you're a parent who has a child with celiac disease, it may be difficult to explain why he or she can no longer have their favorite foods. You may feel uncomfortable about asking your friends or family to make special dishes for you or asking about all the ingredients in the recipes. Going on vacation can be challenging, since all food is usually eaten out. You may also sometimes feel it is just easier to stay home!

The good news is that today there is much more information available to help you follow a gluten-free lifestyle, including organizations, Web sites, and support groups. Supermarkets are starting to carry more gluten-free foods, and more and more companies are producing and selling thousands of gluten-free foods on the internet. There's beginning to be a much greater awareness of celiac disease and non-celiac gluten sensitivity—even many restaurants now have gluten-free options listed on their menus. Receiving a diagnosis of celiac disease can be difficult, but with patience and education, you can lead a normal, happy, and healthier life.

Celiac Sprue vs. Refractory Sprue

A very small percentage of people with celiac disease will not experience improved health even after six months to a year on a strict gluten-free diet. These individuals may have developed refractory sprue. Treatment options may include a combination of therapies such as steroids and immune-suppressive drugs, along with a gluten-free diet.

Refractory sprue is thought to be a malignant condition, and people with this condition are often malnourished and have weakened immune systems. Close monitoring by a physician is necessary, as in many cases malabsorption and malnutrition progress despite treatment, and nutrition may have to be delivered via alternate routes, such as TPN (total parental nutrition)—IV feeding that bypasses the gastrointestinal tract completely and delivers nutrients directly into the bloodstream.

It is unknown why refractory sprue develops. One theory is that since it is usually only found in older adults, it may have developed due to celiac disease having been present and untreated for many years. Left unchecked and untreated, refractory sprue condition can lead to many complications as well as higher risk for cancer. It is thought that something as simple as following a gluten-free diet early after diagnosis on can prevent this condition from developing.

Can Eating Less Gluten Improve Everyone's Health?

There are times you might consider a gluten-free diet even if you are sure you don't have celiac disease. A good number of my patients have reported that they become ill whenever they consume gluten, even though they have been tested many times for celiac disease and nothing has been found. Often this intolerance to gluten is refered to non-celiac gluten intolerance or non-celiac gluten sensitivity. In addition, many parents of autistic children report an improvement in their child's behavior when they put their child on a gluten-free diet. (For more information on autism and a gluten-free diet, see Chapter 15.)

Non-celiac gluten sensitivity is currently not recognized as a disease. However, there may be other forms of celiac disease that are yet to be discovered. We don't know how to test for non-celiac gluten sensitivity, and so today we just call it that, or non-celiac gluten intolerance. Hopefully the future may show us answers to many of these questions.

Why is gluten causing so many problems today? Perhaps because it is a larger protein that is difficult to digest, or maybe because we are adding gluten to so many foods. There is so much more to learn, but it is important to note that following a gluten-free diet can help a lot of people.

Learning the Basics (But Not the Needless Details) of Living Gluten-Free

What Does Gluten-Free Living Really Mean?

The doctor walks in, reporting that the results of your tests have arrived, and it is good news. They have finally identified what has been making you so ill, and it is something that is easy to treat: the root of all your ailments is that you have celiac disease, which, put simply, means that you have a problem digesting the gluten found in food. In a sigh of relief you burst out, "Thank God! Thank you so much—I was so worried. Now, tell me again, what did you say . . . gloo what?"

The doctor repeats, "Gluten—you can't eat gluten. Just stop eating gluten, and you will feel yourself again." He hands you some papers and says, "Here is a list of foods that may contain gluten."

What a relief—it's not as serious as you had feared. It is as if someone removed a huge weight from your shoulders: all you need to do is change your diet. This is something you can live with. You glance down at the list of foods the doctor gave you. Everything on the "do not eat" side are the foods that you do eat. Hardly any of the foods you normally eat are on the list noted as safe. If hardly anything is safe, how can you eat at all? Can having a problem with one little thing like gluten affect everything? *A million questions come to mind, but who can you ask? The doctor didn't give you any instructions except to follow this list, but surely there has to be bigger list of foods you can eat, a list of gluten-free foods?*

In theory you're right. But finding a list of foods that are gluten-free is not as easy as it should be, because gluten is often hidden within many foods. Gluten is used as filler and a flavoring agent and is often mixed

15

D's Dieting Dilemmas

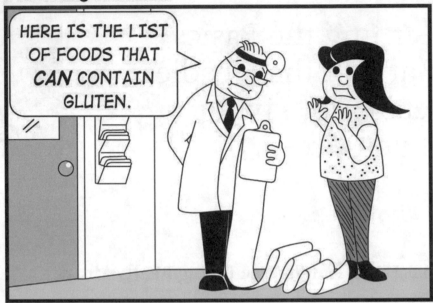

By M Brown Ken Brown and Will Cypser ©

into food during the production process due to cross-contamination. So you can't even always know what is okay to eat and what is not. Every label must be checked and analyzed. But don't despair!

TIP
Getting started is easy as long as you have the right tools.

Getting Started

All you need to know is what to look for on labels, what to ask when calling companies about their products, what to look for when dining out, and how to substitute alternate grains and seasonings in your recipes when needed. As with anything new, acquiring these skills takes a little time. It may seem like a lot of work, but making these changes will be well worth the improvements you'll experience in your health and in your daily life.

Whether you are a great cook or buy all your meals on the run, the tools for success are the same:

- **Shopping:** Buy gluten-free products, and use them in place of your regular breads, bagels, cereals, pizzas, and pastas. Find out which stores in your area carry gluten-free choices, and where these foods and ingredients can be ordered online. There is a large listing of companies that carry gluten-free choices in Chapter 10.

- **Labels:** Start looking at food labels. Gluten may lurk where you least expect it. Ingredients that could contain wheat gluten may include seasonings, modified food starch, and hydrolyzed vegetable protein. Common ingredients that may contain barley gluten may be listed as malt. For more information and details on what to look out for when reading labels, see Chapter 6.

- **Dining Out:** Locate restaurants that have gluten-free menus or those that understand your dietary restrictions and are willing to work with you on making substitutions. This will make your dining experience much more enjoyable. In our resource section I have included a list of restaurants that have already started listing gluten-free choices on their menus. Some restaurants have much more extensive gluten-free choices, so make sure you contact them and review their menu prior to dining out. The most important difficulty with most restaurants is the hidden gluten due to cross-contamination.

- **Events:** Trying to explain your restrictions to a busy wait staff at a crowded noisy function can be uncomfortable. To be sure safe choices will be available when you will be dining at preset functions, such as weddings, large meetings, and conventions, call catering halls ahead of time. By calling in advance, you will know which places can accommodate you, when you need to bring food with you, and where to find the best gluten-free cuisine.

- **Gluten-Free Cooking:** Start developing a list of great gluten-free recipe favorites. I have included many delicious recipes in this book in Chapters 4 and 11, as well as quick and easy mix-and-match meals that are listed in Chapter 5.

- **Support:** Many towns and regions have local celiac support groups. Join one of these and check out events and local functions. Join the listservs such as www.enabling.org/ia/celiac/index.html to help you network on important issues and go to the Celiac Sprue Association Web site at www.csaceliacs.org. In the resource section at the end of this book, you'll find a listing of local celiac organizations in your area, and my own site, www.glutenfree-hasslefree.com, also includes listings of different gluten-related events throughout the country.

- **Family and Friends:** Educate your family and friends about your dietary needs in order for them to understand how careful you need to be. See "Getting Started Living Gluten-Free," in Chapter 13.

Why Can't I Cheat Sometimes?

Most people ask why they can't have gluten just on rare occasions. This is the most common question I get asked, and it seems like a reasonable request; after all, many who are on other types of special diets do "cheat" on occasion. Unfortunately, for those who have celiac disease, this is not an option. Each time gluten is consumed, celiac disease triggers an autoimmune reaction in the body and does damage to the intestinal wall. These negative reactions occur any time gluten is consumed, and once they are started, it may take some time for your body to return to normal. The future may provide some relief; currently ongoing research is exploring the possibility of taking a pill when gluten is consumed, but at present all the kinks are not worked out, so for now, *gluten should never be consumed*. This is, without question, the most difficult part of caring for your condition. But the rewards of a healthier life, having more energy, and really feeling good will certainly outweigh the hardships.

> **TIP**
> If you have celiac disease you can never eat gluten.

It may be hard to believe, but even the smallest amount of gluten can cause a reaction. Those with celiac must be vigilant when it comes to the risk of cross-contamination. Consider this: someone with celiac disease or non-celiac gluten sensitivity cannot even safely use a toaster that has previously been used to toast wheat-containing bread, or a spatula that has been used to turn wheat-containing pancakes. Even a spread such as mayonnaise, mustard, peanut butter, or jelly that has previously been used on bread is no longer safe if the knife was put back into the jar! Just a pinhead's worth of gluten is enough to make someone sick. Left untreated, celiac disease can lead to serious consequences, so it is important for others in your life to understand that you are not being difficult: you really must avoid any trace of gluten, or you will get ill. No exceptions. Again, Chapter 13 provides a list of what others need to know about "Getting Started Living Gluten-Free," and Chapter 7 will give you some suggestions for how to handle your feelings as you adjust to what is most likely a dramatic difference in your diet and lifestyle.

TIP
There are many foods that are naturally gluten-free.

Simple Gluten-Free Eating

Prior to delving into the vast variety of gluten-free foods available from other sources, such as specialty shops, health food stores, and the Internet, it's good to become familiar with what may be available to you in your local grocery. To minimize any sense of being overwhelmed you may be experiencing when newly diagnosed with celiac disease, we'll keep it simple at this stage. Later in this book, more extensive lists of gluten-free choices will be discussed.

Some supermarkets have elaborate gluten-free sections, but others have only a few items located in the refrigerator or health food aisles. This "starter" meal plan is designed around common, familiar, readily available foods—easy to find, easy to prepare, and gluten-free. In Chapter 3, there are more extensive lists of gluten-free choices for those of you who are ready to dive in. "Safe Supermarket Shopping" will give you the tools needed to put meals together from your average supermarket.

> **Every effort was made to check the gluten-free status of the brands listed. Manufacturers may change ingredients from time to time. When in doubt, choose an alternate product or contact the manufacturer.**

In the beginning, reading every label that you pick up at your local supermarket can seem overwhelming. The following includes some brand name suggestions so you can just pick up products and go. Also any product with gluten-free noted on the label can also be used. Since companies often change their formulas, it is important to call companies and to read labels to double check products' gluten-free status. The brands listed below will give you possible choices to include in your starter meal plan. Many other brands contain gluten-free choices as well and can be substituted in this meal plan. There are many gluten-free brands listed in Chapter 10.

Picking Off the Shelf

There are many foods that are safe for those following a gluten-free diet; some are naturally gluten-free, and others require a gluten-free alternative. See Chapter 3 for more detailed listings of gluten-free foods.

Alcohol: All distilled alcohols (such as vodka, gin, and scotch) are considered gluten-free. Beer is not distilled, and it is not gluten-free, since it is made from barley. However, many gluten-free beers are now being produced. Chapter 10 includes a listing of gluten-free beers.

Beans, Tofu, and Soy: Beans are gluten-free, and high in fiber, but on rare occasions gluten may be added to flavored beans. To be safe, buy canned or dried plain, unseasoned beans, or check the packaging to make sure no gluten-containing ingredient was added. Tofu is also gluten-free unless it is baked or marinated in a gluten-containing ingredient, such as soy sauce. Although most soy products are gluten-free, except those containing barley malt or fillers, soy sauce is usually made from wheat, and cannot be used. However, there are some gluten-free varieties of soy sauce available, such as Eden Tamarai, Jade Dragon, La Choy, Panda (carry-out packets), Wal-Mart's Great Value, and SanJ (Organic Tamari Wheat Free Soy Sauce). Most restaurants' soy sauce and teriyaki sauce usually contains gluten unless the restaurant has a gluten-free menu that specifies otherwise.

Chips (Potato and Corn): Most brands are made from just corn or potato with only oil and salt added and are gluten-free. When unsure, pick unflavored chips, which are much less likely to contain gluten. Some brands that are mostly gluten-free include Cape Cod, Fritos, Lay's, Ruffles, Tostitos, UTZ, and Wise.

Cheese: Real cheeses are gluten-free (unless there are gluten-containing ingredients folded into the cheese, as in the cases of blends and cheese spreads). So in the beginning, it is best to pick 100 percent pure cheese products.

Cold Cuts: Many brands have gluten-free choices such as Boar's Head, Hillshire Farms, Hormel, and Wellshire Farms. When you are uncertain, it is safest to pick pure meats that are 100 percent meat, like real roasted turkey or roast beef, with no added fillers. Always ask if it is possible for the machine to be wiped down prior to having your cold cuts sliced, since you cannot be sure if gluten-containing products have been sliced previously on that equipment.

Cereal: Most store brand cereals contain gluten—even some cereals that may appear safe, such as Rice Krispies, have gluten. On occasion you can find a cereal in the supermarket that is safe to eat, such as Rice Chex, Corn Chex, Honey Nut Chex, Chocolate Chex, Cinnamon Chex, grits, cream of rice, and Nature's Path Mesa Sunrise cereal, but in general, most gluten-free cereals will be found in specialty and health food stores.

Corn Tortillas: Most brands are gluten-free, but, again, read the labels to make sure there are no added ingredients. If the label says corn, salt, and oil and there is no warning about possible wheat contamination, it is usually safe to use. Some gluten-free brands of corn tortillas include Don Pancho, Food for Life, La Tortilla Factory (Dark & Ivory Teff Gluten-Free Wraps), Manny's (Corn Tortillas), Mission, Que Pasa, Snyder's of Hanover (Corn Tortillas [White, Yellow]), Trader Joe's (Corn Tortillas, Handmade, Original).

Dairy Products: Milk, half-and-half, cream, cream cheese, cottage cheese, butter, and ricotta cheese are naturally gluten-free. Processed cheese blends, some light sour creams, and many flavored yogurts and other flavored dairy products may contain gluten. Laughing Cow cheese blends and Friendship's light sour cream are gluten-free. Gluten-free yogurt choices are listed later in this chapter.

Desserts: Most ice cream, sherbet, sorbet, popsicles, whipped topping, and egg custards are gluten-free, except those with cookie dough or toppings mixed in (check labels for added fillers).

Many gluten-free desserts are now available; see the recipe selections found in Chapters 4 and 11, and the product listings in Chapter 10. Some examples of gluten-free dessert mixes include those sold by Pamela's Products, 123 Gluten-free, and Bob's Red Mill.

Eggs: All eggs and egg whites, as well as most egg substitutes, are gluten-free.

Fish: All fresh fish is gluten-free, unless it is breaded or in a gluten-containing marinade. Frozen fish needs to be checked for gluten, because it is often marinated or breaded. So, for now, stick with fresh fish, or buy canned gluten-free choices such as plain Bumble Bee, Starkist, or other gluten-free varieties. (Please note, don't choose the flavored or herb choices, or those that come with crackers; they usually contain gluten.)

Gluten-Free Flours, Grains, and Starches: There are many grains and flours that are naturally gluten-free, such as almond, amaranth, bean, buckwheat, coconut, cornmeal, grits, millet, gluten-free oats, potato, quinoa, rice, sorghum, and teff flours, all of which are usually gluten-free (please be careful if flavoring agents or fillers are added, because they may contain gluten; also, be on your guard against grain manufacturing processes contaminated with gluten). When in doubt, look for a gluten-free label on the packaging to be sure it is safe.

There are also many gluten-free cereals, bars, breads, rolls, pastas, muffins, and mixes available. Chapter 10 contains listings of where to find gluten-free grains; today, you can find many gluten-free choices available in supermarkets and health food and specialty stores. Fresh potatoes are always gluten-free, and 100 percent pure potato starch or flakes are safe. A safe grain found in supermarkets is rice, available in a number of varieties: brown, jasmine, instant, long grain, and so forth. However, avoid supermarket rice blends—Rice a Roni, for example, contains gluten.

Ices: Almost all ices are gluten-free, but don't buy ices that have crunchies, sprinkles, or cookie dough folded in. When in doubt, look for gluten-free on the label or check the ingredients to make sure there is no added wheat or barley malt.

Ice Cream: Many ice creams are gluten-free, but it is important to check the labels to make sure that no cookies, wafers, chips, sprinkles, wheat, or barley malt have been added. Most ice creams at ice cream parlors are also gluten-free. However, they are often contaminated with gluten because the same scoop is used for all flavors. Most Edy's and Haagen-Dazs flavors are gluten-free, except those with cookies or crumbs added.

Meats and Poultry: Most are gluten-free except those that are breaded or those that are marinated in a gluten-containing mixture. Poultry that has a self-basting agent or broth added usually also contains gluten. Make sure you use 100 percent pure poultry, beef, and pork to be safe. Look for those that have no additives listed in the ingredients. If you want to marinate foods, do so yourself by using gluten-free marinades and dressings.

Nuts and Oils: Almost all nuts and vegetable oils are gluten-free unless the nuts are coated with a flavoring agent or processed on equipment that has also processed wheat. Butter, margarine, and shortening are also gluten-free.

Oats: In the past, it was thought that those following a gluten-free diet could not consume oats, even though pure oats do not contain gluten. Recent evidence has shown that if oats are grown and processed so that they do not get contaminated with gluten, they should be safe for many who are following a gluten-free diet. When using oats, make sure they are from a gluten-free source (many sources of gluten-free oats are listed in Chapter 10). Before adding oats to your diet make sure you have been successfully following a gluten-free diet and are symptom-free. Only introduce oats in limited quantities—about 50 grams per day for adults (1/2 cup dry) and 20–25 grams per day for children (1/4 cup dry)—to see if it is tolerated. However, some individuals with celiac disease may not be able to include oats in their diets, because even though oats do not contain gluten, they do contain the protein avenin, which may awaken the immune system in certain individuals. It is thus important to introduce oats carefully, with the support of a health care team. Supermarkets generally do not carry gluten-free oats; brands such as Quaker oats are not gluten-free.

Popcorn: Air-popped fresh popcorn using fresh kernels is gluten-free. Flavored popcorn often contains gluten, so double-check each brand for safety. The following brands are usually gluten-free: Newman's Own, Pop Secret, and Jolly Time Popcorn.

Produce: Fresh fruits and vegetables are all gluten-free, and frozen and canned fruits and vegetables are usually gluten-free unless additives, sauces, or fillers that contain gluten are used. Dried fruits and fruit juices are also usually gluten-free. On occasion, dried flavored fruits or dates may have been dusted with flour (to prevent sticking), so look for 100 percent pure fruit.

Pudding: Most flavors in the following powdered and prepared puddings are gluten-free: Hunt's (except tapioca), Jell-O, Kozy Shack, Meijer Brand, Trader Joe's, and Wegman's Brand.

Rice Cakes: Most flavors of Lundberg, Stop and Shop rice cakes are gluten-free. (Quaker rice cakes in the U.S. are not gluten-free.)

Salad Dressings: Many salad dressings are gluten-free, but some brands may add fillers or barley malt, so care should be taken. When in doubt, ask for oil and vinegar. In general, most flavors of the following salad dressings are currently gluten-free: Kraft, Newman's Own, Laura Lynn, Maple Grove, and Walden Farms dressings.

Sauces, Dressings, and Marinades: Many gluten-free choices are available; look for brands that are labeled gluten-free or those that have been checked for gluten-free status. Some marinades that claim to be gluten-free include Annie's Naturals (Organic Smokey Tomato), Emeril's (Basting Sauce & Marinade, Herbed Lemon Pepper), Jack Daniel's EZ Marinader (Honey Teriyaki, Slow Roasted Garlic & Herb), Ken's (Buffalo Wing Sauce, Herb & Garlic, Lemon Pepper), Lawry's (Baja Chipotle, Caribbean Jerk, Havana Garlic & Lime, Mesquite, Tequila Lime), McCormick (Grill Mates, Baja Citrus Marinade, Chipotle Pepper Marinade, Hickory BBQ Marinade, Mesquite Marinade), Wegman's Brand (Chicken BBQ, Citrus Dill, Fajita, Greek, Honey Mustard, Lemon & Garlic, Rosemary Balsamic, Santa Fe, Spiedie, Steakhouse Peppercorn, and Tangy), Zesty (Savory, Thai). See Chapter 11 for homemade marinades that can easily be prepared.

Seasonings: Fresh and dried herbs, all whole spices, and garlic and onion powder are gluten-free and are safe. Seasoning blends can contain a gluten-containing filler, so do not use these unless they are labeled gluten-free or you have checked with the manufacturer first.

Soy Milk: If you are lactose intolerant, you may be using lactaid milk, or soy milk. Some gluten-free brands of soy milk include Silk, Trader Joe's, and Westsoy. Double-check other brands of soy milk for gluten—sometimes gluten is added as barley malt.

Sweeteners: Almost all sweeteners are gluten-free, including sugar, Sweet 'n' Low, Equal, Splenda, Stevia, agave, honey, molasses, and many more.

Vinegars: All distilled vinegars are gluten-free. Vinegars that may contain gluten include malt vinegars and those made with barley, such as rice vinegar (rice vinegar is not distilled and sometimes includes barley).

Yogurts: Almost all flavors in the following brands are gluten-free: Albertson's, Brown Cow, Colombo (Classic, Light), Horizon, Lowes Food Brand, Meijer Brand, Publix, Stonyfield, Tillamook, Trader Joe's, Wegman's, Weight Watchers, and Yoplait. Take care not to select yogurt with sprinkle or candy toppings. (Dannon currently states that only their plain yogurt is gluten-free).

TIP

Most fresh foods are gluten-free.

Easy Start Gluten-Free Meal Plan

Week 1: All you want to know is what can you eat. This is not the time to learn everything there is to know about gluten-free eating and shopping. This quick-and-easy meal plan makes it easy to get started.

You can overcome feeling overwhelmed by keeping things simple at the start. The meal plans found in this book make it easy for you to put together quick gluten-free meals with limited meal preparation. Whether you pick up your food from the supermarket, the specialty stores, or online, a large variety of gluten-free products are now available. Later, if you are someone who likes to cook, try some of the terrific gluten-free recipes found in Chapters 4 and 11.

Breakfast Choices

- Rice Chex or Corn Chex or other gluten-free cereal with milk and blueberries or other fresh fruit

- Corn tortillas, warmed, with scrambled eggs, chopped tomato, and melted cheese

- Gluten-free cream of rice with chopped almonds and milk

- Gluten-free waffles (such as Van gluten-free waffles) with butter and syrup

- Omelet with onions, peppers, and tomatoes, with two soft corn tortillas and ketchup

- Grits with butter and salt

- Cottage cheese and fruit

- Gluten-free pancakes (some brands that have gluten-free pancakes include Arrowhead Mills, Bob's Red Mill, Gluten-Free Essentials, Gluten-free Pantry, Kinnikinnick, Sylvan, and Vans) with butter and syrup

- Gluten-free yogurt (such as Stonyfield) layered with berries and flax

- Ricotta cheese mixed with sugar and layered with berries

- Hard-boiled eggs mixed with mayonnaise, served on toasted corn tortillas

Lunch Choices

- Sliced turkey with lettuce, tomato, and mayonnaise on warmed corn tortillas with baby carrots

- Grilled sliced chicken over mixed greens, with red peppers, sliced tomato, broccoli florets, and chickpeas, served with oil and vinegar or gluten-free salad dressing (such as Paul Newman)

- Toasted gluten-free bread or warmed corn tortillas, with tuna fish made with mayonnaise, chopped onion, sliced tomato, shredded lettuce, and chopped cucumber

- Grilled salmon or tuna served over mixed greens with shredded carrots, chopped tomatoes, and cucumbers. Serve with oil and vinegar, or favorite gluten-free salad dressing, gluten-free rice crackers, and lemon wedges

- Grilled chicken, salmon, or tuna, with shredded lettuce, sliced tomatoes, baby carrots, and gluten-free rice cakes

- Gluten-free ham on gluten-free toast or warmed corn tortillas with mustard and coleslaw

- Cottage cheese with mixed fruit

- Grilled chicken cutlet marinated in garlic, oil, and lemon, served over chopped romaine lettuce, with gluten-free Caesar dressing (such as Paul Newman), parmesan cheese, and gluten-free rice crackers

- Grilled or broiled sirloin burger with lettuce, tomato, sliced onion, catsup, and a gluten-free roll if available—if not available serve over a mixed salad with oil and gluten-free vinegar

- Grilled chicken marinated in garlic, oregano, oil, salt, and pepper, with a sweet potato, butter, and mixed veggies

- Chicken salad made with cooked chicken, mayo, onions, walnuts, and grapes, over a mixed green salad

- Grilled portabella mushroom marinated in garlic and oil, served with mixed green salad

- Peanut butter and jelly on gluten-free rice cakes (such as Lundenberg)

Dinner Choices

- Salmon baked with mustard and honey, served with brown rice and steamed green beans

- Hardboiled egg, sliced, with steamed green beans, baby spinach, sliced cucumber, sliced tomato, and chickpeas with oil and vinegar or gluten-free salad dressing

- Grilled chicken cutlet marinated in garlic, oil, and onion powder, served with cooked brown rice, steamed broccoli, and mixed greens served with oil and vinegar or gluten-free salad dressing

- Cooked kidney beans and brown rice added to chopped onions sautéed in olive oil with garlic, and with chopped tomato, chopped red pepper, and hot pepper added to taste, served with a green salad and gluten-free dressing

- Broiled skirt steak with garlic, onion powder, and a dash of salt, served with steamed cauliflower and a medium baked potato with butter or margarine

- Baked flounder cooked with chopped onions, tomatoes, cilantro, garlic, and onion powder, served with steamed spinach, rice, and a mixed green salad with sliced tomato and cucumber and oil and vinegar or gluten-free salad dressing

- Pork loin cut into two-inch cubes and placed on a skewer with chunks of pineapple, cherry tomatoes marinated in gluten-free

Italian dressing, grilled, and served with steamed broccoli and corn with butter or margarine and a dash of salt

- Roasted chicken with carrots, potatoes, and onions, seasoned with garlic, onion powder, salt, pepper, and Italian herbs

- Grilled or baked chicken, shrimp, or veal, placed in a casserole dish and topped with tomato sauce, mozzarella, and parmesan cheese, served with gluten-free pasta

- Gluten-free rice, corn, or quinoa pasta with tomato sauce and a mixed green salad with favorite gluten-free dressing

- Grilled shrimp over a mixed salad with baby potatoes and favorite gluten-free salad dressing

- Hand-pressed hamburger or turkey burger, with onion and sliced tomato, baked sweet potato fries, and green beans

- Frozen gluten-free pizza baked and served with mixed green salad and gluten-free salad dressing

Snack Choices

- Pear or other fresh fruit

- Canned fruit in its own juice

- Gluten-free yogurt (see page 24)

- Apple sauce with cinnamon

- Baby carrots and snow peas with hummus

- String cheese with dried fruit

- Gluten-free pudding (see page 23)

- Gluten-free rice cakes (see page 23)

- Gluten-free nuts with dried fruit (nuts are naturally gluten-free unless flavored or processed on gluten-containing equipment; check dried fruit labels to make sure no gluten-containing ingredient has been added)

- A cup of strawberries with Cool Whip

- Plain peanuts or almonds

- Gluten-free rice cakes with cream cheese and jam

- Gluten-free frozen ices

- Gluten-free ice cream

Foods and Additives That Contain Gluten

The following items all contain gluten; see Chapters 3 and 5 for lists of gluten-free alternatives.

Gluten-Containing Foods and Ingredients to Avoid

Wheat

Atta*	Kamut**
Bulgur	Matzoh, Matzoh Meal
Couscous	Modified Wheat Starch
Dinkel (also known as spelt)**	Seitan****
Durum**	Semolina
Einkorn**	Spelt (also known as farro
Emmer**	or faro; dinkel)**
Farina	Triticale
Farro or Faro (also known as spelt)**	Wheat Bran
Fu***	Wheat Flour
Graham Flour	Wheat Germ
Hydrolyzed Wheat Protein	Wheat Starch

*A fine whole-meal flour made from low-gluten, soft textured wheat used to make Indian flatbread (also known as chapatti flour)
**Types of wheat
***A dried gluten product derived from wheat that is sold as thin sheets or thick round cakes. Used as a protein supplement in Asian dishes such as soups and vegetables.
****A meat-like food derived from wheat gluten used in many vegetarian dishes. Sometimes called "wheat meat."

Barley

Ale*	Malt**
Barley (Flakes, Flour, Pearl)	Malt Extract/Malt Syrup/
Beer*	Malt Flavoring***
Brewer's Yeast	Malt Vinegar
Lager*	Malted Milk

*Most regular ale, beer and lager are derived from barley which is not gluten-free. However, there are several new varieties of gluten-free beer derived from buckwheat, sorghum, and/or rice which are gluten-free.

**Malt is an enzyme preparation usually derived from sprouted barley which is not gluten-free. Other cereal grains can also be malted and may or may not be gluten-free depending on the additional ingredients used in the malting process.

***These terms are used interchangeably to denote a concentrated liquid solution of barley malt that is used as a flavoring agent.

Rye

Rye Bread	Rye Flour

Oats*

Oatmeal	Oat Flour
Oat Bran	Oats

*Celiac organizations in Canada and the USA do not recommend consumption of commercially available oat products as they are often cross contaminated with wheat and/or barley. However, pure, uncontaminated specialty gluten-free oat products from North America are now available and many organizations allow consumption of moderate amounts of these oats for persons with celiac disease.

From: Shelley Case, RD, 2008, *Gluten-Free Diet: A Comprehensive Resource Guide, Revised and Expanded Edition*, Case Nutrition Consulting, Inc. www.glutenfreediet.ca.

Creating a Gluten-Free Shopping List

When you are just setting up your gluten-free pantry, all you need are enough gluten-free options to get you through a few weeks until you are ready to do more exploring. As you go on, you will begin to establish new staples in place of old so you do not have to feel like you are missing something. Since others in your home may have been spreading their bread with mayo, mustard, peanut butter, and so on, they have contaminated those choices already in your house, so make sure to buy new spreads, and mark them with your name or "GF" so others know not to double-dip in your choices.

Many gluten-free choices can be found in health and natural food stores.

Cereal

Gluten-free cold and hot cereal
Gluten-free bread crumbs
Frozen gluten-free bread, bagels, and pizza crusts
Corn or rice or teff tortillas

Dairy

Butter
Cheese (most cheese is gluten-free, cheese spreads and blends sometimes contain gluten)
Margarine (most brands)
Milk
Gluten-free yogurt

Fats and Oils

Butter, margarine, vegetable oils, and gluten-free salad dressings

Grains and Starches

Amaranth
Beans, bean flours, and soy
Corn, corn starch, cornmeal (naturally gluten-free)

Gluten-free bread, bagels, muffins, wraps, and pizza crusts
Gluten-free crackers, rice cakes
Gluten-free pasta, such as rice, corn, quinoa, buckwheat
Mesquite, millet, and montina flour
Potatoes, potato starch
Quinoa
Rice, unflavored, white, brown, instant, jasmine, basmati, and rice flour
Sorghum and sorghum flour
Teff and teff flour
Xanthan gum, guar gum, expandex

Protein

Eggs and egg substitutes
Poultry (is naturally gluten-free except when found with marinades or when self-basting agents have been added)
Beef and pork (watch out for marinades and fillers)

Produce

All fresh fruits and vegetables are gluten-free
Canned, frozen, and dried fruits and vegetables are gluten-free as long as gluten-containing ingredients have not been added to them

Nuts

Nuts, seeds, and nut butters without added seasonings or coatings are gluten-free

Sauces

Gluten-free catsup, mustard, relish, barbeque sauce, tomato sauce, salsa (soy sauce and teriyaki sauce are usually made with wheat, so only buy those brands that are marked gluten-free)

Soup Bases

Gluten-free bouillon cubes and stocks (note that most soup bases contain gluten)

Sweets

Gluten-free cake, cookie, and brownie mixes (check any candy or chocolate that you usually buy for gluten-containing ingredients)

Snacks

Unseasoned nuts
Gluten-free popcorn (for example, air-popped or gluten-free microwave popcorn, such as Newman's brand)
Gluten-free pretzels (such as Glutino)
Gluten-free corn and potato chips with gluten-free salsa
Gluten-free yogurt (such as Stonyfield)

Spreads, Dips, and Condiments

Catsup
Mustard
Mayo
Gluten-free salad dressing
Syrup
Tartar sauce
Tomato sauce
Vegetable oils
Distilled vinegar

Spices and Herbs

Use only 100 percent pure herbs and spices, and check labels for fillers

Prevent Cross-Contamination

Buy condiments in squeeze bottles or buy separate spreadable products and mark them as gluten-free
Use separate utensils for serving gluten-free foods
Don't use a toaster that has been used with gluten-containing foods
Have separate cooking pans for gluten-free foods
Wipe down cooking surfaces before preparing foods
Safely mark and separate all gluten-free products

Discovering What You Can and Can't Eat

Safe Supermarket Shopping

Now that you have the basic tools for living gluten-free, you are ready to take the next step. Since safe food choices are a must, knowing what is safe at the supermarket will make it easier to find your favorite gluten-free foods. Let's start by shopping around the outside area of the store (the perimeter), as this is where most fresh and gluten-free products can be found. Fruits, vegetables, meats, fish, chicken, and dairy are mostly all gluten-free. After picking up your fresh produce, meat, and dairy, go to the health food aisle. This is where many gluten-free products, such as GF pasta and GF pancake mixes, are located. Then you can go through the rest of the supermarket using the following lists to help make safe choices.

The following is a list of individual foods which have been labeled as either safe, not safe, and those to question.

> **TIP**
> The perimeter of the supermarket is where most gluten-free foods can be found.

What to Eat and What Not to Eat

In the United States, **packaged foods** that contain wheat must state so clearly on the label, but barley and rye do not need to be so listed. Barley is usually listed as barley or malt, and rye is usually only added to wheat-containing foods (which you would be avoiding in any case).

35

Currently, **meats and poultry** are not required to list wheat on their packaging; doing so is completely voluntary (although it is often done). So, even though most meats are gluten-free, it is important to look out for marinades, self-basting poultry, modified food starch, and dextrin as possible hidden sources of gluten (when in doubt, call manufacturers).

The listing **gluten-free with wheat listed in the ingredients** can be confusing. This means that although a product was made with wheat, the gluten-containing proteins in it have been removed, and the product is now gluten-free.

 MONEY-SAVING TIP

To label or not to label? Currently, the gluten-free status of foods is not required to be listed on a label, so there are many gluten-free items on the shelves that do not call attention to that status. You might pay three times as much for a comparable product that is marked gluten-free (like gluten-free vanilla extract) when one on the shelf right next to it may be just as gluten-free but simply not labeled as such. Read carefully, and save money!

Detailed Food Chart

The following charted foods are listed as Safe (S), Questionable (Q), and Not Safe (NS). For specific gluten-free mixes or brands, see the resource section at the end of this book.

	Safe(S)	Not Safe (NS)	Questionable (Q)
Baking			
Baking chocolate (pure)	(S)		
Baking powder, baking soda			(Q) most are GF, but double-check

	Safe(S)	Not Safe (NS)	Questionable (Q)
Baking (Continued)			
Brewer's yeast		(NS)	
Carob chips			(Q) most are GF, but some contain barley malt
Carob and cocoa powder	(S)		
Coco mix			(Q)
Coconut	(S)		
Chocolate chips			(Q) usually GF, but some contain barley malt
Cream of tartar	(S)		
Coconut (flavored or sweetened)			(Q)
Flour (wheat, rye, barley, or gluten-containing flour)		(NS)	
Frosting			(Q) many are GF, but some contain gluten as a filler
Guar gum	(S)		
MSG	(S)		
Vanilla extract	(S)		
Xanthan gum	(S)		

	Safe(S)	Not Safe (NS)	Questionable (Q)
Baking (Continued)			
Yeast	(S)		
CANDY			
Candy			(Q) varies with flavors and brands
Chocolate			(Q)
Licorice		(NS)	
GF Licorice	(S)		
Marshmallows			(Q) some contain gluten
Condiments			
Barbeque sauce, Worcestershire sauce			(Q)
Bouillon cubes (most contain gluten)		(NS)	
Catsup			(Q) most brands GF
Gravy		(NS)	
Plain relish, olives, pickles	(S)		
Honey	(S)		
Salad dressing			(Q) check for malt or wheat
Sauces			(Q)

	Safe (S)	Not Safe (NS)	Questionable (Q)
Condiments (Continued)			
Stuffed olives, pickles			(Q)
Pickles made with wheat flour		(NS)	
Distilled vinegar (apple cider, rice, balsamic, white, grape, wine)	(S)		
Rice vinegar			(Q) may contain barley malt
Malted vinegar		(NS)	
Marinade			(Q)
Miso			(Q) often made with barley
Mustard (yellow)	(S)		
Mustard			(Q) most GF, but some brands may have gluten-containing ingredients
Salsa			(Q) most brands GF
GF soy sauce or GF tamari (must be labeled GF)	(S)		
Tamari			(Q) most GF, but check labels

	Safe(S)	Not Safe (NS)	Questionable (Q)
Condiments (Continued)			
Teriyaki sauce		(NS)	
Soy sauce (made with wheat)		(NS)	
Stocks and broths (when are not homemade)			(Q)
Tomato sauce and paste	(S)		
Flavored tomato products			(Q)
Dairy			
Butter	(S)		
Buttermilk (regular and low-fat)	(S)		
Cheese (hard and soft cheese)	(S)		
Veined cheese (blue cheese, gorgonzola cheese, and silton)	(S)		
Cheese sauce and spreads			(Q) some have gluten-containing fillers
Flavored cheese			(Q)
Cottage cheese	(S)		
Flavored and lower-fat cottage cheese			(Q)

	Safe(S)	Not Safe (NS)	Questionable (Q)
Dairy (Continued)			
Regular cream cheese	(S)		
Lower-fat and flavored cream cheese			(Q)
Eggs	(S)		
Egg substitutes			(Q) most GF, but check labels
Fat-free half-and-half	(S)		
Heavy cream	(S)		
Ice cream			(Q) most GF, but check brands, watching out for added ingredients and cross-contamination
Milk	(S)		
Malted milk		(NS)	
Milk shakes, flavored milk, and drinks			(Q)
Sour cream	(S)		
Low-fat sour cream			(Q) most GF
Frozen yogurt			(Q) most GF, but check flavors and brands

	Safe (S)	Not Safe (NS)	Questionable (Q)
Yogurts			
Flavored yogurt			(Q) some brands contain gluten
Frozen yogurt			(Q) most GF, but check flavors and brands
Plain yogurt	(S)		
Desserts			
Cakes, cookies, cupcakes, pies made with gluten-containing ingredients		(NS)	
GF cakes, cookies, pies, waffle cones	(S)		
Plain gelatin	(S)		
Flavored gelatin	(S)		
Frostings/icing (most are GF)			(Q) some brands do contain gluten
Ice cream and ices without added gluten-containing ingredients	(S)		
Ice cream with added cakes, cookies, muffins, fillers, or other gluten-containing ingredients		(NS)	

	Safe(S)	Not Safe (NS)	Questionable (Q)
Desserts (Continued)			
Sherbet, nondairy whipped toppings, egg custards			(Q)
Milk puddings, custard powder, pudding mixes			(Q)
100 percent dairy whipped topping	(S)		
Drinks			
Unflavored tea, coffee, soft drinks, juice, cider, wine, GF beers, pure liquors, distilled alcohol (such as rum, gin, vodka)	(S)		
Cordials (most types, such as Amaretto and Sambuca, are GF unless a flavoring agent is added after distillation)	(S)		
Instant and flavored teas and coffees, fruit-flavored drinks, chocolate drinks, soy milk, malt, wine coolers			(Q)
Beer, ale, lager, malted beverages		(NS)	
GF beers	(S)		

	Safe (S)	Not Safe (NS)	Questionable (Q)
Fats			
Butter, margarine, lard, vegetable oils, cream, shortening	(S)		
Cooking sprays			(Q)
Lard	(S)		
Mayonnaise			(Q) most GF, but check labels
Salad dressings			(Q) many GF, but check labels
Shortening	(S)		
Suet			(Q)
Fish			
Fish in canned vegetables, broth, or HVP (hydrolyzed wheat protein)		(NS)	
Canned fish			(Q) most GF, but check labels
Fish patties or cakes or croquettes			(Q)
Flavored fish in pouches			(Q)
Fresh and frozen unseasoned fish all varieties	(S)		
Imitation fish products			(Q) often contain wheat

	Safe(S)	Not Safe (NS)	Questionable (Q)
Fish (Continued)			
Stuffed, breaded, and marinated fish		(NS)	
Fruits			
Dates			(Q) some are dusted with flour
Fruit with starches added			(Q)
Fresh, frozen, unflavored dried, canned, and juiced fruits	(S)		
Fruit jams and jellies	(S)		
Canned and frozen fruit			(Q) most are GF, but double-check labels
Fruit pie fillings, dried fruits that have been seasoned			(Q)

Grains and Starches

The grains marked safe below are naturally gluten-free, but they can be contaminated with gluten in the fields or during the manufacturing process. To be doubly safe, check the grains you buy to make sure they are marked gluten-free. One grain that is often contaminated with gluten is oats—make sure all oats you use are marked gluten-free.

Amaranth	(S)		
Arrowroot	(S)		

	Safe (S)	Not Safe (NS)	Questionable (Q)
Grains and Starches (Continued)			
Artichoke flour			(Q) often mixed with other flours; make sure all ingredients are GF
Barley and barley malt, barley grass		(NS)	
Beans			
Beans (all plain beans, including dai, black beans, chickpeas, fava, lentil, and lima)	(S)		
Baked beans			(Q) some contain gluten, so check labels
Besan	(S)		
Bran			(Q) can be wheat, rye, oat, corn or rice— be sure to check GF status
Bread			
Bread/bagels/ biscuits/breadcrumbs/ cornbread/crackers/ doughnuts/English muffins/phyllo/pizza crust/stuffing/wraps containing wheat, rye, barley, spelt or other gluten-containing grains		(NS)	

	Safe (S)	Not Safe (NS)	Questionable (Q)
Bread (Continued)			
GF breads/bagels/ biscuits/breadcrumbs/ cornbread/crackers/ doughnuts/English muffins/phyllo/ pizza crust/stuffing/ wraps	(S)		
(GF choices usually contain grains such as amaranth, arrowroot, bean (legume flours), buckwheat, corn, flax, millet, potato, quinoa, rice sago, sorghum, soy, tapioca, teff, xanthan gum [note some brands may be manufactured in plants that may contain gluten, so double-check labels])			
Buckwheat (100 percent pure)	(S)		
Kasha			(Q) double-check labels; some brands may contain other ingredients
Bulgur		(NS)	
Cassava	(S)		

	Safe (S)	Not Safe (NS)	Questionable (Q)
Cereals			
Cold cereal (GF cold cereals may include amaranth, puffed amaranth, puffed buckwheat, puffed corn, puffed millet, rice, rice flakes, soy, and teff)			(Q) there are not many cold GF cereals available; carefully check labels
Hot cereal (GF hot cereals are available, but check labels to make sure they come from GF facilities and fields; GF hot cereals may include amaranth, cornmeal [grits], cream of buckwheat, cream of rice, GF oats, quinoa, soy grits, and teff)	(S)		
Hot cereal such as cream of wheat, barley, regular oats, rye, triticale, or cereals made with malt		(NS)	
Channa	(S)		
Chestnut	(S)		
Coconut flour	(S)		
Communion wafers		(NS)	
GF Communion wafers	(S)		

	Safe(S)	Not Safe (NS)	Questionable (Q)
Corn			
Corn (fresh, corn starch, plain corn chips, corn syrup)	(S)		
Corn (canned, frozen)			(Q)
Corn (flavored corn chips, grits, tortillas, cereal)			(Q)
Corn, corn arepas, corn malt, corn starch, corn tortillas if 100 percent corn)	(S)		
Corn tacos shells, corn cakes			(Q)
Cottonseed	(S)		
Couscous		(NS)	
Dasheen flour	(S)		
Dinkle or spelt	(S)		
Durum or durum wheat		(NS)	
Egg roll and dumpling wrappers		(NS)	
Einkorn		(NS)	
Emmer		(NS)	
Farina		(NS)	
Faro/farro		(NS)	

	Safe(S)	Not Safe (NS)	Questionable (Q)
Corn (Continued)			
Flavoring			(Q)
Flax	(S)		
Flour, wheat		(NS)	
Fu		(NS)	
Gliadin		(NS)	
Glutenin		(NS)	
Graham crackers		(NS) unless marked GF	
Grits, hominy			(Q) double-check for cross contamination
Hemp			(Q)
Hydrolyzed wheat protein		(NS)	
Job's tears	(S)		
Kamut		(NS)	
Kasha			(Q) double-check for cross contamination at plant
Kudzu	(S)		
Malt			(Q) can be barley (gluten) or corn (GF)
Malt extract, malt flavoring syrup		(NS)	

	Safe(S)	Not Safe (NS)	Questionable (Q)
Corn (Continued)			
Malt vinegar		(NS)	
Matzo, matzah meal		(NS)	
Mesquite	(S)		
Millet	(S)		
Milo	(S)		
MIR		(NS)	
Modified food starch			(Q) could be wheat, corn, potato, or tapioca
Montina	(S)		
Oats			(Q) only oats, oat bran, and oats from GF sources can be used (see Chapter 10)
Pancakes			
Pancakes and waffles and waffle mixes, when made with gluten-containing ingredients		(NS)	
GF pancakes, waffles (frozen, homemade, or mix, or as GF restaurant selection)	(S)		
Potato and potato products	(S)		

	Safe(S)	Not Safe (NS)	Questionable (Q)

Pancakes (Continued)

Potatoes that have been flavored or have added sauces or fried potatoes (not safe if fried in oil that cooked gluten-containing foods)			(Q)

Pasta and Pizza

Pasta/orzo/ramen noodles or pizza made from wheat, wheat starch, spelt, or other gluten-containing ingredients		(NS)	
GF pasta or pizza crust (usually made from buckwheat, beans, corn, rice, sorghum, quinoa)	(S)		
Buckwheat pasta			(Q) check to make sure it is either marked GF or 100 percent buckwheat
Wheat or corn noodles			(Q)
Quinoa or quinoa pasta	(S)		

	Safe (S)	Not Safe (NS)	Questionable (Q)
Rice			
Rice, plain, Arborio, rice bran, black, brewer's, brown, calrose, Carolina, della, glutinous, japonica, jasmine, paddy rice, pearl, polished, popcorn, red, risotto, rosematta, white, wild	(S)		
Flavored rice and rice pilaf			(Q)
Rice noodles that are 100 percent rice	(S)		
Risotto mixes			(Q)
Rye		(NS)	
Sago	(S)		
Seitan		(NS)	
Semolina		(NS)	
Sorghum	(S)		
Soba noodles			(Q) some brands contain wheat
Soy and soybean flour	(S)		
Spelt		(NS)	

	Safe (S)	Not Safe (NS)	Questionable (Q)
Rice (Continued)			
Spring roll wrappers			(Q) some are not 100 percent rice or are fried in oil with gluten-containing foods
Sweet potato flour	(S)		
Taco shells			(Q)
Tabbouleh		(NS)	
Tapioca	(S)		
Taro	(S)		
Teff	(S)		
Tortillas, wheat		(NS)	
Tortillas, corn, rice	(S)		
Triticale		(NS)	
Water chestnut flour	(S)		
Wheat berries		(NS)	
Wheat, wheat bran, wheat flour, wheat germ, wheat grass, wheat starch		(NS)	
Wheat nuts		(NS)	
Wonton, and wheat eggroll and dumpling wrappers		(NS)	

	Safe(S)	Not Safe (NS)	Questionable (Q)
Meat and Meat Substitutes			
Beef jerky, dried meats, and imitation bacon bits			(Q)
Breaded or flour-coated meats		(NS)	
Deli meats, including bacon, sausages, and pates			(Q) most GF, but some do have added fillers
Ham			(Q)
Meat extenders			(Q)
All meats that do not have marinades or seasonings added	(S)		
Meat patties			(Q)
Meatloaf			(Q)
Meat substitutes such as seitan		(NS)	
Tempeh			(Q)
Plain tofu	(S)		
Flavored tofu			(Q) many seasoned with wheat-containing soy sauce
TVP (texturized vegetable protein)			(Q) can be made from wheat or soy

	Safe (S)	Not Safe (NS)	Questionable (Q)
Meat and Meat Substitutes (Continued)			
Vegetable burgers			(Q) most contain gluten
Veggie crumbles, hot dogs, and sausage			(Q) most contain gluten
Nuts			
Chestnuts	(S)		
Unseasoned nuts, all varieties	(S)		
Seasoned or dried roasted nuts			(Q)
Other			
Anything breaded		(NS)	
Sauces and gravies made from GF ingredients	(S)		
Sauces and gravies made with wheat or other gluten-containing ingredients		(NS)	
HVP/HPP			(Q) often the source is wheat
Poultry			
Breaded or floured chicken		(NS)	
Poultry patties			(Q)

	Safe (S)	Not Safe (NS)	Questionable (Q)
Poultry (Continued)			
Fried chicken			(Q) check the coating, and whether the oil is dedicated for GF frying
Plain turkey, chicken, or other poultry that does not have gluten-containing ingredients added	(S)		
Poultry cooked in broth		(NS)	
Stuffed poultry		(NS)	
Turkey, chicken, or other poultry that has had a self-basting product added to it (such as hydrolyzed wheat protein)		(NS)	
Sauces			
Cocktail sauce			(Q)
Tarter sauce	(S)		
Tomato sauce	(S)		
Soy sauce		(NS)	
GF soy sauce or tamari	(S)		
Snacks			
Most snack and cereal bars contain gluten unless they are labeled GF		(NS)	

	Safe(S)	Not Safe (NS)	Questionable (Q)
Snacks (Continued)			
Chips that contain wheat, rye, or barley		(NS)	
Rice cakes			(Q) some brands contain gluten
Plain 100 percent corn, potato, or rice chips	(S)		
Seasoned potato, taco, corn, or rice chips			(Q)
Multigrain chips		(NS)	
Air-popped popcorn, GF pretzels	(S)		
Rice crackers (that are 100 percent rice)	(S)		
Soups			
Packaged broths, soup mixes, and bouillon cubes (these often contain gluten)		(NS)	
Canned and frozen soups			(Q) most contain gluten, only okay when labeled GF
Restaurant soups			(Q) unless homemade base, most will contain broths or bouillon cubes with gluten

	Safe(S)	Not Safe (NS)	Questionable (Q)
Soups (Continued)			
Homemade broths that do not have bouillon cubes or gluten-containing ingredients added	(S)		
Spices			
Fresh herbs and spices	(S)		
Seasoning mixes and blends			(Q)
Dried pure herbs and spices	(S)		
Extracts			(Q) most GF, but check labels
Monosodium glutamate (MSG)	(S)		
Vegetables			
Fresh, frozen, and canned vegetables and juices	(S)		
Salad kits			(Q) watch out for dressings and croutons
Scalloped potatoes, batter-dipped vegetables		(NS)	
Flavored canned vegetables			(Q)

	Safe(S)	Not Safe (NS)	Questionable (Q)
Vegetables (Continued)			
Squashes	(S)		
Sprouted wheat and barley		(NS)	
Vegetables fried in oil in which other foods have also been fried, or vegetables coated in batter or flour		(NS)	
Vegetables, seasoned or in sauce			(Q)
Wheat grass and wheat grass juice		(NS)	

Basic Gluten-Free Foods and Where to Find Them

Most supermarkets have dedicated sections or aisles where they stock their health or specialty foods, but some stores have larger sections than others. It is these dedicated sections that often carry gluten-free choices such as pastas, cereals, flour blends, and crackers. Throughout the rest of the store there may be products that are gluten-free as well, some of which are labeled as such, and some of which are not.

Now that you have a list of safe gluten-free foods and have started checking your local stores and some Web sites, you will be able to put together a more extensive gluten-free meal plan.

Simple Choices, 30-Day Meal Plan

Day 1

Breakfast: Mesa Sunrise cereal or other GF cereal with 1% milk and a small banana

Snack: 1 medium pear

Lunch: GF sliced turkey with lettuce, tomato on GF flat bread or corn tortilla with mayonnaise with 1 cup of baby carrots

Snack: GF yogurt

Dinner: Grilled sliced chicken over mixed greens with 1 cup sliced red peppers, 1 medium sliced tomato, 1 cup broccoli florets, ½ cup chickpeas, oil and vinegar or GF salad dressing, and a sprinkle of parmesan cheese

Snack: ½ cup apple sauce with cinnamon

Day 2

Breakfast: Two 6" corn tortillas, warmed, with scrambled eggs and a slice of low-fat cheese

Snack: GF yogurt

Lunch: GF tortilla, 3 oz. white meat tuna with mayonnaise, sliced tomato, onion, shredded lettuce, and chopped cucumbers

Snack: ½ cup baby carrots, ½ cup hummus

Dinner: Steak kabob with onions, tomatoes, mushrooms, marinated in favorite GF dressing, served over brown rice

Snack: string cheese and a medium sliced pear

Day 3

Breakfast: GF cream of rice with cinnamon, sweetened to taste, and chopped almonds with 1% milk

Snack: 6 oz. fruit in its own juice

Lunch: Roast beef on GF bread with catsup, shredded lettuce, 1 cup baby carrots and chopped tomato

Snack: A medium apple

Dinner: Roasted chicken cooked with butter, garlic, and onion powder over brown rice with steamed broccoli

Snack: GF fat-free pudding

Day 4

Breakfast: GF oats with 1 Tb chopped almonds, 2 Tb raisins, cinnamon, and brown sugar

Snack: GF yogurt

Lunch: Cooked salmon, mixed with mayonnaise, mustard, and dill, served with shredded lettuce and sliced tomato in a gluten-free teff wrap, with baby carrots and sliced cucumber on the side

Snack: String cheese with a medium apple

Dinner: Quick beans and rice: sauté chopped onions in olive oil with garlic, add chopped tomato, chopped red pepper, cayenne pepper, and kidney beans; serve with brown rice and a salad with GF salad dressing

Snack: 10 almonds and a medium apple

Day 5

Breakfast: GF Rice Chex or Corn Chex with 1% milk and strawberries

Snack: GF yogurt

Lunch: GF sliced turkey on GF toast with mustard; also, coleslaw

Snack: Mixed green salad with mandarin orange wedges and GF salad dressing

Dinner: Baked chicken cutlet with garlic and onion powder with steamed cauliflower and a medium sweet potato with butter, brown sugar, and cinnamon

Snack: Strawberries with whipped cream

Day 6

Breakfast: Egg whites sautéed in olive oil with chopped green onions and chopped red pepper, served with two toasted soft corn tortillas

Snack: GF yogurt

Lunch: American cheese melted on GF toast with sliced tomato and roasted red pepper

Snack: Grapes

Dinner: Broiled flounder cooked with GF salsa, steamed green beans, and brown rice

Snack: A medium pear and 5 almonds

Day 7

Breakfast: Cream of rice with 2 Tb raisins, 1 tsp cinnamon with brown sugar, and 1% milk

Snack: GF fruit yogurt

Lunch: Cottage cheese with melon

Snack: GF rice cakes

Dinner: Baked skinless chicken cutlet, topped with GF honey mustard with steamed asparagus, a baked potato, and sour cream

Snack: GF vanilla ice cream with mini M&Ms

Day 8

Breakfast: GF waffles with butter and syrup and 1% milk

Snack: Small banana with peanut butter

Lunch: Greek salad with lettuce, tomatoes, cucumbers, feta, olives, onions, and chickpeas, served with GF salad dressing

Snack: GF yogurt

Dinner: Grilled hamburger with sautéed onions, lettuce, tomato, and onion, and baked sweet potato fries

Snack: GF pudding

Day 9

Breakfast: Poached eggs over toasted GF English muffin with cheddar cheese

Snack: Jell-O

Lunch: GF ham and Swiss with mustard on corn tortilla

Snack: GF snack bar

Dinner: 2 hardboiled eggs, sliced, with ½ cup green beans, steamed and then chilled, 2 cups chopped spinach, half a cucumber, sliced, a small boiled potato, peeled and sliced, and a medium sliced tomato, served with oil and vinegar or GF salad dressing

Snack: GF chocolate pudding

Day 10

Breakfast: GF cereal with 1% milk and blueberries

Snack: Hummus with baby carrots

Lunch: Tuna melt: gluten-free tuna with mayonnaise over GF toast with sliced tomatoes and melted mozzarella

Snack: Fruit salad

Dinner: Grilled salmon with dill, and cooked millet with steamed green beans

Snack: GF chocolate chip cookies and 1% milk

Day 11

Breakfast: GF pancakes with sliced banana, whipped butter, and syrup
Snack: GF rice cakes
Lunch: Large mixed salad with grilled chicken, chickpeas, roasted peppers, parmesan cheese, and GF dressing
Snack: GF rice pudding
Dinner: Roasted pork loin, baked with GF honey mustard, corn, and steamed broccoli
Snack: GF whipped cream with blueberries

Day 12

Breakfast: GF oatmeal with raisins, cinnamon, brown sugar, and 1% milk
Snack: GF ice pop
Lunch: Broiled or grilled hamburger with cheddar over mixed greens with sliced onion and tomato
Snack: GF snack bar
Dinner: Flounder with garlic, onion, oregano, and lemon over cooked amaranth with mixed vegetables
Snack: Baked apple with cinnamon and brown sugar

Day 13

Breakfast: Scrambled eggs with Canadian bacon and toasted GF corn tortillas
Snack: Grapes
Lunch: Stuffed tomato with tuna fish and GF brown rice crackers
Snack: GF yogurt
Dinner: Chicken, red pepper, and onion kabob, marinated in GF Italian dressing and grilled over cooked millet
Snack: GF ice cream

Day 14

Breakfast: GF cereal with 1% milk and mixed berries
Snack: GF rice cakes
Lunch: GF turkey and cheddar on GF wrap with mustard
Snack: GF bar

Dinner: Roasted chicken with garlic and rosemary with new potatoes and green beans
Snack: GF ices

Day 15

Breakfast: GF grits with shredded cheese and butter
Snack: GF yogurt
Lunch: Turkey burger over a salad with GF salsa and GF corn chips
Snack: GF three-bean salad
Dinner: Grilled pork and pineapple with GF barbeque sauce, corn, and green salad
Snack: GF cookies and milk

Day 16

Breakfast: GF cereal with 1% milk and sliced peaches
Snack: GF rice cakes
Lunch: Deviled eggs with a mixed green salad and GF dressing
Snack: GF yogurt
Dinner: Stuffed peppers with beef, rice, onion, garlic, and tomatoes
Snack: Mixed fruit salad

Day 17

Breakfast: Frittata with sliced potatoes, egg, cheese, tomatoes, onions, and mushrooms
Snack: GF ice pop
Lunch: GF potato pancakes with sour cream and applesauce, with a mixed salad and GF dressing
Snack: GF yogurt
Dinner: GF chicken enchiladas with rice and beans
Snack: GF cookies and milk

Day 18

Breakfast: GF French toast with butter, syrup, and sliced banana
Snack: Half a grapefruit with brown sugar
Lunch: Fresh cold shrimp platter over salad with lemon and GF cocktail sauce

Snack: Sliced apple with peanuts
Dinner: Roasted turkey with cranberry sauce, sweet potato with butter, and green beans
Snack: GF pudding

Day 19

Breakfast: Cooked hot teff cereal with dried berries, flax seeds, and maple syrup
Snack: Peaches in their own juice
Lunch: Chicken salad served with toasted corn tortillas
Snack: GF snack bar
Dinner: Cornmeal-crusted catfish with mixed vegetables, and baked potato with butter
Snack: GF ice cream

Day 20

Breakfast: Ricotta cheese, layered with berries and GF cereal
Snack: String cheese
Lunch: GF roast beef and GF horseradish sauce with GF crackers
Snack: 1 oz. plain mixed nuts
Dinner: Chicken fajitas with GF salsa, sour cream, and warmed corn tortillas
Snack: Cappuccino (no flavoring agents)

Day 21

Breakfast: GF waffles with peanut butter, raisins, and 1% milk
Snack: Fruit smoothie
Lunch: GF turkey rolled with Swiss cheese in lettuce leaves with mustard
Snack: GF snack bar
Dinner: GF pizza with salad and GF dressing
Snack: GF ice pops

Day 22

Breakfast: Polenta with melted mozzarella cheese and sliced tomato
Snack: GF yogurt

Lunch: Cornmeal-crusted chicken fingers with apricot preserves
Snack: Baked apple with cinnamon, walnuts, and brown sugar
Dinner: Chicken breast stuffed with spinach and blue cheese, with a sweet potato topped with melted butter
Snack: Fruit kabob

Day 23

Breakfast: GF oats with sunflower seeds, raisins, and brown sugar
Snack: GF pudding
Lunch: Grilled cheese on GF bread with baby carrots
Snack: GF rice cakes
Dinner: Grilled chicken cutlet with tomato sauce and melted mozzarella with GF pasta
Snack: GF cookies and milk

Day 24

Breakfast: GF toasted bagel with cream cheese, onion, tomato, and lox
Snack: Jell-O
Lunch: GF tuna salad over roasted red peppers and sliced cucumbers with brown rice crackers
Snack: GF three-bean salad
Dinner: Grilled tuna with GF soy sauce, ginger, and garlic over cooked millet with mixed vegetables
Snack: GF ice cream

Day 25

Breakfast: GF blueberry muffin with 1% milk
Snack: Sliced peaches and cottage cheese
Lunch: GF chili in a baked potato with a mixed green salad and GF dressing
Snack: GF snack bar
Dinner: Beef, onion, tomato, and mushroom kabobs marinated in GF Italian dressing with minced garlic, broiled or grilled and served over brown rice
Snack: GF coffee cake and milk

Day 26

Breakfast: GF pumpkin pancakes with butter, syrup, and 1% milk
Snack: GF rice cakes
Lunch: GF cheese enchiladas with rice and beans
Snack: Pea pods and hummus
Dinner: Grilled chicken with GF honey mustard, on a GF roll with lettuce and tomato
Snack: GF chocolate cake with 1% milk

Day 27

Breakfast: GF cornbread with 1% milk
Snack: Mixed dried 100 percent fruit and unseasoned nuts
Lunch: Grilled eggplant with melted mozzarella and a mixed green salad with GF dressing
Snack: GF yogurt
Dinner: Roasted chicken with brown rice and mixed vegetables
Snack: GF pudding

Day 28

Breakfast: GF cereal and 1% milk with sliced strawberries
Snack: GF fruit rollups
Lunch: Baked potato stuffed with broccoli florets and melted cheddar
Snack: GF snack bar
Dinner: Grilled steak with sautéed mushrooms and onions, with oven baked fries
Snack: GF pudding

Day 29

Breakfast: Hot teff cereal with dried berries, maple syrup, and cinnamon
Snack: GF yogurt
Lunch: GF pasta with mixed vegetables, black olives, baby shrimp, and GF Italian salad dressing
Snack: GF rice pudding
Dinner: GF hot dogs with sauerkraut and GF baked beans
Snack: GF ice cream

Day 30

Breakfast: Cantaloupe stuffed with 1% cottage cheese
Snack: GF snack bar
Lunch: GF turkey rolled with coleslaw, Swiss cheese, and mustard, served with GF crackers
Snack: Dried apricots
Dinner: GF pasta with tomato sauce, ricotta cheese, and grilled zucchini
Snack: GF chocolate chip cookies and 1% milk

Essential Dos and Don'ts

DOS	DON'TS
Find restaurants with gluten-free menus	Stop going out because it is more difficult to find gluten-free choices
Find delicious gluten-free combos to replace gluten-containing choices	Start eating plain, boring, repetitive meals because you are confused about what to eat
Be excited about all the new interesting food choices you are making	Start feeling depressed because you can't do things exactly as you are used to
Bring gluten-free dining out cards to your favorite restaurants so they will know how to accommodate you	Try to just pick things off a menu without letting the restaurant know of your special needs
Stock up on gluten-free choices at home	Let gluten-free supplies run low at home
Bring gluten-free snacks, crackers, and choices with you on the go	Go on trips and to events without packing some gluten-free choices
Have a dedicated toaster and dedicated spreads and dips for your gluten-free eating	Use the same toaster or spreads as other family members
Have a special shelf to store your gluten-free staples at home	Mix your gluten-free choices in with all other family foods, making them difficult to find (or fair game to be eaten by someone else browsing for a snack)
Choose more whole grains and higher-fiber gluten-free choices like legumes	Use only prepackaged gluten-free blends (typically low in fiber and high in fat)
Pay attention to labels for serving size, fat, calories, carbohydrates, and fiber	Stop reading labels because you have too much to do already
Pick foods higher in calcium, like milk and gluten-free yogurt; take gluten-free supplements if you don't get adequate dairy	Continue using products you have before without checking to make sure they are GF

Planning and Cooking Simple Gluten-Free Meals

Tips for Gluten-Free Cooking

Eating gluten-free does not mean complicated, boring, or tasteless. But getting familiar with an array of completely new or modified favorite recipes may present a bit of a learning curve.

Having delicious gluten-free meals is easy when you used these tips to get started:

- Start with recipes that don't usually contain gluten; this way, you won't have to make any modifications.

- Or, begin with those recipes that only need a small amount of changes so you will have a better chance of success. For example, substitute a gluten-free broth for regular broth, or use rice flour or potato starch as a thickener in place of wheat flour—these are easy modifications that are sure to work.

- Keep a tabbed notebook or a folder on your computer with information on gluten-free ingredients and sources for quick access to information.

- Check sauces, dressings, and seasoning agents to ensure that they are gluten-free.

- Make sure you mark spreads such as peanut butter, butter, margarine, mayonnaise, and jam so that others don't accidently double-dip and cross-contaminate your food.

- Use a designated gluten-free toaster or toaster bags (as found in the resource section), and cover cooking surfaces with aluminum foil to help prevent cross-contamination.

- Store gluten-free products on top shelves so gluten-containing foods don't accidently get mixed into safe foods.

- Have dedicated colanders and measuring utensils for your gluten-free cooking.

- Put together labeled containers with scoops to keep your gluten-free ingredients easier to access.

- Premix your own gluten-free flour blends for easy use, or buy already-mixed blends and keep them on hand for quick recipe development.

- Sign up for gluten-free cooking classes. You'll save a lot of time and money by learning the right way to work with gluten-free grains right from the start.

- Get involved with local celiac support groups and trade recipes with others.

Stocking a Gluten-Free Kitchen

- Keep gluten-free ingredients on hand for easy-to-prepare meals.

- Stock up on gluten-free grains, as well as staples such as gluten-free pasta, polenta, and rice.

- Keep a supply of favorite gluten-free broths, sauces, and dressings.

- Make sure packaged rice, corn, and potato products are from gluten-free sources.

- Have gluten-free crackers, breads, and chips available.

- Stock gluten-free cereals for quick coatings for fish and chicken and as an easy-to-use base for pie crusts.

- Have gluten-free flours available, such as amaranth, bean flour, brown rice flour, corn flour, corn meal, buckwheat flour, millet, nut flours, sorghum, and teff (make sure you keep them refrigerated or in the freezer to help them stay fresh longer).

- Keep gluten-free starches on hand, such as arrowroot, cornstarch, potato starch, and tapioca flour to be used as thickening agents.

- Keep your freezer stocked with gluten-free breads, bagels, bread-crumbs, waffles, and pizza crusts.

- Purchase premade gluten-free frozen meals (for quick meals when you don't have the time).

- Have premixed gluten-free mixes, such as cake, cookie, and flour blends.

Easy Gluten-Free Recipes

If you're looking for ways to throw together quick meals, these recipes can be prepared quickly for easy, delicious, gluten-free meals.

Breakfast Recipes:

- Banana Pancakes

- Quick and Easy Coconut Pancakes

- Cornmeal Breakfast Cakes

- Toasty Cinnamon Sticks

- Ricotta Surprise

- Yogurt Parfait

Banana Pancakes   **Serves 4**

A yummy, delicious pancake, perfect for those Sunday brunches.

1 cup brown rice flour
¼ cup tapioca flour
2 tsp gluten-free baking powder
½ tsp gluten-free baking soda
2 Tb sugar
1 tsp cinnamon powder
¼ tsp nutmeg
2 eggs
¼ cup 1% buttermilk
2 bananas, sliced
Gluten-free cooking spray

1. Sift all dry ingredients together in a large mixing bowl.

2. Beat eggs and buttermilk together in a small bowl.

3. Add wet ingredients to dry ingredients and stir until well combined.

4. Coat a hot griddle with cooking spray or vegetable oil.

5. Drop batter by ¼-cupfuls onto hot griddle. Place banana slices carefully onto pancakes.

6. When bubbles begin to form, flip pancakes and continue cooking until browned on the bottom.

Nutritional information per serving: 205 calories, 6 grams protein, 40 grams carbohydrates, 3 grams fat, 72 milligrams cholesterol, 263 milligrams sodium, 2 grams fiber, 104 milligrams calcium, <1 milligram iron

Tip: Sprinkle with pecans and serve with warm maple syrup.

Quick and Easy Coconut Pancakes   Serves 4

¾ cup skim milk
2 Tb melted butter
1 egg
¾ cup all-purpose gluten-free baking blend (such as those sold by Bob's Red Mill)
¼ cup coconut flour
2 tsp baking powder
2 Tb sugar
½ tsp salt
Gluten-free cooking spray (or cooking oil)

1. In a large bowl, mix together milk, butter, and egg.

2. In a small bowl, mix together all dry ingredients.

3. Blend dry ingredients into wet.

4. Spray a skillet with cooking spray and heat over a low heat.

5. Ladle pancake mix onto griddle.

6. Cook until brown on one side and bubbling. Turn pancakes.

7. Serve with butter and syrup.

Nutritional information per serving: 261 calories, 6.1 grams protein, 39.3 grams carbohydrates, 9 grams fat, 69 milligrams cholesterol, 492 milligrams sodium, 2 grams fiber, 110 milligrams calcium, 1 milligram iron

Tip: Coconut flour adds a nice flavor to pancakes; another great gluten-free flour that can be used in place of coconut flour is mesquite flour (it has a sweet, nutty flavor).

Cornmeal Breakfast Cakes   Serves 4

A simple to prepare, rustic breakfast cake that you are sure to love.

1 cup gluten-free yellow cornmeal
½ tsp salt
¾ cup 1% milk
1 Tb honey
1 Tb butter
2 egg whites
Gluten-free cooking spray (or vegetable oil)

1. Mix cornmeal and salt in a large bowl.

2. In a small saucepan, heat milk, honey, and butter to a low simmer.

3. Pour mixture over cornmeal; stir to combine. Let sit for 5 minutes.

4. In an electric mixer, beat egg whites in a small bowl until stiff white peaks form. Gently fold egg whites into the cornmeal mixture.

5. Coat a hot griddle with cooking spray or vegetable oil. Pour batter by ¼-cupfuls and spread to ¼ inch thick.

6. Cook for 2–3 minutes on each side until golden brown.

Nutritional information per serving: 203 calories, 6 grams protein, 44 grams carbohydrates, 3.5 grams fat, 10 milligrams cholesterol, 336 milligrams sodium, <1 gram fiber, 57 milligrams calcium, 1 milligram iron.

Tip: Serve with butter and syrup or honey or agave, or make a maple butter whip: take 2 parts butter or margarine, softened, and blend with 1 part honey or syrup. (Also great with cinnamon.)

Toasty Cinnamon Sticks   Serves 3

Kids will love these—or make them as a treat for the kid inside you!

6 pieces of gluten-free bread, with crust removed
2 eggs
¼ cup skim milk
1 tsp vanilla extract
2 tsp cinnamon
2 tsp butter melted
Gluten-free cooking spray (or vegetable oil)
2 tsp powdered sugar
¼ tsp cinnamon
Optional toppings (maple syrup or jam)

1. Cut each piece of bread into 3 strips each.

2. Mix together eggs, skim milk, vanilla, cinnamon, and butter.

3. Lightly soak breadsticks in egg mixture until well coated.

4. Spray a large skillet with cooking spray or coat with vegetable oil.

5. When skillet is hot, place cinnamon sticks on pan and brown on both sides.

6. Sprinkle with sugar and cinnamon and serve with a little maple syrup or jam.

Nutritional information: 251 calories, 6.6 grams protein, 29 grams carbohydrates, 11.7 grams fat, 48 milligrams cholesterol, 107 milligrams sodium, 1.6 grams fiber, 93 milligrams calcium, 2.5 milligrams iron

Tip: Delicious served with fresh berries or sliced bananas.

Ricotta Surprise   Serves 2

If you like Italian dessert fillings like those found in Italian pastries, you will love these. What a great way to start the morning.

1 cup skim ricotta cheese
2 Tb light cream cheese
2 Tb sugar
½ cup favorite gluten-free cereal
1 cup mixed berries
¼ tsp cinnamon

1. Mix together ricotta cheese, cream cheese, and sugar until smooth.

2. Layer cheese mixture, cereal, and berries in two parfait glasses.

3. Sprinkle with cinnamon.

4. Chill till ready to serve.

Nutritional information: 309 calories, 16.5 grams protein, 32.8 grams carbohydrates, 12.5 grams fat, 46.5 milligrams cholesterol, 252 milligrams sodium, 1.3 grams fiber, 382 milligrams calcium, 3.4 milligrams iron.

Tip: This is quick, easy, and delicious. It can be prepared in paper cups ahead of time for a quick grab-and-go breakfast.

Yogurt Parfait   Serves 2

Light, quick, and delicious. Perfect for those mornings when you don't have a lot of time but want a special start for the day.

2 (6-oz) containers gluten-free lite vanilla yogurt (such as Stonyfield)
1 small banana, sliced
½ cup blueberries (or other favorite berry)
2 Tb gluten-free whipped topping (such as Cool Whip)
2 gluten-free cookies such as gluten-free animal crackers or gluten-free graham crackers crumbled (optional)

1. Place a piece of cheesecloth over a medium cup and hold in place with a rubber band.

2. Pour yogurt in cheese cloth and leave in refrigerator for a few hours, or overnight, if possible. Save creamy part of yogurt and discard liquid in the cup.

3. Layer yogurt with gluten-free cookies, blueberries, and banana, top with whip cream, and serve.

Nutritional information: 225.6 calories, 8 grams protein, 44.7 grams carbohydrates, 2.5 grams fat, 5 milligrams cholesterol, 101 milligrams sodium, 4.4 grams fiber, 305.1 milligrams calcium, <1 milligram iron.

Tip: Any kind of fruit and gluten-free cookie or cereal can be used to make a delicious parfait. The creamy part of the yogurt, also known as yogurt cheese, makes a great spread.

Breads:

- Popovers
- Socca
- Stuffed Arepas

Popovers   Serves 6

These are light, crispy, and custardy in the middle. Delicious with fruit-flavored butter or fresh preserves.

3 eggs
¾ cup nonfat milk
¾ cup gluten-free flour blend (see basic flour blends, formula 1)
1 tsp salt
1 tsp xanthan gum
3 Tb butter (or reduce the amount of fat by using light butter or light trans fat–free margarine)

1. Preheat oven to 375 degrees.

2. Separate butter equally in each popover tin, and place popover pan in the oven to heat.

3. Beat eggs, and blend into milk.

4. Mix flour with salt and xanthan gum.

5. Blend flour mixture into egg mixture.

6. Fill each popover tin about 2/3 full (do this quickly, taking care not to let the pan cool too much during the process).

7. Bake for about 30–35 minutes, until puffed.

8. To keep the popovers from falling, don't open the oven while baking.

9. Remove from the oven and poke popovers with a fork to keep from them from falling.

Nutritional information: 171 calories, 5.5 grams protein, 18.8 grams carbohydrates, 8.6 grams fat, 121.6 milligrams cholesterol, 489 milligrams sodium, <1 gram fiber, 73 milligrams calcium, <1 milligram iron.

Tips: Make sure you use a popover pan—it is much deeper than a typical muffin pan. Although you can make a popover in a different pan, you won't get that extra puff or height. These are also delicious with honey butter: softened butter or margarine processed with honey.

Socca   Serves 4

Found in Nice, France, or Northern Italy, socca are a real treat. Not only are they quick and easy to make, but they have fabulous taste and texture.

1 cup chickpea flour
1 cup water
2 Tb olive oil
½ Tb rosemary, freshly chopped
½ tsp salt
¼ tsp pepper
¼ cup onion or shallots, sliced thin (optional)
Gluten-free cooking spray (or vegetable oil)

1. Mix together chickpea flour, water, 1 Tb olive oil, rosemary, salt, pepper, and shallots, and let mixture it sit for about ½ hour, covered, at room temperature. (Mixture will resemble a thick cream.)

2. Preheat oven to broil.

3. Spray a 9½-inch round nonstick skillet with cooking spray (or coat with vegetable oil) and heat on low until hot.

4. Pour about ½ cup batter into pan and swirl around to coat pan like a crepe in a nice round shape (use a rubber spatula to loosen up the sides).

5. Cook socca until crispy on one side, slide onto a cookie sheet or a pizza pan, drizzle with ¼ Tb olive oil, and brown under the broiler until crispy.

Nutritional information: 153 calories, 5.2 grams protein, 14.3 grams carbohydrates, 8.3 grams fat, 0 milligrams cholesterol, 306 milligrams sodium, 2.7 grams fiber, 14.3 milligrams calcium, 1.2 milligrams iron.

Tips: Although socca is traditionally made on a different type of pan and in a much hotter oven, cooking it this way cuts the fat in half and works easily for home cooks. Socca can be used as a flatbread with dips or can be topped with any of your favorite toppings. If you wish to add toppings, broil until it just starts to crisp, lightly sprinkle with cheese or tomato or other favorites, and put back under the broiler to finish. Keep toppings light so you don't drown out the flavor of the socca.

Stuffed Arepas   Serves 4

Delicious Hispanic flatbread, often served as a sandwich for eggs or cheese. It can be made from precooked corn or masa harina, as below—a great find!

1 cup instant gluten-free masa harina (precooked cornmeal)
1½ cups boiling water
½ tsp salt
Gluten-free cooking spray (or vegetable oil)
2 Tb parmesan cheese
2 oz hard provolone cheese
4 pieces roasted red pepper

1. In a medium bowl, mix together masa harina, boiling water, and salt until well combined. Let mixture sit for about 5 minutes.

2. Preheat oven to 350 degrees.

3. Wet your hands with cold water and separate mixture into 4 balls; flatten these with your hands into patties.

4. Spray a large skillet with cooking spray (or coat with vegetable oil) and heat it over medium heat until hot.

5. Place each patty in the skillet and cook for 5–7 minutes on each side until it browns and puffs up a little and the center is mostly set (the middle will be a little soft, like polenta).

6. Sprinkle top of each arepa with parmesan cheese.

7. Slice each arepa open and fill it with provolone and red pepper. Place on a baking sheet and bake at 350 degrees until the cheese melts.

Nutritional information: 176 calories, 7.6 grams protein, 24.4 grams carbohydrates, 5.7 grams fat, 12 milligrams cholesterol, 456 milligrams sodium, 3.5 grams fiber, 178 milligrams calcium, 2.3 milligrams iron.

Tip: Arepas are easy to prepare and make a quick easy sandwich bread.

Appetizers:

- Artichoke Cheese Dip
- Baked Vidalia Onion Dip
- Black Bean Mango Salsa
- Black Bean Dip with Corn Chips
- Cold Sesame Noodles
- Cornmeal Crusted Chicken Tenders
- Hot Crabmeat Dip
- Layered Taco Dip

Artichoke Cheese Dip   **Serves 20**

This is a terrific lower fat version of a classic party favorite.

1 cup grated parmesan
12 oz part skim shredded Mozzarella cheese
1 cup low-fat mayonnaise
1 can (14 oz) artichoke hearts, drained
1 tsp garlic powder
Gluten-free crackers or veggie sticks

1. Preheat oven to 400 degrees.

2. Blend all ingredients together in a food processor.

3. Pour into a 1-quart casserole dish.

4. Bake for about 25 minutes, until bubbly.

5. Serve with veggie sticks or gluten-free crackers.

Nutritional information: 110 calories, 6 grams protein, 3.5 grams carbohydrates, 7.8 grams fat, 17 milligrams cholesterol, 284 milligrams sodium, <1 gram fiber, 169 milligrams calcium, <1 milligram iron.

Tip: Add some gluten-free breadcrumbs to this mixture, and stuff the uncooked mixture into mushroom caps and bake until the mushrooms are cooked for a yummy stuffed mushroom appetizer.

Baked Vidalia Onion Dip   Serves 12

So simple to prepare that it will disappear as quickly as you can make it—a cheesy treat!

2 large finely minced Vidalia onions
2 cups shredded Swiss cheese
2 cups low-fat mayonnaise
1 cup parmesan cheese
Veggies sticks and gluten-free crackers

1. Preheat oven to 400 degrees.

2. Mix all ingredients together.

3. Place all ingredients in a casserole dish.

4. Bake for about 20–25 minutes, until bubbling.

5. Serve with gluten-free crackers and veggie sticks.

Nutritional information: 240 calories, 8 grams protein, 6 grams carbohydrates, 19 grams fat, 29 milligrams cholesterol, 466 milligrams sodium, <1 gram fiber, 285 milligrams calcium, <1 milligram iron.

Tip: Any kind of cheese can be used in this recipe—it's a sure party hit!

Black Bean and Mango Salsa   Serves 12

This salsa gives a fresh, colorful, finished touch to any meal. A real crowd pleaser.

2 (10½-oz) cans black beans, drained and rinsed
1 ear of corn, kernels only (about 1 cup frozen corn, if fresh is unavailable)
1 mango, chopped
Juice of 2 limes
1 jalapeno pepper, chopped
1 red pepper, chopped
1 red onion, chopped
¼ cup cilantro, chopped

1. Mix all ingredients together.

2. Refrigerate mixture until ready to use.

Nutritional information: 63 calories, 3 grams protein, 13.2 grams carbohydrates, <1 gram fat, 0 milligrams cholesterol, 99 milligrams sodium, 2.9 grams fiber, 20 milligrams calcium, <1 milligram iron.

Tips: Great served over chicken or fish! To remove the kernels from an ear of corn, remove husk from the corn and run a knife down each side of the corn over a small bowl, removing and saving all kernels.

Black Bean Dip with Corn Chips   Serves 6

A great party dip that is loaded with flavor and fiber—leftovers work great as a sandwich spread.

2 Tb olive oil
1 large onion, chopped
1 Tb minced garlic
1 tsp dried oregano
1 tomato, chopped
10.5 oz can black beans, drained and rinsed
2 Tb lime juice
1 Tb gluten-free hot sauce (to taste)
1 tsp ground cumin
1 tsp chili pepper
¼ cup cilantro, chopped

¼ cup (2 oz) gluten-free vegetable broth (such as Pacific Brand)
1 tsp salt
1 tsp pepper
6 oz 100% corn chips

1. Heat oil and sauté onion, garlic, and oregano together until onion starts to brown.

2. Add to that tomato, black beans, lime juice, hot sauce, cumin, chili pepper, cilantro, and vegetable broth. Cook for about 5–10 minutes; if too dry, add a little water. Then add salt and pepper.

3. Put all ingredients through a food processor until very smooth.

4. Refrigerate overnight before serving.

5. Serve with corn chips.

Nutritional information: 236 calories, 4.4 grams protein, 29 grams carbohydrates, 12.7 grams fat, 0 milligrams cholesterol, 741 milligrams sodium, 5 grams fiber, 91.7 milligrams calcium, 1.5 milligrams iron.

Tip: Beans are a great way to increase the fiber in your diet. Bean dips can keep well refrigerated for about a week.

Cold Noodles in Sesame Sauce   Serves 6

This is a rich, delicious side dish that can stand alone as a meal or work great as part of an appetizer buffet selection.

1 pound of brown rice linguini
2 Tb gluten-free light soy sauce (such as LaChoy)
1 tsp hot sauce
1 Tb sesame oil
1 Tb cider vinegar
1 tsp sugar
1 clove minced garlic (about 1 tsp)
1 Tb peanut or vegetable oil
4 Tb toasted sesame seeds
6 scallions, chopped

1. Cook linguini until just cooked; rinse thoroughly under cold water. Make sure pasta is dry before mixing with other ingredients.

2. Combine all remaining ingredients and toss with pasta.

3. Chill until ready to use. Serve cool or at room temperature.

Nutritional information: 368 calories, 7.2 grams protein, 61 grams carbohydrates, 7.5 grams fat, 10 milligrams cholesterol, 200 milligrams sodium, 1.7 grams fiber, 71.3 milligrams calcium, 3 milligrams iron.

Tip: These are great served warm or cold or with a chopped cucumber salad and grilled chicken breasts.

Cornmeal-Crusted Chicken Tenders   Serves 4

Chicken fingers are always a hit. Make them ahead of time and freeze them so you can always have a batch ready to go.

1 pound uncooked plain chicken tenders
2 Tb potato starch
¼ tsp salt
¼ tsp pepper
2 eggs
¼ cup instant mashed potato flakes (most are GF, but double-check the label!)
¼ cup cornmeal
2 tsp grill seasoning blend (see tip)
2 Tb vegetable oil

1. Place chicken, potato starch, salt, and pepper in a gallon-size zipper bag. Shake to coat chicken.

2. Beat eggs in a shallow dish.

3. In a separate shallow dish, mix potato flakes, cornmeal, and grill seasoning.

4. Remove chicken from bag, dip it in the egg mixture, and roll it in the cornmeal mixture until it is well coated.

5. Heat oil in a large nonstick skillet over medium high heat. Place chicken in skillet and cook for 3–4 minutes on each side until cooked through. (Turn chicken often to prevent burning.)

6. Remove from skillet and place on paper towel–lined plate to drain.

Nutritional information per serving: 286 calories, 30 grams protein, 17 grams carbohydrates, 11 grams fat, 171 milligrams cholesterol, 205 milligrams sodium, <1 gram fiber, 29 milligrams calcium, 2 milligrams iron.

Tips: Serve with gluten-free honey mustard dressing (see sauce recipes in this book, or buy premade gluten-free choices). Also, if you are unsure about the gluten-free status of your grill seasoning blend, make your own by combining dehydrated garlic and onion, salt, black pepper, sage, thyme, rosemary, red pepper, dehydrated parsley, dehydrated orange peel, paprika, dehydrated green bell peppers (when making your own seasoning blend, it is handy to make extra and keep it in a jar in your spice cabinet).

Hot Crabmeat Dip   Serves 4

This crabmeat dip makes the perfect start for a great evening of entertaining. It can be made with baby shrimp or lobster in place of the crab if so desired.

2 cans (6 ounces each) lump crabmeat (but see tip*)
4 oz gluten-free low-fat cream cheese
¼ cup light mayonnaise
1 Tb minced dried onions
1 tsp gluten-free red curry paste (such as Taste of Thai)
1 tsp dried parsley flakes

1. Preheat oven to 375 degrees.

2. Drain and rinse crabmeat.

3. Mix drained crabmeat with remaining ingredients and place in a 1-quart oven-safe baking dish.

4. Sprinkle with parsley.

5. Bake for 20 minutes, until bubbly.

6. Serve with favorite gluten-free crackers or gluten-free chips.

Nutritional information per serving: 167 calories, 16 grams protein, 5 grams carbohydrates, 9 grams fat, 96 milligrams cholesterol, 467 milligrams sodium, 0 grams fiber, 68 milligrams calcium, 1.2 milligrams iron.

Tips: For added crunch, top with any kind of chopped nuts before baking. *Make sure you use real crabmeat—imitation crabmeat often contains gluten.

Layered Taco Dip   Serves 12

This dip includes many favorite Mexican toppings, is easy to make, and is very inexpensive. Put it together, refrigerate it, and pull it out when your guests arrive. Leftovers work great as part of a homemade taco salad.

16-oz jar gluten-free salsa
1 cup shredded low-fat cheddar cheese
1 cup shredded lettuce
2 green onions, chopped
8 oz gluten-free fat-free sour cream
16 oz can gluten-free refried beans
15.5 oz can black beans (drained)
7 oz can corn kernels drained
2 tomatoes, chopped
2 avocados, peeled and chopped
2 oz can black olives, sliced (drained)

1. In a glass bowl no more than 6 inches thick, layer ingredients as desired.

2. Serve with veggie sticks, or gluten-free corn chips.

Nutritional information: 187 calories, 8.7 grams protein, 22 grams carbohydrates, 8.5 grams fat, 11.5 milligrams cholesterol, 604 milligrams sodium, 6 grams fiber, 228 milligrams calcium, 1.7 milligrams iron.

Tip: This is yummy if just warmed in the microwave for about a minute. If you like things spicy, add some chopped jalapeno peppers or hot sauce while layering.

Soups, Salads, and Sandwiches

- Italian Tuna Salad

- Portabella Mushroom Burgers

- Shrimp Salad–Stuffed Tomatoes

- Easy Chicken and Rice Soup

- Cheddar Quesadillas

- Turkey Avocado Melt

- Roasted Peppers and Tomato Salad

Italian Tuna Salad   Serves 2

Most people think of tuna as something that you find at the local deli. But this tuna fish salad is so different and so delicious that you won't want to leave a bite.

6 oz canned gluten-free solid white tuna in water, drained
½ cup pitted green olives, chopped
¼ cup red onions, chopped
2 Tb good-quality olive oil
1 Tb capers
2 Tb lemon juice
2 gluten-free teff wraps (such as La Tortilla gluten-free wraps—or 4 toasted corn tortillas)
1 tomato, chopped
1 cup lettuce, shredded
1 cucumber, chopped

1. Drain tuna and place in a bowl; break into small pieces with a fork.

2. Add olives, onions, oil, capers, and lemon juice to the tuna and blend well.

3. Serve in teff wraps or corn tortillas with tomato, lettuce, and cucumber.

Nutritional information: 474 calories, 25 grams protein, 42 grams carbohydrates, 2.3 grams fat, 36 milligrams cholesterol, 910 milligrams sodium, 6.5 grams fiber, 69 milligrams calcium, 2.3 milligrams iron.

Tip: This recipe works great with salmon as well.

Portabella Mushroom Burgers   Serves 4

If you have never had portabella mushrooms before, you will be surprised and thrilled by how wonderful they truly are. Leftovers work great in salads and wraps and mixed into spreads.

4 portabella mushroom caps
½ tsp salt
½ tsp pepper
2 crushed garlic cloves
2 Tb olive oil
1 Tb balsamic vinegar
1 tomato, sliced
4 slices roasted red peppers
4 thin slices red onion
4 lettuce leaves

1. Rinse and dry mushroom caps.

2. Mix mushrooms with salt, pepper, garlic, olive oil, and balsamic vinegar, and marinate in a zipper bag for about ½ hour.

3. Preheat oven to 350 degrees.

4. Place mushrooms gill-side down on a baking sheet and bake for about 10–15 minutes, until cooked through.

5. Serve each mushroom with sliced tomato, roasted red pepper, red onion, and lettuce leaves.

Nutritional information: 121 calories, 5 grams protein, 10.7 grams carbohydrates, 10.7 grams fat, 0 milligrams cholesterol, 305 milligrams sodium, 3.4 grams fiber, 79 milligrams calcium, <1 milligram iron.

Tip: Portabella mushrooms have a meaty, satisfying texture that makes a nice sandwich. (Great on your favorite toasted gluten-free roll)

Shrimp Salad–Stuffed Tomatoes   Serves 4

Tomatoes make a perfect food for stuffing, especially fresh-picked summer tomatoes. And there is no better filling than shrimp salad. You can also use cherry tomatoes, cut in half, as a perfect appetizer size.

4 medium tomatoes
8 oz precooked shrimp, shells and tails removed and cut into ½-inch pieces
1 celery stalk, chopped
4 Tb green onion, chopped

4 Tb reduced-fat gluten-free mayonnaise
1 Tb catsup
2 Tb parsley, chopped
¼ tsp salt
¼ tsp pepper
1 Tb lemon juice or hot sauce
Parsley to garnish

1. Cut tops off tomatoes and hollow out, reserving pulp and discarding liquid.

2. Mix tomato pulp thoroughly with all remaining ingredients except parsley garnish.

3. Refrigerate all ingredients overnight to allow the flavors to blend.

4. Stuff filling into tomatoes; garnish with parsley and serve.

Nutritional information: 127 calories, 13 grams protein, 6 grams carbohydrates, 5.4 grams fat, 113 milligrams cholesterol, 407.6 milligrams sodium, 1.7 grams fiber, 42 milligrams calcium, 2.2 milligrams iron.

Tip: Use lemon juice or hot sauce to taste.

Easy Chicken and Rice Soup   Serves 10

Quick chicken soup like mom used to make is always something that warms you from the inside out. This soup is so good that no one will believe that you were able to just throw it together.

Gluten-free cooking spray (or vegetable oil)
1 large onion, chopped
4 celery stalks, sliced thin
1 cup baby carrots, sliced
1 potato, cut into ¼-inch pieces
96 oz (3 [32-oz containers]) low-sodium gluten-free chicken broth (such as Pacific Brand)
2 (6-oz) boneless skinless chicken breasts
1 cup cooked brown rice

1. Spray a large pot with cooking spray (or coat with vegetable oil), and sauté veggies.

2. Add chicken stock and simmer for about 1 hour.

3. Cut chicken cutlets into 2-inch pieces and add to simmering broth, along with cooked rice, until chicken is just cooked.

4. Serve hot.

Nutritional information: 94 calories, 9.8 grams protein, 11 grams carbohydrates, 1 gram fat, 16 milligrams cholesterol, 194 milligrams sodium, 1.3 grams fiber, 14.5 milligrams calcium, <1 milligram iron.

Tip: Leftover gluten-free pasta or cooked beans works great in place of the brown rice in this soup as well.

Cheddar Quesadillas   Serves 2

These are the best quesadillas I've ever had. You won't miss the typical flour tortillas at all.

2 (6-inch) corn tortillas
2 Tb shredded light gluten-free cheddar cheese
¼ avocado, sliced
½ jalapeno pepper, chopped (optional)
2 Tb black olives, chopped
½ cup drained gluten-free salsa (a mini strainer works)
2 Tb fat-free sour cream

1. In a sauté pan, heat both sides of the tortillas.

2. While each tortilla is still in the sauté pan, place ½ cheese, avocado, jalapeno, and olives on one side of each tortilla.

3. When cheese starts to melt, place salsa and sour cream on same side and fold tortilla in half.

4. Heat several minutes more and serve.

Nutritional information: 139.5 calories, 5.1 grams protein, 20 grams carbohydrates, 5.4 grams fat, 6.4 milligrams cholesterol, 516 milligrams sodium, 4 grams fiber, 164.5 milligrams calcium, <1 milligram iron.

Tip: Wrap in aluminum foil for a quick grab-and-go meal.

Turkey Avocado Melt   Serves 2

Avocado and cheddar give a nice, creamy texture and a burst of flavor to this terrific sandwich. Pickles, roasted peppers, and bacon are also great additions to this sandwich.

4 slices whole-grain gluten-free bread
2 Tb gluten-free brown mustard
4 oz gluten-free honey turkey (such as Boar's Head), sliced thin
⅛ avocado, peeled and sliced
1.5 oz shredded reduced-fat gluten-free cheddar cheese
2 slices red onion
2 slices tomato
Gluten-free cooking spray

1. Toast bread in a gluten-safe toaster.

2. Spread mustard on bread.

3. Make up each sandwich with turkey, avocado, cheddar, red onion, and tomato.

4. Spray a skillet with cooking spray and brown each sandwich on each side until cheese melts, then serve.

Nutritional information: 362 calories, 19.8 grams protein, 39.7 grams carbohydrates, 14.1 grams fat, 35 milligrams cholesterol, 1094 milligrams sodium, 2.3 grams fiber, 366 milligrams calcium, 3.3 milligrams iron.

Tip: Many people don't realize that they can be as careful as possible with their gluten-free foods and then turn around and contaminate them with gluten in a toaster that has previously toasted regular wheat bread. To protect your food, have a dedicated gluten-free toaster, use toaster-safe bags, or use your oven with aluminum foil on the rack.

Roasted Peppers and Tomato Salad   Serves 4

This summer salad makes the perfect side dish for a barbeque.

2 cucumbers, sliced
2 cups cherry tomatoes, cut in half
¼ cup red onion, chopped
½ cup roasted peppers, chopped (if jarred, rinse and drain)
2 Tb basil, freshly chopped

Dressing:
1½ Tb olive oil
2 tsp wine vinegar
1 tsp gluten-free Dijon mustard
1 tsp oregano, freshly chopped (or ¼ tsp dried)
2 tsp brown sugar

1. Whisk together all dressing ingredients.

2. Toss all ingredients together with dressing, and refrigerate until ready to serve.

Nutritional information: 100 calories, 2 grams protein, 12.3 grams carbohydrates, 5.4 grams fat, 0 milligrams cholesterol, 39 milligrams sodium, 2.3 grams, fiber, 38 milligrams calcium, <1 milligram iron.

Tip: For a sensational taste, make your own roasted peppers. To roast peppers, put them on a baking sheet that has been covered with aluminum foil, and put them into a 450 degree oven and cook until the peppers start to turn black on the outside. Cool and then peel and discard seeds and skin. Roasted peppers can be refrigerated for several days and stored in a glass jar in the refrigerator.

Entrees

*   Chicken in Vodka Sauce with Mushrooms

*   Blackened Mahi Mahi

*   Asian Rubbed Flank Steak

*   Eggplant Rollatini

Chicken in Vodka Sauce with Mushrooms   Serves 4

This Italian favorite is perfect served with gluten-free pasta. See tips for making extra vodka sauce.

2 Tb light margarine
2 Tb garlic, chopped
1 pound of chicken tenders
¼ cup brown rice flour

½ tsp salt
⅓ cup vodka
14 oz can diced tomatoes
8 oz mushrooms, sliced
4 Tb fat-free half-and-half
2 Tb parmesan cheese

1. Combine rice flour and salt in a medium bowl.

2. Melt margarine in a large skillet over medium heat.

3. Sauté garlic in margarine for 2–3 minutes.

4. Meanwhile, toss chicken in rice flour and salt.

5. Brown chicken in skillet on both sides until just cooked, and remove from pan.

6. Remove pan from heat, add vodka, and then return to heat.

7. Add diced tomatoes with liquid and simmer.

8. Add mushrooms and simmer until mushrooms are cooked. Add chicken back to pan, and add half and half with Parmesan cheese. Simmer for a few minutes until sauce starts to thicken, and serve.

Nutritional information: 457.7 calories, 21 grams protein, 34 grams carbohydrates, 21.2 grams fat, 49.4 milligrams cholesterol, 1,064 milligrams sodium, 3 grams fiber, 118 milligrams calcium, 2.4 milligrams iron.

Tip: To make vodka sauce separately, (1) melt margarine in a large skillet and sauté garlic for 2–3 minutes; (2) add about 1 Tb of rice flour and salt and stir until thickened; (3) add vodka and diced tomatoes, with their juice, and stir until all ingredients are combined; (4) add half-and-half and Parmesan cheese and continue stirring; (5) simmer for a few minutes, until the sauce starts to thicken; (6) serve immediately. You can use vodka sauce with any pasta dish, or over grilled shrimp or other fish—delicious!

Blackened Mahi Mahi   Serves 4

This spicy favorite will take you right back to the islands.

1 Tb lemon pepper
½ tsp cayenne pepper

1 tsp oregano
1 tsp thyme
1 tsp white pepper
3 Tb butter (or trans-fat free margarine), melted
16 oz (4 [4-oz each]) mahi mahi fish fillets
Gluten-free cooking spray (or vegetable oil)

1. In a small bowl, mix together lemon pepper, cayenne pepper, oregano, thyme, and white pepper.

2. Spray a heavy cast iron skillet with cooking spray (or coat with vegetable oil) and heat over medium-high heat until very hot.

3. Brush each fillet with melted butter and sprinkle with pepper spice mix on both sides. Press mixture into fish with hands.

4. Place fish in skillet. Cook until fish has a charred appearance—about 2–3 minutes. Turn fish over and continue to cook until fish is blackened and easily flakes with fork.

Nutritional information: 181 calories, 21 grams protein, <1 gram carbohydrate, 9 grams fat, 106 milligrams cholesterol, 401 milligrams sodium, <1 gram fiber, 27.4 milligrams calcium, 1.5 milligrams iron.

Tips: Make sure you have good ventilation and the fan on when cooking this fish—it will smoke!

Asian Rubbed Flank Steak   Serves 4

This recipe is a barbecue favorite, easy to make and loaded with flavor.

1 lb flank steak

Marinade:
¼ cup gluten-free soy sauce (such as La Choy)
3 Tb pineapple juice
¼ tsp black pepper
1 clove garlic, minced
½ tsp ginger, freshly chopped

Dry Spice Rub:
½ tsp cinnamon

¼ tsp ground cloves
¼ tsp dry ginger
¼ tsp allspice
½ tsp garlic salt
1 Tb black peppercorns, crushed
1 tsp anise seeds, crushed

1. Mix all marinade ingredients in a gallon zipper bag. Add flank steak and turn to coat. Seal bag and place in refrigerator for 1–2 hours.

2. Mix dry rub ingredients in a small bowl.

3. Preheat broiler.

4. Remove steak from marinade. Discard marinade.

5. Press dry rub onto both sides of steak and place on broiler pan.

6. Place under broiler and cook for 3–4 minutes on each side, or to desired doneness.

Nutritional information: 204 calories, 25 grams protein, 2 grams carbohydrates, 10 grams fat, 48 milligrams cholesterol, 503 milligrams sodium, <1 gram fiber, 18.7 milligrams calcium, 2.4 milligrams iron.

Tip: This recipe works great with any steak.

Eggplant Rollitini   Serves 4

Grilling the eggplant cuts down the amount of fat used in the traditional recipe and saves time, since you skip the breading step.

1 medium eggplant
1 Tb olive oil
½ cup water
1 tsp garlic powder
¾ cup skim ricotta cheese
3 Tb basil, freshly chopped
4 oz skim mozzarella (shredded)
2 cups tomato sauce
2 Tb grated parmesan cheese

1. Pre-heat oven to 350 degrees.

2. Peel eggplant and slice lengthwise into 8 pieces.

3. Mix together olive oil, water, and garlic powder.

4. Dip eggplant slices in liquid mixture.

5. Grill eggplant until just cooked on both sides.

6. Mix chopped basil with ricotta.

7. Roll eggplant with 1½ Tb ricotta mixture in each piece of eggplant.

8. In a casserole dish, pour ½ cup tomato sauce, and place each eggplant roll in a single layer on top of the sauce.

9. Top with the rest of the sauce, cover with sliced or shredded mozzarella cheese, and sprinkle with parmesan cheese.

10. Bake for about 15–20 minutes, until cheese is melted and hot.

Nutritional Information: 241 calories, 16.2 grams protein, 18 grams carbohydrates, 12.7 grams fat, 34.6 milligrams cholesterol, 914 milligrams sodium, 6.5 grams fiber, 407 milligrams calcium, 1.9 milligrams iron.

Tip: Can be made as either an appetizer or a main dish.

Desserts

- Yogurt Pie

- Quick and Easy Cheesecake

- Chocolate Dream Treats

- Bananas Foster

- Frozen Banana Cream

Yogurt Pie   Serves 8

What a wonderful way to get some extra calcium in your diet, a dessert that is easy and inexpensive to make

1 8-oz package gluten-free ginger snaps, crushed
2 Tb butter, melted
1 small banana, sliced

2 (6-oz) 90 calorie gluten-free fruit yogurts (such as Stonyfields)
1 (3-oz) packet gluten-free cherry Jell-O
8 oz fat-free cool whip

1. Mix cookie crumbs with butter and press into a 9-inch pie plate.

2. Arrange banana slices over pie crust.

3. Blend together yogurt, Jell-O, and Cool Whip and pour in pie crust.

4. Freeze pie until set, then serve.

Nutritional information: 289 calories, 2 grams protein, 42 grams carbohydrates, 11.8 grams fat, 8 milligrams cholesterol, 66 milligrams sodium, <1 gram fiber, 106.5 milligrams calcium, <1 milligram iron.

Tip: Any fruit-flavored yogurt works well in this pie.

Quick and Easy Cheesecake   Serves 10

Any cheesecake recipe can easily be made gluten-free. Using a gluten-free cereal makes the crust a snap.

1 cup Rice Chex (finely ground)
2 Tb slivered almonds
2 Tb dark brown sugar
½ tsp cinnamon
¼ tsp nutmeg
3 Tb melted butter
2 (8-oz) packages reduced-fat cream cheese
¾ cup sugar
2 eggs
½ cup reduced-fat sour cream
1 tsp almond extract

Crust:

1. In a food processor, blend Rice Chex, almonds, brown sugar, cinnamon, and nutmeg until finely ground.

2. Add butter and blend until mixed.

3. Press into a 9-inch pie pan to form crust.

Filling:

1. In a large bowl, beat cream cheese, sugar, eggs, sour cream, and almond extract until smooth and well mixed.

2. Pour into prepared shell.

3. Bake at 350 degrees for 45–55 minutes or until set.

4. Allow to cool completely before serving.

Nutritional information: 250 calories, 6.9 grams protein, 24 grams carbohydrates, 14.2 grams fat, 80 milligrams cholesterol, 212 milligrams sodium, <1 gram fiber, 89 milligrams calcium, 2.1 milligrams iron.

Tip: This is a delicious, easy-to-prepare cheesecake recipe. Why not top it with your favorite fruit preserves or fold in some jam or gluten-free chocolate chips for a nice addition?

Chocolate Dream Treats   Serves 30

Everyone loves candy, and these creamy, decadent treats will make you savor every bite.

1 (4.4-oz) bar gluten-free milk chocolate (like Hershey's)
1 (4.25-oz) bar gluten-free dark chocolate (like Hershey's)
1 (8-oz) container gluten-free mascarpone cheese
1 tsp gluten-free vanilla extract
1 shot gluten-free liquor (cordial, such as Amaretto)

1. Melt chocolate in top of a double boiler (or in the microwave).

2. Remove from heat and stir in cheese, vanilla, and liquor.

3. Pour chocolate into molds or pour about 1 Tb each into mini-muffin paper cups dusted with cocoa or powdered sugar.

4. Refrigerate to set and serve.

Nutritional information per serving (serving size 1 treat): 56 calories, 1 gram protein, 4.6 grams carbohydrates, 3.5 grams fat, 5.6 milligrams cholesterol, 32.5 milligrams sodium, <1 gram fiber, 11.1 milligrams calcium, <1 milligram iron.

Tip: If desired, top with shredded coconut and dried fruit.

Bananas Foster Serves 4

This simple to prepare bananas Foster is a lightened-up version of that traditional New Orleans favorite.

2 Tb lite butter or margarine
2 bananas, sliced
1 tsp cinnamon
2 Tb brown sugar
2 Tb dark rum
2 cups low-fat vanilla ice cream

1. Melt butter or margarine in a skillet over medium heat.

2. Add bananas, cinnamon, brown sugar, and rum to the skillet, and heat until the bananas start to caramelize—about 5 minutes; add a tiny bit of water if pan gets too dry.

3. You can keep the banana mixture refrigerated until ready to use, just microwave it before serving.

4. Serve ice cream topped with caramelized bananas.

Nutritional information: 221 calories, 3.7 grams protein, 37.4 grams carbohydrates, 5.2 grams fat, 17.5 milligrams cholesterol, 109 milligrams sodium, 2 grams fiber, 107 milligrams calcium, <1 milligram iron.

Tip: Traditionally, this recipe is made with a lot of butter and brown sugar and then set on fire when the rum is added, then ladled over ice cream. It is naturally gluten-free and is a decadent way to have your ice cream.

Frozen Banana Cream Serves 4

Cool, light, delicious, and easy to prepare.

4 small bananas (peeled, cut into 2-inch pieces, and frozen)
2 cups strawberries (frozen)
2 Tb strawberry jam
$\frac{1}{8}$–$\frac{1}{4}$ cup water
4 mint sprigs (optional)

1. Puree bananas, strawberries, and jam in a food processor.

2. Gradually add water until desired texture is achieved, but be careful not to add too much water.

3. Garnish with mint or some berries and serve immediately.

Nutritional information: 156 calories, 1.8 grams protein, 39.4 grams carbohydrates, .6 grams fat, 0 milligrams cholesterol, 4.6 grams fiber, 19.4 milligrams calcium, <1 gram iron.

Tip: Any berry or jam works well in this recipe. To make it easier to use the bananas, peel them before freezing, then package them in a freezer bag. Bananas are hard to peel after they are already frozen!

Quick and Easy Substitutions

Finding Quick Substitutes for Your Favorite Foods

We are all creatures of habit, and we like to keep things exactly the way we are used to them. Our habits follow us everywhere—especially the ways we like our food. Many people will say that their mom's lasagna is the best, but everyone's mom can't have the best lasagna. But it is the lasagna, or pot roast, or chicken soup that you have always eaten, that is at the heart of your soul, that is the one you are looking for.

Thus, the hardest part of changing your diet will always be finding ways to have your favorite foods the way you like them, and if you can't do this, you will always feel like you are missing something. So whether you cook, grab-and-go, or dine out, you need to stay gluten-free while finding wonderful substitutes for the foods you love.

Consider the foods that you normally eat that contain gluten: breads, pastas, and desserts. For some of these, you can find good substitutes, and in others the key will be tweaking the ingredients in favorite recipes so that they still work while eliminating the gluten that makes you sick. Learning how to work with gluten-free grains will help you achieve better textures and flavors in your recipes. You'll want to stock up on dried and frozen gluten-free pasta or try some homemade pasta recipes like those in Chapter 11. Pick up gluten-free breads, bread crumbs, flat breads, bagels, cereal, crackers, pancakes, muffins, and waffles—both frozen and mixes—and keep them stocked at home.

Make sure your spices, seasonings, condiments, and packaged foods are all gluten-free. Carry gluten-free bars, chips, fruits, nuts, and snacks with you when you are out and need something quick to eat. The trick is being prepared, so that you won't ever feel deprived by whatever choices (or lack of choices) may be available wherever it is that you are.

Thinking like a Great Gluten-Free Cook

Start by picking recipes that are naturally gluten-free or those that need very few changes. When preparing new recipes always use fresh, flavorful ingredients and stick with small changes to give you a better chance of success. Add new flavors to your meals by learning how to work with gluten-free grains in place of wheat, rye, and barley. In Chapter 3, you learned which grains were gluten-free, but now you need to know how to use them.

Some gluten-free grains, especially the flours, have a shorter shelf life than wheat flours, so it is best to keep them in a cool, dry place, in an airtight container, to help extend their freshness. Storing them in a freezer may help to extend the shelf life even longer.

TIP
Keeping gluten-free grains in the freezer helps keep them fresh longer.

Gluten-Free Grains

Some of the most commonly used gluten-free grains are

Amaranth: This is one of the ancient grains. Its tiny seeds are high in fiber, iron, and protein. They are easy to use and are found as seeds, puffed, or ground into flour.

Arrowroot Flour: This is a starch that can be used in equal amounts in place of cornstarch in recipes and is a great alternative for those who cannot have corn.

Bean Flours: High-protein flours like bean flours help provide a better texture to baking blends. Try them in desserts, bread, and homemade pasta blends. Since some people are allergic to beans, it is always important to let others know when you include them in your recipes. Note that some people lack the enzyme to digest fava beans (a condition called favism); they will get anemia when they consume fava beans. These individuals, mostly men of Mediterranean descent, must avoid fava beans.

Buckwheat: Buckwheat, contrary to its name, is not from the wheat family but from the rhubarb family, and it is gluten-free. It is found as whole groats, such as kasha, and as a flour, is great for making pancakes, breads, and crêpes. Buckwheat is full of flavor and nutrients.

Corn: Corn is naturally gluten-free, is widely available in many forms, and is used in most Hispanic dishes. It is a versatile and inexpensive grain.

Corn Flour: Corn flour is often used in corn bread, tortillas, and muffins.

Cornmeal: Ground dried corn, found in many Mexican dishes. Precooked cornmeal is also available, such as masa harina, which is great for dishes such as arepas and corn empanadas (breads and patties often served stuffed with cheese and meat).

Cornstarch: A starch made from corn, often used in Asian cooking and in puddings, sauces, and baking.

Expandex: A modified food starch made from tapioca that can be used in breads and baked products for a texture similar to gluten-containing baked foods.

Guar Gum: A powder made from a plant that works well to provide texture to baked products. It has a high fiber content, so you need to take care not to use too much in recipes because it can cause stomach problems for those who have sensitive stomachs.

Mesquite: Ground mesquite pods make a delicious gluten-free flour addition with a mocha coffee aroma and a taste of cinnamon and chocolate.

Millet: A delicious small grain with a sweet taste that is quick and easy to prepare. It comes whole, puffed, and as flour.

Nut Flours: Nut flours are made from ground nuts and work great in baked recipes and when added to the flour blends are especially flavorful in desserts. Some nice GF flour blends will include almond, hazelnuts, and chestnut. Since nuts are usually a common allergen, it is important to alert others about the ingredients when serving nut-based flour products.

Potato: All potatoes are gluten-free, and potato flours and starches are often used in gluten-free cooking.

Potato Starch: When added to gluten-free flour blends, it helps lighten up baked products.

Potato Flour: This is a heavier product than potato starch and has a strong potato taste. When buying premade potato products, double-check to make sure the manufacturer hasn't added gluten to the product.

Rice: All rice is generally gluten-free unless it has become contaminated by other foods. It is important to double-check any flavored rice products, or rice that has been produced in a plant that handles gluten-containing grains. Rice flours are great when added to almost all flour blends, because they don't overpower the flavors in the recipe, and they have nice texture. Rice flours come in both fine and medium grinds; heavier grinds will require more liquid in recipes. One-hundred percent rice paper is also a great choice for dumplings and stuffing.

Sweet Rice Flour: Sweet or sticky, or glutinous, rice does not contain gluten. It works well in sauces and is sometimes called sweet rice flour. Make sure you check mixes that include glutinous rice to make sure that other gluten-containing ingredients are not added.

Sorghum: A small, round grain about the size of barley. Sorghum takes on the flavor of other ingredients found in recipes and is ideal for putting together gluten-free flour blends. Available whole and as a flour. When whole sorghum is toasted it will puff like tiny popcorn kernels, with a sweet, nutty taste.

Soy Flour: This flour has a nutty taste and is higher in fat and protein. Soy flour works great with other grains, especially when combined with stronger-flavored ingredients like chocolate, dried fruit, and nuts, and it is often found in gluten-free cookies and mixes. Soy has a short shelf life, so only buy it when you are going to use it. Some people with celiac disease are often sensitive to soy proteins. Often the soy found in baked goods is soy lecithin, or the fat component of the soy, which does not usually include the soy protein.

Tapioca Flour or Tapioca Starch: Tapioca is a very light starch and is often added to baked goods in flour blends. It keeps well and gives a nice crispy texture and golden color to breads.

Teff: Teff is a tiny grain that is high in iron and that is available as both a light and dark grain. It is great in flour blends and delicious cooked whole as a hot cereal. It has a nice sweet aroma when cooking.

Quinoa: Quinoa is a high-protein grain loaded with nutrients. It needs to be rinsed three times before cooking to remove its outer coating, unless it is purchased prerinsed. Quinoa is delicious and hearty and works well in stews, casseroles, and pasta flour blends. When cooking it whole, wait until the small tail-looking end pops out—then you'll know it's done.

Xanthan Gum: A product that has been produced by the fermenting of corn sugar. Xanthan gum can be used as a thickener or to produce a texture similar to that which gluten gives to bread recipes.

Cooking with Gluten-Free Grains

Now that you know what some ingredients are, you will need to know how to measure, combine, and cook them. If you have trouble finding any ingredient, see Chapter 10 and the resource section at the end of this book for sources of gluten-free grains.

When working with gluten-free grains, difficulties come when you try to work with them the same way you would work with wheat. Wheat has specific properties that are not found in other single grains, so knowing how to combine different flours and enhancers can make the difference between a dense, tasteless product and a delicious treat.

Gluten-Free Thickeners

In order to thicken a sauce or a stew, use gluten-free thickening agents:

- Arrowroot
- Cornstarch
- Gelatin
- Gluten-free flours
- Potato starch
- Tapioca flour

Baking Powder

Baking powder sometimes contains gluten. When gluten-free baking powder is unavailable, make your own at home: 1 part baking soda +1 part starch +2 parts cream of tartar = homemade baking powder.

Substitutes for Small Amounts of Flour in Recipes

When a recipe is calling for just a few tablespoons of flour as a coating or part of the recipe, any of the following flours can be used:

- Bean
- Rice

- Millet
- Sorghum
- Tapioca

The next section will give you some ideas about how to make your own flour blends, as well as teaching you what ingredients work well together to obtain better textures.

You can work to achieve your own favorite flour blend or use some of the combinations suggested here. I am indebted to Carol Fenster, whose flour blends have been the inspiration and starting place for many of these flour blends.

Gluten-Free Baking Blends. *The following are some all-purpose flour combinations that can be used in many recipes throughout this book. For recipes that require some extra texture, such as breads and pasta, add 1 tsp of xanthan gum, guar gum, or expandex for every 2–3 cups of blend.*

Gluten-Free Flour Blend #1   Makes 4½ cups

Works well in any basic recipe—if it is a little too wet when blending into a dough, add some rice flour.

1½ cups sorghum flour
1½ cups potato starch or cornstarch
1 cup tapioca flour
½ cup chickpea, corn, almond, or hazelnut flour
Printed with permission from *Gluten-Free 101* by Carol Fenster (Savory Palate, 2008).

Gluten-Free Flour Blend #2   Makes 5½ cups

Great in gluten-free pasta and bread recipes.

1 cup sorghum
¾ cup brown rice flour
2 cups potato starch
1 cup tapioca starch
½ cup garbanzo bean flour

Gluten-Free Flour Blend #3   *Makes 5 cups*

Gives a nice golden crispy texture to baked foods.

1 ½ cups sorghum flour
½ cup brown rice flour
1 ½ cups potato starch or corn starch
1 cup tapioca flour
½ cup chick pea or almond flour or corn flour

Baking Combinations: Combos of these flours make great baked products.

Base Flours

Combine with modifiers and starches for improved texture.

- Buckwheat

- Chestnut

- Rice

- Sorghum

Texture-Enhancing, Flavorful Grains

HP means higher protein (provides stability).

- **(HP)** Bean and nut flours
- Amaranth
- Buckwheat
- Corn
- Flax
- Job's Tears
- Mesquite
- Millet
- Teff
- Quinoa

Modifiers and Starches

Lightens product and provides crisper crust.

- Arrowroot
- Cornstarch
- Potato starch
- Glutinous or sweet rice flour
- Tapioca flour and starch

High-Protein Additions

HP choices provide better consistency by holding together well.

- **(HP)** Bean and nut flours
- **(HP)** Eggs (powder or whole)
- **(HP)** Cheese
- **(HP)** Milk
- **(HP)** Beans (flours, or puréed)
- **(HP)** Nuts (flours, or butters)

Fruit Blends

These help provide good texture and stability to baked products.

- Fruit butters
- Fruit sauce or purees (such as apple, and pear)
- Mashed bananas

Leavening Agents

Reduces crumbling, helps products rise, very small amounts of these are added to recipes.

- Xanthan gum (add to dry ingredients) (usually 1–2 tsp for every 2–3 cups flour blend)
- Guar gum (add to dry ingredients)
- Expandex (add to dry ingredients)
- Gelatin (soften in water, use twice as much as the gums above)

Cooking Beans and Gluten-Free Grains

Grain or Bean	Amount of Grain	Amount of Water	Cooking Time	Yield
Amaranth (whole)	1 cup	3 cups	20–25 minutes	3 cups
Black beans	1 cup	4 cups	1½ hour	2¼ cups
Brown rice	1 cup	2½ cups	40–50 minutes	3 cups
Buckwheat groats	1 cup	2 cups	15 minutes	2½ cups
Chickpeas	1 cup	4 cups	2–3 hours	2 cups
Kidney beans	1 cup	3 cups	1½ hours	2¼ cups
Lentils	1 cup	2¼ cups	20 minutes	2¼ cups
Lima beans	1 cup	4 cups	1 hour	2 cups
Millet	1 cup	3 cups	20–30 minutes	3½ cups
Navy beans	1 cup	3 cups	1 hour	2⅔ cups
Pinto beans	1 cup	3 cups	2 hours	2½ cups
Polenta (corn grits)	1 cup	4 cups	10–15 minutes	2½ cups
Quinoa	1 cup	2 cups	10–15 minutes	2¾ cups
Gluten-free rolled oats	1 cup	3 cups	5–8 minutes	3½ cups
Sorghum (whole)	1 cup	3 cups	50–60 minutes	4 cups
Soybeans	1 cup	4 cups	3+ hours	3 cups
Split peas	1 cup	4 cups	45 minutes	2 cups
Teff	1 cup	3 cups	20 minutes	3½ cups
White rice	1 cup	2 cups	20–30 minutes	3 cups
Wild rice	1 cup	3 cups	40 minutes	4 cups

Converting Measures

When converting recipes it is important to know how to alter measurement amounts.
When working with dry ingredients,

3 tsp = 1 Tb
4 Tb = ¼ cup
16 Tb = 1 cup

When working with wet ingredients,
2 Tb = 1 oz.
1 cup = 8 oz.
2 cups = 16 oz. (1 pint)
4 cups (32 oz.) = 1 quart
4 quarts (128 oz.) = 1 gallon

Mixing It Up: Combining Gluten-Free Dishes and Ingredients

Sometimes all you need to know is how to combine foods and you can have a delicious meal. If you run out and do not feel safe using the prepared salad dressings and barbeque sauces available, why settle for eating your food plain? Improvise! Mixing together available safe condiments can spice up your meal. The following suggestions show how to combine common seasonings to give you familiar toppings. In Chapter 11 you'll find recipes for specific sauces and seasonings, but here are the quick fixes when you do not have your kitchen available to you. Thankfully, most of these choices are available in most restaurants.

Sauces and Seasonings

Always carry a safe seasoning blend. Store it in an old plastic spice jar, and keep it in a zip lock bag just in case it opens. Mix together garlic powder, onion powder, paprika, salt, pepper, and some dried herbs, such as basil, oregano, thyme, and parsley. Keep this with you to spice up food whenever needed. Mix up combinations below to your taste. Lea & Perrins Worcestershire is only GF in the U.S.

Barbeque Sauce: Mix together catsup, mustard, vinegar, sugar, hot sauce, a little jelly or jam (if available), and spice blend to taste.

Cheese Sauce: Mix mayonnaise with a crumbly strong-flavored cheese (such as blue or feta), use milk to thin, add Worcestershire sauce (use a safe choice like Lea & Perrins), add a squeeze of lemon, and spice blend to taste.

Cranberry Glaze: Mix cranberry sauce with oil, vinegar, and spice blend to taste.

Fra Diavlo Sauce: Mix tomato sauce, hot sauce, and wine with spice blend to taste.

French Dressing: Mix catsup, oil, vinegar, and sugar with GF Worcestershire (use a safe choice like Lea & Perrins).

Honey Mustard: 2 parts mustard, 1 part honey; thin with water or apple juice. To make creamy honey mustard, add mayonnaise, plain yogurt, or sour cream until desired texture is achieved.

Lobster Sauce: Mix melted butter with spice blend and lemon.

Louis Sauce: Mix mayonnaise, catsup, spice blend, chopped onion, and hot sauce to taste; use heavy cream to thin, and add a dash of salt and pepper and GF Worcestershire (use a safe choice like Lea & Perrins).

Mustard Sauce: Mix GF Dijon mustard, vinegar, chopped onions or shallots, GF hot sauce, sugar mayonnaise, and spice blend to taste.

Olive Sauce: Mix chopped olives, onions, tomatoes, capers, olive oil, and spice blend to taste.

Salsa Topping: Ask for a side of tomatoes and onions, and chop it up. Add hot sauce or lime juice to taste (if fresh herbs like cilantro are available, that's just an added bonus!).

Steak Sauce: Mix catsup, mustard, vinegar, GF Worcestershire (use a safe choice like Lea & Perrins), salt, pepper, sugar, and a little bit of spice blend to taste.

Sweet-and-Sour Sauce: Mix vinegar, water, sugar, and spice blend to taste (or add mayonnaise to make it creamy).

Sweet-and-Spicy Sauce: Mix jam, vinegar, and hot sauce to taste.

Tahini Sauce: Mix sesame seed paste, olive oil, water, and spice blend to taste.

Tartar Sauce: Mix mayonnaise, lemon juice, pickle relish, salt, and pepper to taste.

Thousand Island Salad Dressing: Mix catsup and mayonnaise—add pickle relish if available.

Yogurt Sauce: Mix plain yogurt or sour cream with spice blend, lemon juice, and chopped onions.

TIP: QUICK-AND-EASY GLUTEN-FREE COATINGS

Looking to make breaded cutlets or fish but out of gluten-free bread crumbs? No problem! Process gluten-free cereal, corn chips, or potato chips in a food processor and mix together with seasonings such as garlic, onion power, and dried herbs, and you're ready to go.

Mix-and-Match Desserts

Most restaurants have ice cream, and most plain vanilla ice cream is gluten-free. Unfortunately, it really seems pretty boring while everyone else is diving into a chocolate mud pie. Some yummy toppings or gluten-free cookies or bars can really jazz things up:

- Crushed gluten-free cookies swirled into ice cream
- Gluten-free chocolate bar broken into pieces and mixed into ice cream, with ordered liquor poured over the top
- Gluten-free brownie bar or M&Ms
- Chocolate-chip cookies dipped in single-serve peanut butter tubs along with your ice cream
- Individual gluten-free caramel sauce (available at restaurant supply stores)—a terrific ice cream topping
- Mini ice cream sandwiches made from gluten-free cookies

Easy Mix-and-Match Meals

Someone said to me once, "I don't have time to cook—I'm lucky if I find the time to boil rice noodles." People who are following a gluten-free diet are doing it because they have to. Some love to cook, some hate to cook, and some have no time to cook. Since the diet needs to be followed at all times, finding easy ways to throw meals together is essential for everybody.

Looking at what food you have on hand and combining it with seasonings or sauces makes meal planning a breeze. The following chart teaches you how to combine foods in three steps for easy mix-and-match meals. When you open your refrigerator, you will see all the possibilities for a meal.

Mix-and-Match Food Chart

The following combos give you choices from many food groups. The possibilities are endless—add your own!

1. Pick from food choices from different categories.

2. Combine your selections with seasonings, sauces, or sweeteners.

3. Heat and serve.

Starches

- Cooked gluten-free: Pasta, oats, grits, corn, amaranth, beans, buckwheat, flax seed, millet, polenta, potatoes, quinoa, rice, polenta, teff, potato/sweet potato (baked, grilled, fried), plantains (baked, frilled or fried), pumpkin, butternut squash, chili

- Gluten-free cereals (both hot and cold)

- Gluten-free breads, wraps, pancakes, waffles, crackers, pizza crust, rice cakes, corn tortillas, chips, and arepas

Fruits and Vegetables

- Fresh, frozen, canned, or dried fruit

- Fresh, frozen, canned, or dried vegetables, squash, and mixed greens

- Grilled fruits or vegetables (e.g., eggplant, onions, zucchini, peppers, apples, pears, papaya, pineapple)

- Shredded or cubed vegetables (e.g., carrots, beets, zucchini)

- Fruit and vegetable juices

Proteins (cubed, sliced, strips, or shredded)

- Chicken, turkey, fish, tofu, beans, beef, pork

- GF deli meats, cheese, (hard and soft), eggs, milk, buttermilk

- Nuts, nut butters, and seeds

- Yogurt (plain and GF flavored)
- Hummus or bean dips

Sauces/Seasonings/Fats

- GF salad dressing, catsup, mustard, syrup, honey, molasses, agave, relish, sugar, oils, distilled vinegars, soy sauce, barbeque sauce, yogurt sauce, tomato sauce, garlic sauce, cheese sauce, tahini, hot sauce
- Jams and jellies
- Fats and oils (such as olive, soy, peanut, corn, walnut, almond, hazelnut, canola, and vegetable), butter, margarine and avocado, GF broths and stocks, half-and-half
- Wines and distilled liquor
- Herbs (e.g., basil, oregano, thyme, sage, rosemary, mint)
- GF spices (e.g., garlic and onion powder, pepper, mustard, paprika, and salt)
- GF olives, capers, pickles, salsa

Ideas for Mix-and-Match Meals

These combinations are different from the standard meal plans provided earlier because all these suggestions are based what you have on hand and require little cooking or preparation. The purpose here is to see what you have in your refrigerator or cabinet and then to combine choices in order to have a quick and easy gluten-free meal. Use the mix-and-match food chart to give you ideas of how to combine foods. For example, if you looked in your refrigerator and found a baked potato, some grilled onions, a cooked hamburger, shredded cheese, and salsa, you could make salsa-stuffed potato skins. Cut the potato open and scoop out the center and mash the potato with the leftover hamburger and stuff it back into the shell (it will be a little overstuffed). Top the stuffed potato with grilled onions, salsa, and shredded cheese, then microwave until the potato is hot and the cheese is bubbling. There are so many possibilities! The following combos provide many ideas for breakfast, lunch, and dinner.

Breakfast Combos

- GF waffles or pancakes with butter and syrup or peanut butter and raisins

- Cottage cheese and mixed fruit

- Corn grits with melted cheese

- Toasted corn tortilla, folded and filled with scrambled eggs and cheddar

- GF cereal (such as Rice Chex, Corn Chex, or Mesa Sunrise) with skim milk and berries or sliced bananas

- GF rice cakes spread with peanut or almond butter and raisins

- GF cooked leftover teff with maple syrup and berries or dried fruit

- Instant quinoa cereal

- GF oatmeal with cinnamon, honey, and toasted walnuts

- Scrambled eggs served over toasted corn tortillas with GF salsa

- GF French toast with butter and syrup

- GF yogurt and GF cereal or flax topping

- Scrambled eggs and cheese with leftover GF fries

Lunch Combos

- Baked potato with broccoli florets and melted cheddar cheese

- Store-bought GF pizza crust with tomato sauce, shredded mozzarella, and sliced mushrooms

- GF wrap with roasted turkey, lettuce, tomato, and mayonnaise

- GF bread toasted with peanut butter and jelly

- GF instant polenta with tomato sauce and goat cheese

- Toasted corn tortilla with guacamole and salsa

- Grilled chicken breast with GF barbeque sauce on a toasted GF roll

- Leftover rice mixed with chopped onions, tomatoes, feta cheese, leftover shrimp or chicken, and GF salad dressing

- GF ham and Swiss cheese with mustard on a GF roll or tortilla

- Leftover GF pasta with mixed veggies, cheese, olives, and GF Italian salad dressing

- Hummus with corn chips and Greek salad

- Tuna with mayo, and pickle relish with chopped lettuce and tomato and GF crackers

- Large salad, with chickpeas, leftover tuna or chicken, and GF salad dressing

Dinner Combos

- Use leftovers to create kabobs, such as tuna, chicken, or beef with a combo of tomato, onion, and pepper kabob marinated in GF salad dressing

- Chili stuffed in a baked potato

- Leftover grilled burger or chicken breast with salsa and shredded cheese

- Leftover pork or chicken with GF barbeque sauce on a roll with a salad

- Leftover GF pasta with tomato sauce and ricotta cheese

- Roasted chicken with leftover brown rice or millet and mixed vegetables

- Large salad with veggies—toss with salmon or tuna and GF salad dressing and chickpeas

- Leftover GF breaded chicken breasts, heated with tomato sauce and mozzarella cheese

- Any baked fish with GF salad dressing, served with salad and leftover rice or potatoes

- Grill a steak and serve with salad or veggies and GF baked beans

- GF premade soup with a salad

- Leftover GF sausage, sautéed with onions and peppers

- Leftover shrimp with GF mayonnaise and chopped onions with corn tortillas

Reading and Translating Labels

6

What You Need to Know about Reading Labels

Food labels provide us with necessary information about the foods that we eat. Along with the name of the food, ingredients, and serving size, they also might include a suggested recipe, or maybe something designed to appeal to us, such as "New and Improved Flavor" or "Supports a Healthy Heart." In order to ensure that labels and claims on foods are accurate, the government has stepped in. However, in spite of laws, labels still can be confusing to understand. Figuring out whether a product contains gluten or not used to be especially tricky, since numerous individual ingredients may contain it.

Additives and Flavoring Agents

There are many ingredients that could be made from starch, such as caramel color, dextrin, glucose syrup, maltodextrin, and modified food starch. Fortunately, in the United States, when wheat is the source of starch, most food labels must say so. However, when it comes to meat, poultry, and egg products, wheat is not yet required to be listed, so on these types of products, make sure to check the labels for caramel, maltodextrin, glucose syrup, modified food starch, dextrin, marinade, or self-basting poultry agents, because they *could* contain hidden traces of wheat. If a product contains caramel, it is most likely not a concern, because caramel is usually made from corn, and when it is made from wheat it rarely contains intact gluten (but, to be safe, if you are not sure, it's better to avoid it).

Natural flavoring agents could be made from rye or barley, but barley is usually listed as malt, and when rye is used, it is mostly found in bakery products.

Pure herbs and spices are always gluten-free, provided no anti-caking ingredients have been added to them; even when they are, most do not contain gluten. However, seasoning agents that are blends can often contain gluten as an added ingredient and always need to be checked.

Understanding Current Labeling Laws in US and Canada

The Food and Drug Administration (FDA) of the U.S. government has made it easier for you to identify some of the foods that have ingredients that contain gluten.

In 2004, the Food Allergen Labeling and Consumer Protection Act, known as FALCPA, stated that by January 1, 2006, food manufacturers had to identify in plain English any ingredient from a list of eight major food allergens. This means that if the food contains milk, eggs, fish, crustacean shellfish, tree nuts, peanuts, wheat, or soybeans, the label is required to say so. The law allows this to be done in one of two ways – either by listing it in the ingredients or by adding a "contains" statement at the end of the ingredient list. Here's an example of the former:

> Ingredients: Enriched flour (wheat flour, malted barley, niacin, reduced iron, thiamin mononitrate, riboflavin, folic acid), sugar, partially hydrogenated soybean oil and/or cottonseed oil, high fructose corn syrup, whey (milk), eggs, vanilla, natural and artificial flavoring, salt, leavening (sodium acid pyrophosphate, monocalcium phosphate), lecithin (soy), mono- and diglycerides (emulsifier).

In this option, if an ingredient contains a food an allergen, it says so in plain English in parentheses next to the food. "Enriched flour" has a parenthesis next to that clearly states wheat, "whey" has a parenthesis next to it that clearly says milk, and eggs are also clearly listed. (Parentheses are not needed—eggs are eggs!) Using the second option, the list of ingredients would not have these clarifications in parentheses. It would simply conclude the list with the statement:

> Contains Wheat, Milk, Eggs, and Soy

This does ease reading the food label since as soon as you see the word wheat or a "contains" statement with wheat in it you know it has gluten. However, gluten is not found only in wheat. Also, as discussed in the previous chapter, cross-contamination can happen in the manufacturing or packing of processed foods, just as it can happen in your own home. Manufacturers will sometimes use a plant to make more than one kind of food. So if a company produces a food that contains gluten—for example, bread—and then also produces a gluten-free food (such as gluten-free cookies), there could be a risk of gluten cross-contamination. This means that you first must check the ingredients list for foods, other than wheat, that have gluten (since wheat will be clearly indicated). These include rye (not a common ingredient) and barley, which is used more often and might be listed as barley, barley malt, malt, or, sometimes, a flavoring. The good news is that the Food and Drug Administration is trying to make this easier, too—more on this soon. Keep an eye on gluten-free labeling in the United States at www.fda.gov/Food/LabelingNutrition/FoodAllergensLabeling/ GuidanceComplianceRegulatoryInformation/default.htm. Updates will also be periodically listed at www.glutenfreehasslefree.com under the expanded resources section.

The contamination issue is a little more complicated, because it falls under what the FDA calls "advisory labels." This means manufacturers will now give consumers more information about whether their product was in contact with a food that is one of the top eight allergens. For instance, you might see "This food was manufactured in a plant that also processes peanuts," or "May contain wheat."

Although the FDA also is currently trying to make label reading easier for those of us who need to avoid foods that contain gluten, this is not as easy as you might think. First, there currently is no set standard for an allowable amount of gluten that is safe for someone with celiac disease or non-celiac gluten sensitivity, and second, the methods used to identify the amount of gluten in foods are not often accurate or consistent. These issues have taken some time to resolve, but as of January 2007, the FDA has proposed a definition, allowable amount, and method of detection. Let's first look at the proposed definition:

- Gluten is defined as the proteins that naturally occur in a prohibited grain and that may cause adverse health effects in people with celiac disease.

A prohibited grain is any of the following or related grains:
- Wheat (triticum)
- Rye (secale)
- Barley (hordeum)
- Crossbreeds of wheat, rye, or barley (for example, triticale, a cross between wheat and rye)

Thus, if something is labeled gluten-free, it would mean that a food bearing this claim would not contain any one of the following:

- An ingredient that is a prohibited grain
- An ingredient derived from a prohibited grain that has not then been processed to remove gluten
- An ingredient that is derived from a prohibited grain that has been processed to remove gluten, if the use of that ingredient results in the presence of 20 parts per million (ppm) or more gluten in the food

20 ppm is so small that it is one of the lowest detectable amount of gluten —which is why it is the set number. Gluten is difficult to detect in smaller amounts, so the government decided that it would be difficult to regulate anything smaller than that. But just so you can think about it with a little more clarity . . .

One part per million is equal to

- One penny in $10,000

- One minute in two years

- One dime in a one-mile-high stack of pennies

It's taken a long time to get this resolution, because it was important to first determine an allowable amount. Zero gluten is difficult to obtain and even more difficult to measure. Safety studies continue to be performed to evaluate the 20 ppm limit. Identifying gluten in foods has not been easy, and there are several methods that are used—some better than others. Right now, the FDA is suggesting that testing be performed using the ELISA method, since it is this method that seems to produce the most consistent data. It also acknowledges that in the future a better method may be discovered that allows us to find gluten more easily at less than the 20 ppm level.

Compliance would be monitored by the FDA through review of food labels, on-site inspections of food manufacturers, and analysis of food samples. Manufacturers of foods that are found to contain gluten at more than the 20 ppm levels would face the charge of misbranding. Some manufacturers, in preparation for this proposed ruling, have removed the gluten-free claim from their labels, while some have added advisory statements and others have actually added wheat to avoid the issue altogether.

Also, at this writing, the rule is voluntary. This means that if a manufacturer meets all of the proposed definitions listed above, it can put a gluten-free claim on its label if it chooses to do so—but it is under no obligation to do so. Therefore, you will find that some foods are gluten-free even though they do not claim that they are. All of these problems stem from the fact that these rules are only currently *proposed*. Unfortunately, a final rule has not yet been set. Hopefully, a final decision will help eliminate some of the confusion for the manufacturers and make buying gluten-free easier.

Additionally, the above only pertains to all foods under FDA rule, but the FDA doesn't govern all foods. The United States Department of Agriculture (USDA) regulates meats, poultry, and egg products, and at this time it has not yet initiated the same rules. So these foods are not required to indicate the most common allergens on their labels. Many of these companies have elected to list allergenic ingredients on their labels, and regulations are being considered for the future, but labeling of these allergens is not mandatory under USDA regulations at this time.

In Canada, the agencies that enforce labeling are Health Canada (HC) and the Canadian Food Inspection Agency (CFIA). In order to label a food gluten-free, Canada currently requires, under food and drug regulation #B.24.018, that "No person shall label, package, sell or advertise a food in a manner likely to create an impression that it is gluten-free unless the food does not contain wheat, including spelt and kamut, or oats, barley, rye or triticale or any part thereof."

For foods that are not labeled gluten-free, there are proposed regulations that will make it easier for those trying to identify the hidden gluten on the ingredient panel of the food labels. As of July 2008, these proposed amendments were posted in the *Canada Gazette* Part 1, requiring that manufactures of all food products declare on their labels the

10 major food allergens, and gluten sources and sulphites, when added as ingredients or part of ingredients. Currently these amendments are under review, so at this time the HC and CFIA strongly urges manufactures to declare these allergens and hidden sources of gluten and sulphites on their food labels until the final version is complete and the law is passed.

Gluten-Free Certifications

There are celiac organizations that have established criteria that they would like used when a product is labeled gluten-free. If a company meets these standards, then it may be eligible to post the organization's logo on its product. For specifications make sure to check each Web site:

Certified Gluten-Free Certification Organization (GFCO Mark)
www.gfco.org
253-218-2956
The Celiac Sprue Association (CSA)
www.csaceliacs.org
877-CSA-4-CSA
The Coeliac Society of Australia
www.coeliacsociety.com.au
(02) 948788 50
Asociacion Celiaca Argentina in Buenos Aires
www.celiaco.org.ar

What the Future Holds

The certification of gluten-free products can at least help provide some quality standards. The future will see many regulations passed and, in the United States, manufacturers will be using gluten-free on their labels, and you the consumer will feel more confident that those foods are really safe for you to eat. In Canada, any food that contains gluten or protein derivatives will be listed on the label in the ingredient list or after it in a statement much like what we see now in the United States. Since the regulations are under consideration at this time, there may be some changes in the specific details. You can keep current on any updates by using the Web sites as noted in the resource section at the end of this book.

When There Are No Labels, Part 1: Gluten-Free on the Run

It is impossible to plan for every situation where there will be food selections to choose from. In many cases, it will even be hard to find out your how your food was prepared. So what do you do? Going hungry isn't the answer. A solid knowledge base will help make it possible for you to find safe foods wherever you are. The basics found in Chapter 2 provide you with many food choices that are naturally gluten-free. As an added tool, why not make a copy of the chart of safe foods found in Chapter 3 so you can quickly review your options at any time? When in doubt, always opt for fresh choices such as fruits, veggies, plain meats, chicken, eggs, dairy, and fish. Carry gluten-free salad dressings, crackers, and seasoning packets with you to help spruce up your meals. Carry gluten-free trail mix, dried fruit, nuts, and cheese with you so you can have something quick when you aren't able to easily find something to eat. Bring a favorite entree and dessert with you to parties and events so you'll have something both safe and special. Carry the dining out sheets in Chapter 12 to make things easier in ethnic restaurants. Call ahead to restaurants and catering halls so you do not have to figure out everything in front of a group of people or a busy staff.

The most important thing to do is to be prepared. Even when you are not in an ideal situation, you can have always have delicious food choices available to you.

When There Are No Labels, Part 2: Gluten-Free at the Deli and in Fast-Food Restaurants

There are many times you may be on the road or in a hurry when you will want to grab something quick to eat. Although you may not like eating fast food, some circumstances may dictate this as the only choice. Knowing what to buy at the deli or in a fast food restaurant will make these times so much easier.

In the Deli

Although we usually think of a deli as a sandwich stop, there are many choices for the gluten-free diner as well. Why not pick up a fresh salad? Tuna, chicken, and egg salad are good choices, as long as bread is not added to the recipe to extend the salad—and be sure to ask whether the same scoops and spatulas are used when spreading on wraps and bread to avoid cross-contamination. Grilled chicken can be a good choice if the marinade is gluten-free and the grill is covered with aluminum foil to protect your food. Fresh fruit, canned and dried fruits, and packaged gluten-free chips and nuts are available in most delis. Many brands of cold cuts are gluten-free, as are most cheeses, so if you carry gluten-free crackers, you can throw together a quick meal. **Below is a listing of many gluten-free products typically found at delis:**

- Applegate Farms GF organic deli meats and cheese

- Boar's Head deli meats, cheeses, and condiments

- Carl Buddig deli meats

- Foster Farms deli meats

- Hebrew National salami, bologna, and hot dogs

- Hormel Natural choice deli meats

- Hormel cure 81 ham

- Jennie-O deli meats

- Thumann's GF deli meats, cheese, condiments, and pickles

* Please note that many other brands may also be gluten-free—make sure to check with the manufacturer.

TIP
Be careful of cross-contamination from the meat slicer and grill. Ask to have the slicer wiped down before your meat is sliced, and for the grill to be covered with aluminum foil before your food is cooked.

Brands that sometimes contain gluten include

- Dietz & Watson

- Organic Valley

This is a partial listing; if in doubt on a particular brand, be sure to contact the manufacturer.

Also question all condiments, salads, and soups—they may contain bouillon cubes, seasoned mustards, malt vinegars, and salad dressings that are not gluten-free.

Avoid Dietz & Watson scrapple, bockwurst, fat-free beef franks, and gourmet lite franks.

* Note that many brands may contain gluten; double-check by calling or e-mailing a manufacturer whenever you are trying a new brand or product.

When you encounter a new brand of deli meat, call the manufacture or see if you can check the label. Avoid any deli meat that contains hydrolyzed vegetable protein, modified food starch, or wheat.

TIP

Always ask the deli manager if he or she can provide you with a list of ingredients on questionable products. If you use the same deli on a regular basis, go during slow times, when staff may be available to answer your questions.

At Fast-Food Restaurants

Many chains regularly change their menu items, so make sure you look for regular updates by calling their headquarters or checking their Web sites to make sure your food choices are safe. Some chains specify wheat-free but not gluten-free, so their offerings may not be safe to consume. In general, watch out for French fries, which are often fried in the same oil as breaded products. Fries are only safe if made in a dedicated fryer.

Arby's
www.arbys.com/nutrition/
1 (800) 487-2729 x 4315
Arby's posts allergen information on its site listing gluten-free options. Check regularly for updates.

Baja Fresh
www.bajafresh.com/nutritionals.php
1 (877) 225-2373
Allergen information is not posted on the site, but the company recommends that you e-mail any questions concerning allergens.

Baskin Robbins
www.baskinrobbins.com/Nutrition/
1 (800) 859-5339
Many Baskin Robbins products are classified as wheat-free but not gluten-free. And even if a flavor is gluten-free, it can be cross-contaminated by a shared ice cream scoop, so it should be avoided unless a fresh container of GF ice cream is being scooped using a clean scoop. All ice cream with gluten-containing ingredients such as cookies or crumbles should always be avoided.

Boston Market
www.bostonmarket.com
1 (800) 365-7000
Boston Market has a large listing of gluten-free items on its Web site.

Burger King
www.bk.com/
1 (305) 378-3535
Burger Kings lists wheat-free products on its Web site but does not make a gluten-free statement. Therefore the gluten-free status of these choices is in question. French Fries, however, are listed as wheat-free and in a dedicated fryer.

Carvel's
www.carvel.com
Carvel's lists many of its ice creams as gluten-free on its Web site. Make sure to avoid sprinkles, crunchies, and any gluten-containing cookie or crumb toppings.

Chick Fil A
www.chickfila.com
Chick Fil A's Web site states that several items may fit into your gluten-free diet per their suppliers, but this is not guaranteed and should only be used as a guide when making selections.

Chili's
1 (800) 983-4637
Chili's Web site provides a listing of "Suggested Menu and Beverage Options for Wheat/Gluten Allergies" monthly at **www.chilis.com/ menu/default.asp.** Allergy statements are available at **www.brinker. com/gr/allergens/Chilis%20Allergen.PDF.**

Dunkin Donuts
www.dunkindonuts.com
1 (800) 859-5339
Gluten-free items are not listed on the Web site, but a few items are listed as wheat-free.

Hardee's
www.hardees.com
1 (877) 799-STAR
Hardee's web site provides a list of product ingredients. The company also claims that some food items are "wheat- and wheat gluten-free," although this is not an acceptable method for listing gluten-free foods. Many foods may be wheat-free yet contain other forms of gluten, so you need to ask questions in order to be safe.

Jack in the Box
www.jackinthebox.com
1 (800) 955-5225
The Jack in the Box Web site lists products as wheat-free but not as gluten-free. However, the full ingredient panel is available for you to check for other sources of gluten such as barley and rye.

Kentucky Fried Chicken
www.kentuckyfriedchicken.com
1 (800) 225-5532
Kentucky Fried Chicken does have an allergy listing on its Web site that indicates wheat, gluten, and other common allergens.

Long John Silver's
www.ljsilvers.com/nutrition/
Long John Silver's has an allergy listing on its web site that lists wheat/gluten-free items and items containing other common allergens, as well as an ingredient listing.

McDonald's
www.mcdonalds.com
1 (800) 244-6227
McDonalds provides "ingredients statements" on its Web site and lists products as wheat-free but not as gluten-free.

Panera Bread
www.panerabread.com
At this time Panera bread does not provide gluten-free information on its Web site.

Starbuck's
www.starbucks.com
At this time Starbucks does not provide gluten-free information on its Web site.

Subway
www.subway.com
Subway has an allergy listing on its Web site that indicates wheat, gluten, and other common allergens.

Taco Bell
www.tacobell.com
1 (800) TACOBELL
Taco Bell has its gluten-free menu items listed on its Web site.

Wendy's
www.wendys.com/
1 (614) 764-3100
Wendy's has a large listing of gluten-free menu items listed on its Web site.

White Castle
www.whitecastle.com
At this time allergen information is not readily available on the White Castle Web site.

Handling Your Feelings—and Knowing You're Not Alone

It's Okay to Get Upset

Never! The word seems to carry its own special punishment. If you're like most people, being told that you can never have something only makes you want it more. If you have ever given up your favorite foods for Lent, or leavened bread for Passover, you know how hard it can be to completely abstain from something you love to eat.

Of course, Lent and Passover eventually come to an end, and then you can start eating the forbidden foods again. But with celiac disease and non-celiac gluten sensitivity, that's not an option. You can't eat foods containing gluten for the rest of your life.

It's important to understand that when you can't eat gluten, it's not just one food that you can't have. Anything with even a little wheat or rye or barley is totally off-limits.

This is why being gluten intolerant can be emotionally painful, especially at first. It's no fun having to be careful about every little thing you put in your mouth, especially while everyone around you is happily eating whatever they want.

If you're like most people who can no longer eat gluten, you will particularly miss wheat. Those of us who live in the Western world eat wheat at nearly every meal and use it in almost all recipes. Foods containing wheat are served at parties, at family gatherings, in restaurants and bars, at work, and in classrooms. You literally can't avoid it. You can find entire communities that are children-free or pet-free, but try to find a single block anywhere in the world that is totally gluten-free, and you're out of luck.

Now for the good news: there's nothing special or natural about eating wheat. People in many cultures eat little or none of it. Over thousands of years, we have learned how to cultivate it, harvest it, mill it, and cook it so that it is tasty to most people. But because it is not especially well suited to human digestion, some of us simply can't tolerate it. This brings us to another piece of good news. You are anything but alone. Although you may feel lonely and isolated when you first learn that you are gluten intolerant, remember that more than 1 in 100 people share this problem.

This book is dedicated to helping you find foods that you fully enjoy while living a sane and healthy gluten-free life. In this chapter, we'll focus on the feelings that can arise for people who can no longer eat gluten.

These feelings are very common. Who wouldn't have strong reactions to suddenly learning that for the rest of their life they have to live with so many restrictions?

This chapter offers useful strategies for handling your feelings about your gluten sensitivity when you're angry, bored, depressed, embarrassed, hurt, or overwhelmed.

Dealing with Anger

It's not fair! Everyone else is munching on the bread and splitting appetizers I can't touch, while I just sit here biting my nails. Why do people who are supposed to be my friends always order only one appetizer I can have, like grilled shrimp, and then pass everything around the table, leaving me with only one shrimp? Don't they remember that I can't eat any of those other things? Don't they see that I'm just sitting here, starving?

If I give up and order my own separate appetizer, it's obvious that some of them think I'm being petty or neurotic—and half the time it arrives five minutes after my entrée.

I know it's not their fault that I'm gluten intolerant, but they seem completely blind to my situation, even though I've told them about it a thousand times. It makes it hard to enjoy going out to eat with a group. Sometimes I get really mad at them for not noticing my dilemma or making it easier for me.

Why did this have to happen to me?

It's okay to get mad. It isn't fair that you have to be so careful about what you eat. You didn't choose to be gluten intolerant, and your condition isn't the result of something you did or any decision you made.

It's also important to express your anger, but in a healthy and nonthreatening way—and at an appropriate time and place (not during dinner, perhaps!). Maybe afterward, on your way home, you can say, "I know this is nobody's fault, but sometimes I get angry when people seem to completely forget that I can't eat certain foods. They wouldn't forget if I needed a wheelchair or a seeing-eye dog, would they?" Don't hold your anger in, or you could end up exploding and fighting with family or friends about something else entirely simply because you need to vent.

You can also avoid these situations by being proactive. When a get-together with family or friends is being planned, ask to help plan the meal or choose the restaurant. Suggest or select a restaurant that offers gluten-free choices. Or, if someone suggests a restaurant you haven't been to before, check its Web site before you go, or call ahead to find out what choices you can have. (Make sure there are at least two good entrées for you, so that if one isn't available that day, you won't have to go hungry.) If your options include foods you really enjoy, you will be far less likely to get angry.

If your dining companions want to share their food, don't be afraid to order your own separate appetizer and/or entrée. If need be, explain why, simply and briefly.

If you are going to a wedding or some other catered event, call the caterer a few days before, explain your dietary limitations, and ask them to create something special for you. Unless the caterer is brand-new, they will be very familiar with cooking for people who are gluten-intolerant.

Dealing with Culinary Boredom

A lot of my family favorites have ingredients I can't eat. I've learned how to make gluten-free variations of some of those dishes, and I've created a few of my own gluten-free recipes. But, truth be told, I am not that creative a cook. Now that so many of my favorite ingredients are off-limits, I have a hard time making many dishes that I like anymore. There are a few items that I prepare very well, but I can't eat these same few things every day.

Then when I go out to eat, I either can't figure out what's okay to order, or the limited choices I have to pick from the menu are very plain or tasteless. I am just about bored to death. I wish I could find some more interesting foods to eat.

The urge for variety is simply human nature. Discovering that you are gluten intolerant does not make this human urge go away! To spice up your plate, start with the recipes in this book, in Chapters 4 and 11.

You'll be surprised at how creative, delicious, and simple gluten-free eating can be.

For further gluten-free culinary excitement, go on a gluten-free vacation or take a gluten-free culinary tour. (Yes, there are such things—more of them than you probably realize. See the resource section at the end of this book for some groups to contact.) Dine out at some gluten-free restaurants. More of these open literally every week, and they work hard to please the palate as well as offer healthy selections.

Join a local support group for people with celiac disease and non-celiac gluten sensitivities. Trade recipes with other group members and ask them for recommendations for great gluten-free dishes and restaurants in your area. Other group members will surely have dealt with the same culinary boredom and will be able to offer a variety of tips and solutions.

Dealing with Depressed Feelings

It's no fun going out to eat anymore. Even weddings and parties, which I used to find exciting, have become humdrum, because either I can't eat anything they serve, or they serve me something gluten-free that's also dry and taste-free.

I try my best, but I'm getting to the point where I'd rather just stay home, watch TV, and make myself something to eat. Staying home can be easier than having to explain my situation to every single person I see, or being served something that tastes like it came out of a hospital kitchen—but it's also lonely, and I feel like I'm missing all the fun.

Many people live their lives accommodating one or more physical challenges. It's not always possible to be cheerful about it, but it's important not to give in to a victim mentality, or to allow yourself to retreat into isolation. Don't be afraid to be assertive. Yes, it's a pain to have to explain the same thing over and over—but the results will be tastier food and better health.

Furthermore, as more and more people ask for gluten-free choices, chefs, caterers, and cooks will catch on. The result will be an ever-wider variety of even tastier gluten-free options.

Remember how just a few years ago, it was hard to find organic food in restaurants and supermarkets? Or, a few years before that, how few vegetarian options there used to be at most restaurants and events? Gluten-free eating is starting to follow the same curve.

Here are some easy ways to be assertive:

When you are invited to a party, explain your food restrictions and offer to help the host plan the menu. This isn't being pushy—it's being helpful. Chances are your host will feel relieved, because you're making it easier for him or her to accommodate you.

Also feel free to bring some of your favorite foods with you to the gathering. Depending on the circumstances, it might be a little awkward—but if you needed to take medication, you'd bring that with you, wouldn't you?

Understandably, there will still be some times when you feel it's not worth the trouble and would rather stay home. At those times, make sure you prepare yourself a wonderful, delicious meal of your favorite gluten-free foods.

The trick is to take the lead so that whether you go out or stay home, you get to eat food that's healthy and that you enjoy.

Dealing with Embarrassment

I've never liked to make a big deal out of what restaurant to go to or what to order. For most of my life, if I was given the wrong dressing or side dish, I'd usually just eat it. I didn't want to be a food prima donna, and it would embarrass me when other people made a fuss if their food wasn't exactly the way they ordered it.

Now that I know I'm gluten-intolerant, almost everything has changed. I have to explain my diet to every waiter, chef, friend, relative, or person who's eating with me. The one thing that hasn't changed is how I feel about it. All that calling attention to myself and all those special requests make me want to crawl under the table. I feel as though everyone around me is looking at me like I have two heads. I get even more embarrassed when I have to explain it all.

The worst is when I'm at an event like a wedding, and the servers are trying to deliver food to 150 people all at once, and I ask, "Does the gravy have flour in it?" If the server doesn't speak a lot of English, I might as well forget about eating at all. It makes me want to just eat whatever everyone else is eating, even if it makes me sick.

Few of us want to be the center of attention when it comes to our health. And who wants to be referred to in the restaurant kitchen as "the pain in the butt at table 4?" If you don't want to make a fuss, that's fine. You don't have to do anything that goes against your nature. Here's how you can be proactive without calling undue attention to yourself:

Whenever possible, pick restaurants that already have gluten-free choices on the menu. Then you don't have to explain anything to anyone; just order from the gluten-free options. If possible, call restaurants ahead of time (preferably when they're not busy) to see what they can do for you. It's also best to dine out when the restaurant is not as busy so that chefs and cooks will have an easier time accommodating you.

Photocopy the dining-out sheets in Chapter 12 and carry them with you. (Or, if you prefer, go to www.glutenfreehasslefree.com/facts/living/cards.asp and print them out.) These simple pages explain living without gluten in clear, easy-to-understand language, and then list those foods that you can't eat. Simply hand a list to your server, and ask that the chef use it when preparing your meal.

These cards are included in fourteen languages—English, Arabic, Traditional Chinese, French, German, Greek, Hebrew, Hindi, Italian, Japanese, Spanish, Polish, Thai, and Vietnamese—so they can be used in a wide range of ethnic restaurants, as well as with servers who do not speak much English.

Dealing with Hurt Feelings

When I go to a family event, they don't even try to make this easy for me. They just serve whatever foods they please. Doesn't anyone even care? It's like my childhood all over again: I'm invisible and my needs are completely ignored.

D's Dieting Dilemmas

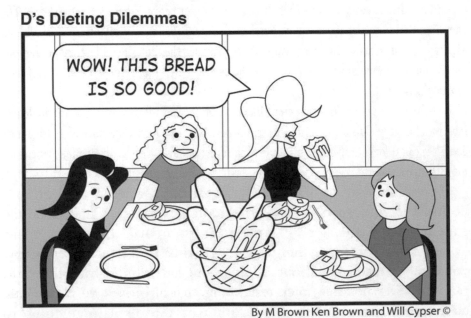

By M Brown Ken Brown and Will Cypser ©

My relatives put out crackers with soft cheese already on them. They toss croutons into the salad, dip the meat in breading, and sprinkle breads crumbs over the vegetables.

When I ask them to just skip the breadcrumbs for once, or serve the croutons or crackers separately, they get mad at me. They say, "Just scrape it off," or "Come on, a little won't hurt you. Don't make such a big deal about it." They don't even try to understand. It's like they blame me for making their lives more difficult. It really hurts.

Believe it or not, most people who act this way aren't trying to be hurtful. They just don't understand how important it is that you follow a gluten-free diet at all times. Many simply don't believe that a tiny amount of gluten can harm your health.

Most people think that celiac disease and non-celiac gluten sensitivities are like diabetes or high blood pressure. Many folks with diabetes can have sugar sometimes, and those with high blood pressure can occasionally have salty food. As a result, a lot of people think that people who don't eat gluten can have a small amount on special occasions. They just assume you're making too big a deal about your dietary restrictions. They may even think you're trying to draw attention to yourself.

You can't always get people to change what they believe, but sometimes you can wake them up by showing them the words of a respected authority. One option is to photocopy "Getting Started Living Gluten-Free" in Chapter 13, as well as the cover of this book. Give these to your relatives and say, "I brought you this. It explains the whole gluten-free thing much better than I can." If you prefer, send them the web link to "Getting Started Living Gluten-Free"—www.glutenfreehasslefree.com/facts/living/living.asp—or go to that page and print it out for them (it's also found in Chapter 13).

If that doesn't help, then you may simply need to accept that your family will never change. Whatever their motivations are, you can't make them act differently—so don't try. Bring your own foods to family events. If you like, bring gluten-free dishes that anyone would want to eat. If people make fun of you for eating something different, take your plate into a different room—and limit your visits in the future.

Dealing with Feeling Overwhelmed

I already have so much to do each day. I can barely keep the house together and get to work on time. I don't have the time to exercise as much as I'd like. Plus, I'd love to catch up on projects I've had on hold for years. I'm already overcommitted, and I feel so tired at the end of each day.

And now this. How can I possibly find the time to plan and cook special meals for myself while taking care of my family, too? I wish I could clone myself so someone else could shop and cook for me.

Most people feel overwhelmed when they first learn they're gluten intolerant. But most of us feel equally overwhelmed when we first begin an exercise program or have our first child or take a new job or go back to school.

So let yourself feel overwhelmed! It's a completely normal and natural feeling.

But remind yourself that this is not the only, the first, or the most difficult challenge that life will throw your way. Also keep in mind that this feeling will go away over time. Once gluten-free living has become a habit, you'll discover that it's not very time-consuming at all. In fact, because it will greatly improve your health, you'll have more energy and less downtime because of illness. You'll naturally feel less overwhelmed and more able to accomplish everyday tasks, with juice left for your favorite leisure activities.

Part of making a gluten-free lifestyle hassle free is making changes in steps rather than all at once. Start with changes that are easy to make, and make only a few of them at a time. Get familiar with the basic gluten-free foods. Make a gluten-free shopping trip to the supermarket. Start with a few gluten-free recipes and a simple meal plan. Don't try to completely change your life overnight. You'll discover that once you have the first step or two behind you, you'll begin to experience some positive changes, and these in turn will make you excited about incorporating others.

Before you know it, you will find that living a gluten-free life is a lot easier than you thought it would be.

PART II: MAKING GLUTEN-FREE LIVING SIMPLE

Finding the Hidden Gluten in Food

From Toothpaste to Lipstick

Following a gluten-free diet doesn't just stop with food. Anything that you breathe in, or ingest (including vitamins, medications, toothpaste, and lipstick) can contain gluten and can make you ill. Sometimes the rubber bands used for children's braces are packed with flour to keep them from sticking together. So knowing where the hidden gluten is can be critical to staying well. Do you know how many lipsticks a typical women will consume in one year?

So where do you start? Any product that contains gluten that touches your lips or that is in the air you breathe can make you ill, so all such items must be checked.

Gluten particles are too large to be absorbed through the skin, but everything that touches your hands has the potential to go into your mouth, so use good handwashing techniques, especially if you use a gluten-containing lotion, shampoo, or sunscreen. Remember, kids will put anything in their mouths, so gluten-free school supplies are a must for a child with celiac disease.

> **Please note that product formulas change regularly; this list is only a guide. Double-check gluten-free status with each of the manufacturers of the brands you use prior to use.**

D's Dieting Dilemmas

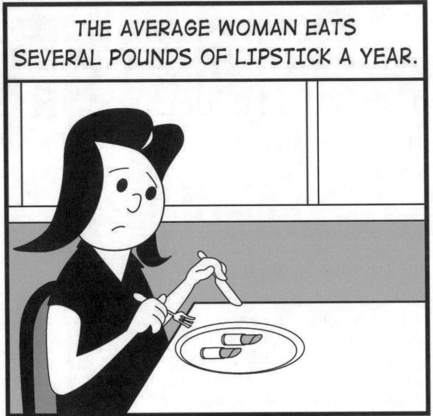

THE AVERAGE WOMAN EATS
SEVERAL POUNDS OF LIPSTICK A YEAR.

By M Brown Ken Brown and Will Cypser ©

Many common household and personal items can contain gluten, including

- Lipstick, lip balm, shampoo, soap, cosmetics, and skin lotion

- Mouthwash and toothpaste: Crest Pro Health Rinse, Crest Whitening Rinse, Listerine, Fixodent, Sensodyne, Orabase B Gel, Super Plygrip Powder

- Household products such as cleaning solutions and detergents

- Vitamins and medicines: pills may be dusted in flour, capsules may contain gluten in the oil inside the capsule (check out glutenfreedrugs.com for an overview of medications and supplements)

- Latex or rubber gloves: used to wash dishes and used for food preparation, but may be dusted with wheat or oat flour; be sure to also ask your dentist, doctor, orthodontist, and periodontist to use unpowdered gloves

- School and art supplies such as face paints, markers, glue and glue sticks, paste, tape, hand stamps, Play-Doh, Crayola clay, Nickelodeon's Floam, and Goop

- Sunscreens and some self-adhesive bandages

- Toothbrushes that are kept in the same holder as other family members

---

TIP

Your pharmacist may be able to tell you if your medication is gluten-free, but you may need to call the manufacturer or pharmaceutical company to be absolutely sure.

Some products that are safe to use include:

- **Cosmetics and lip balm:** Lancome, Burt's Bees, AVEDA, Estée Lauder, Maybelline, Chapstick, Blistex (Afterglow Cosmetics has an entire line of gluten-free products)

- **Sunscreens and self-tanners:** Banana Boat children's sunscreen, Lancome Flash Bronzer Glow 'n Wear Gel, AVEDA Sun Source

- **Soaps, shampoos, and laundry detergent:** Arm and Hammer baking soda detergent, Kirkman Labs' Kleen Products soap and shampoos, Colgate-Palmolive softsoaps, Suave, Dove, Pampers Baby Wipes, Purell and Germ-X instant hand sanitizers

- **Dental products:** Aquafresh, Colgate, and Crest toothpaste, Whitestrips, and Night Effects, Gleem toothpaste, Glide dental floss, Polident tablets, Rembrant, Tom's of Maine, Ultrabrite, Anbesol baby, Anbesol Cold Sore Therapy Gel, Oasis moisturizing mouth spray, Oral B Prophy Paste Stages Tooth and Gum Care

- **School Supplies:** Crayola Silly Putty, ColorWonder Fingerpaints, paints, crayons, pencils, markers, modeling clay, glue, glitter glue, and chalk; Elmer's glue, glue sticks, crayons, paints, and watercolors; Roseart stickers; Scotch Magic Tape; Palmer Paint; Prang Paints

- **Other:** Johnson and Johnson Band-Aids, Kleenex tissues with lotion and anti-viral tissues, Puffs with lotion, Cold-eeze All Natural Lozenges, Kanga Vits vitamins, Nicorette gum

> **TIP**
> Always read ingredient lists or check with manufacturer to confirm that a product is gluten-free.

How to Gluten-Proof Your Home

In the beginning of this chapter, you learned that gluten can be consumed from nonfood items—just by using everyday products. But these are not the only ways you can accidently take in gluten. It can actually get into your food from hidden sources in your kitchen and around your house. Since most meals are eaten at home, you must gluten-proof your home to prevent contaminating your food choices every day. This is especially important when others are bringing gluten-containing grains into the same areas where you will be having your foods.

Equipment

Using pans and equipment in your kitchen that others use for gluten containing foods can contaminate your foods. Use a separate toaster or protect your food with toaster bags (www.toastitbags.com). Protect your food from gluten by having a separate tray for your toaster oven, or make sure you cover it with aluminum foil if it is not dedicated gluten-free. Make sure you don't put food directly on the bottom of the microwave, where gluten can be lurking, without a protective plate. Thoroughly clean your grill or cover the surface with aluminum foil. Have separate colanders, tongs, spatulas, and sheet pans for your gluten-free cooking. Make sure these cooking utensils look different from the others in your house so they don't accidently get mixed up.

Storing Ingredients

It isn't enough to just buy gluten-free foods; you need to store them safely in your home. Make sure your condiments are marked separately from those that the rest of the family uses. This includes mayo, mustard, butter, margarine, jam, peanut butter, and any food item you use a spoon or knife to spread. It isn't that you can't use the same condiments as others (most are gluten-free), it's that most people double-dip with the knife after using it to touch bread and can cross-contaminate these foods. Having your own spreads and marking them helps prevent this from happening.

Wipe down all cooking surfaces before preparing your gluten-free foods. Some gluten-containing residues, such as flour, can stay in the air for hours and then settle on working surfaces.

When it comes to storing your gluten-free flours, pastas, crackers, and cereals, keep them in airtight containers stored on upper shelves. Storing them on lower shelves may lead to some gluten-containing ingredients accidently falling in from residues on the shelves above them.

How to Be Gluten-Free at Work

Work environments can be tricky because you don't always have the resources and control that you would have at home. You may not have a refrigerator, toaster, and microwave to store and heat your gluten-free foods. There may be meetings, trade shows, and workshops that include set catered menus. You may not have the opportunity to bring in food, so find out what the menu is ahead of time, and question anyone about the ingredients. It is not only that it may not be easy to control your food here, but in a working business situation it may not always be in your best interest to ask and talk too much about the food. You are conducting business, not out for a good time (as some might put it).

Sometimes asking lots of little questions can be perceived by some business associates as a negative part of your personality, or just being neurotic. They think you are making a big deal about little things. So how do you deal with this? As before, simply plan. Usually business meetings are booked ahead of time, so you can figure on covering your meals for that day. Carry things with you that are easy to bring into your meetings so you can pull out your food when breaks or meals are taken. Some examples include gluten-free bars, fresh fruit, dried fruit and nuts, yogurt, and gluten-free crackers. In some cases you can even pack a gluten-free sandwich as long as you package the meat and bread separately (it is important to pack the bread separately from the filling, since gluten-free bread can get soggy pretty easily). There may be some safe food choices that you can pick up at the meeting, and combining them with the foods you brought with you gives you a complete meal. The most important thing is getting through your meeting while still being able to have safe foods throughout the day.

Gluten in the Air

Gluten can be lurking in places you would never expect, and there have been cases where bakery workers with celiac disease have gotten ill by breathing flour. There is a lot of flour in the air in bakeries and pizzerias where dough is made from scratch. The flour gets puffed into

D's Dieting Dilemmas

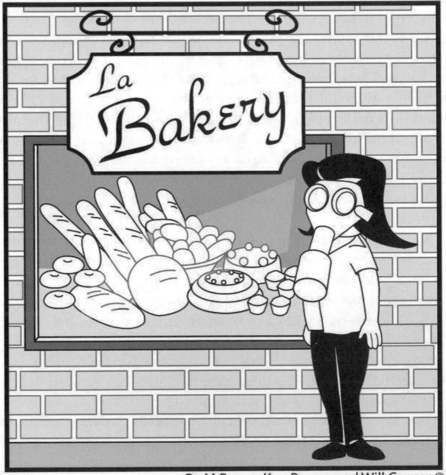

By M Brown Ken Brown and Will Cypser ©

the air, and the particles go everywhere. If you touch something and then your mouth, or if you breathe gluten in (the gluten in the nose will eventually be swallowed), you have consumed gluten. The amount of gluten consumed is so small that it might not cause a reaction in some people (based on tolerance levels), but others who are extremely sensitive may get sick from being in this environment for even a short time. Also, for those who work in that environment every day the effect can be cumulative, catching up to them in time. There is also a danger if you are trying to live gluten-free but live in a home where someone bakes with gluten-containing ingredients. Gluten-containing flour may be unavoidable in this case and may result in the necessity for another family member learning to cook gluten-free, even when they themselves are not ill.

Eating a Balanced Gluten-Free Diet

Easy Replacements for Missing Nutrients

When you are following a gluten-free diet, you are giving up many foods that have important nutritional value. This means that you are no longer taking in some nutrients that are important for your body. This chapter will explore the nutrients that you are missing and how to get them in other ways, as well as extra supplements that may be beneficial. Lastly, since food intolerances do not occur in a vacuum, this chapter will try to help those of you who are dealing with more than one food intolerance at a time.

In addition, if you have just started a gluten-free diet, you might already have mild nutritional deficiencies due to your intestine's inability to absorb all the nutrients in the foods you were consuming. It is important for you to make up for those losses and rebuild the missing stores in your body. Then, after you have recovered, there are still going to be nutrients that are more difficult to get due to the limitations in the foods you can consume. This is why these nutrients are being listed separately, and then the diet given as a whole. To see the USDA current recommendations for vitamins and nutrients, go to www.nutrition.gov.

Vitamin A

Vitamin A is a vitamin that is associated with eye health. A person with celiac disease who has steatorrhea (fatty diarrhea from fat malabsorption) can be deficient in vitamin A. The reason for this is that vitamin A is what is called "fat-soluble." This means that vitamin A likes fat—not water.

Deficiency of this vitamin is rare. If you have or have had steator-rhea, have your doctor check you for a vitamin A deficiency. Correction of this deficiency comes by supplementation of the vitamin. Getting it in the diet thereafter is easy, since we can make vitamin A from caroti-noids. Carotinoids are the yellow, orange, and red colors we see in our fruits and vegetables. This is why carrots are good for your eyes.

Vitamin B1 (Thiamin)

Thiamin or vitamin B1 is found naturally in the hull of grains. In the United States, we started to see deficiencies of this vitamin with the invention of white bread. The process of making bread "white" also stripped off the valuable nutrients hiding in the hull—thiamin, ribofla-vin, niacin, and fiber, to name a few. The FDA made it a requirement that thiamin be added back into the grain after it was refined. This pro-cess is called enrichment. Since it was mainly wheat and rice that were refined, the enrichment program was focused on those grains. Many gluten-free baked products are refined and are currently not enriched, making them very poor sources of many nutrients.

Now if you start putting the pieces together, you see that on a gluten-free diet, with the removal of wheat products, it is very possible to have a thiamin deficiency. Grains that are used as gluten replacements have not been part of the enrichment program in the past. Today, we are seeing many of these manufacturers now including these replacement grains in their enrichment program—but not all. So getting sufficient amounts of thiamin, for example, in your diet means eating a varied diet.

Generally foods that are a good source of thiamin include beans, soy milk, and pork. The following list includes some other foods and the amount of thiamin in each of the servings listed.

Flours, Grains, Beans, Seeds	Serving Size	Thiamin (mg)
Sunflower seed flour	1 cup	2.0 mg
Corn flour (masa), white or yellow	1 cup	1.6 mg
Soy flour	1 cup	0.7 mg
Rice bran	1 cup	3.2 mg
Rice, white, long-grain, enriched	1 cup	1.3 mg

Flours, Grains, Beans, Seeds (Continued)	Serving Size	Thiamin (mg)
Rice, white, medium grain, enriched	1 cup	1.1 mg
Rice, white, short grain, enriched	1 cup	1.1 mg
Rice, white, long-grain	1 cup	0.9 mg
Lentils	1 cup	1.7 mg
Soybeans	1 cup	1.6 mg
Navy beans	1 cup	1.6 mg
Sesame seeds	1 cup	1.5 mg
Peas, split	1 cup	1.4 mg
Pinto beans	1 cup	1.4 mg
Great northern beans	1 cup	1.2 mg
Kidney beans, all kinds	1 cup	1.1 mg

Nuts, Seeds, Protein

Brazil nuts	1 oz	0.2 mg
Flaxseed, whole	1 Tbsp	0.2 mg
Pistachio nuts	1 oz	0.2 mg
Macadamia nuts	1 oz	0.2 mg
Pecans	1 oz	0.2 mg
Hazelnuts	1 oz	0.2 mg
Pork, all kinds	3 oz	0.9 mg
Pompano	3 oz	0.5 mg
Tuna	3 oz	0.4 mg

Vegetables

Sun-dried tomatoes	½ cup	0.15 mg

Vitamin B2 (Riboflavin)

Riboflavin was once called vitamin B2. It, too, is found in the hulls of grains and is thus part of the enrichment program. Riboflavin is even easier to get than thiamin, because it is more common in foods.

Generally, foods that are a good source of riboflavin include meats and dairy. The following list includes some other foods that are good sources in riboflavin.

Flours	Serving Size	Riboflavin (mg)
Soy flour, full fat	1 cup	1.0 mg
Corn flour (masa), white or yellow	1 cup	0.9 mg
Legumes, Nuts, Seeds		
Soybeans	1 cup	1.6 mg
Almonds	1 oz	0.3 mg
Sesame seed butter, tahini	2 Tbsp	0.2 mg
Meat, Fish		
Pork, all kinds	3 oz	0.6 mg
Mackerel	3 oz	0.5 mg
Dairy, Eggs, Cheese, Vegetables		
Milk	1 cup	1.4 mg
Eggs	1 large	0.2 mg
Feta cheese	1 oz	0.2 mg
Roquefort cheese	1 oz	0.2 mg
American cheese	1 oz	0.1 mg
Shitake mushrooms, dried	½ cup	0.4 mg

Vitamin B3 (Niacin)

Niacin was once called vitamin B3. It is a vitamin that we can make in our body, but not in large enough amounts. In order to make it, we need protein foods in our diets that contain an amino acid called tryptophan. Thus, meat, poultry, fish, and dairy foods, all of which contain tryptophan, are good sources. Tryptophan is also found in the enrichment program, for the same reasons thiamin and riboflavin are. Generally, good sources of niacin are some meats, nuts, and yeasts. The following table lists of some good sources of niacin.

Flours, Grains	Serving Size	Niacin (mg)
Peanut flour	1 cup	16.2 mg
Corn flour (masa), white or yellow	1 cup	11.2 mg
Rice flour, brown	1 cup	10.0 mg
Buckwheat flour	1 cup	7.4 mg
Potato flour	1 cup	5.6 mg
Sunflower seed flour	1 cup	4.7 mg
Rice flour, white	1 cup	4.1 mg
Sesame seed flour	1 cup	3.7 mg
Soy flour	1 cup	3.6 mg
Chickpea flour	1 cup	1.6 mg
Grains		
Millet	1 cup	9.4 mg
Rice, brown	1 cup	9.4 mg
Buckwheat groats (kasha)	1 cup	8.4 mg
Rice, white, long grain	1 cup	6.7 mg

Grains (Continued)	Serving Size	Niacin (mg)
Teff	1 cup	6.5 mg
Corn, white or yellow	1 cup	6.0 mg
Rice, wild	1 cup	2.1 mg
Legumes, Seeds, Nuts, Protein		
Peas, split	1 cup	5.7 mg
Lentils	1 cup	5.0 mg
Navy beans	1 cup	4.6 mg
Peanuts	1 oz	4.5 mg
Kidney beans	1 cup	3.9 mg
Black beans	1 cup	3.8 mg
Sunflower seeds	1 oz	3.7 mg
Chickpeas	1 cup	3.1 mg
Soybeans	1 cup	3.0 mg
Peanut butter	2 Tbsp	2.3 mg
Tuna	3 oz	15.9 mg
Chicken, all kinds	3 oz	12.3 mg
Veal, all kinds	3 oz	10.7 mg
Swordfish	3 oz	10.0 mg
Mackerel	3 oz	9.1 mg
Pork, all kinds	3 oz	8.7 mg
Salmon	3 oz	8.6 mg
Beef, all kinds	3 oz	7.5 mg

Legumes, Seeds, Nuts, Protein (Continued)	Serving Size	Niacin (mg)
Turkey, all kinds	3 oz	7.5 mg
Halibut	3 oz	6.1 mg
Tilapia	3 oz	3.9 mg
Haddock	3 oz	3.9 mg
Pompano	3 oz	3.2 mg
Octopus	3 oz	3.2 mg
Crab	3 oz	3.1 mg
Clams	3 oz	2.9 mg
Soymilk	1 cup	8.0 mg

Vegetables, Fruit

Portabella mushrooms	1 cup	7.2 mg
Maitake mushrooms, raw	1 cup	4.6 mg
Shitake mushrooms, dried	1 oz	3.9 mg
Tomatoes	1 cup	3.7 mg
White mushrooms, cooked	½ cup	3.5 mg
Potato, white, with skin	1 small	3.5 mg
Peas, green	1 cup	3.0 mg
Potato, sweet	1 cup	3.0 mg
Sun-dried tomatoes	½ cup	2.5 mg
Tomatillo	1 cup	2.4 mg
Prunes	1 cup	4.0 mg
Apricots, dried, halves	1 cup	3.4 mg

Vitamin B9 (Folate)

Folate, also known as folic acid, is a water-soluble B vitamin that is very important to our health. A deficiency will lead to anemia. Even before a woman knows she is pregnant, folic acid is needed to ensure that the cells of the fetus will divide properly. Since this vitamin is important in the very early stages of pregnancy, the United States added it to the enrichment program. Folate is easily lost in the cooking process, since it is water-soluble. The best way to get folate is to increase folate-containing foods in your diet. If you are trying to get pregnant or are pregnant, a supplement is recommended, but generally folate can be found in vegetables. The table below provides a list of foods that are good sources of folate.

Flours, Grains, Beans	Serving Size	Folate (mcg)
Chickpea flour	1 cup	402 mcg
Soy flour	1 cup	361 mcg
Corn flour (masa), white or yellow	1 cup	266 mcg
Peanut flour	1 cup	149 mcg
Buckwheat flour	1 cup	64.8 mcg
Cornmeal	1 cup	342 mcg
Quinoa	1 cup	313 mcg
Rice, white, long grain	1 cup	261 mcg
Millet	1 cup	170 mcg
Amaranth	1 cup	158 mcg
Rice, wild	1 cup	152 mcg
Teff	1 cup	45.4 mcg
Chickpeas	1 cup	1114 mcg
Pinto beans	1 cup	1013 mcg

Flours, Grains, Beans (Continued)	Serving Size	Folate (mcg)
Lentils	1 cup	920 mcg
Great northern beans	1 cup	882 mcg
Navy beans	1 cup	757 mcg
Kidney beans	1 cup	725 mcg
Lima beans	1 cup	703 mcg

Seeds, Nuts, Protein, Vegetables, Fruits

	Serving Size	Folate (mcg)
Sunflower seeds	1 cup	319 mcg
Sesame seeds	1 cup	173 mcg
Flaxseeds	1 cup	146 mcg
Peanut butter	2 Tbsp	119 mcg
Conch	3 oz	91.2 mcg
Mussels	3 oz	64.6 mcg
Crab	3 oz	43.4 mcg
Edamame	1 cup	482 mcg
Brussels sprouts	1 cup	157 mcg
Beets, raw	1 cup	148 mcg
Asparagus, cooked	½ cup	134 mcg
Turnip greens, raw	1 cup	107 mcg
Mustard greens, raw	1 cup	105 mcg
Broccoli, cooked	½ cup	84.2 mcg
Endive, raw	1 cup	71 mcg
Spinach, raw	1 cup	58.2 mcg

Seeds, Nuts, Protein, Vegetables, Fruits (Continued)	Serving Size	Folate (mcg)
Boysenberries	1 cup	83 mcg
Guava	1 cup	81 mcg
Pineapple juice	1 cup	80 mcg
Orange juice	1 cup	74.4 mcg
Oranges, Valencia	1 cup, sections	70.2 mcg
Papaya	1 cup	53.2 mcg
Plantains	1 cup	40 mcg

Vitamin B12

Vitamin B12 is a very important vitamin for the health and proper functioning of your nervous system. Additionally, when deficient in this vitamin, you can get an anemia. This vitamin is only found in animal products, so vegetarians that exclude all animal products (vegans) need to work on getting this vitamin elsewhere. This vitamin is absorbed in the lower part of the small intestine, and absorption can be affected by damage to the villi in this area. The following table shows some foods that are good sources of vitamin B12.

Fish, Beef, Poultry	Serving size	Vitamin B12 (mcg)
Clams	3 oz	84.1 mcg
Oysters	3 oz	29.8 mcg
Mussels	3 oz	20.4 mcg
Mackerel	3 oz	16.1 mcg
Herring	3 oz	11.6 mcg

Fish, Beef, Poultry (*Continued*)	Serving size	Vitamin B12 (mcg)
Tuna	3 oz	9.2 mcg
Sardines	3 oz	7.5 mcg
Beef, all parts	3 oz	5.3 mcg
Salmon	3 oz	4.9 mcg
Turkey, all parts	3 oz	1.2 mcg
Pork, all parts	3 oz	1.2 mcg
Chicken, all parts	3 oz	0.6 mcg
Dairy and Eggs		
Yogurt	1 cup	1.4 mcg
Milk	1 cup	1.3 mcg
Swiss cheese	1 oz	0.9 mcg
Mozzarella cheese	1 oz	0.6 mcg
Eggs	1 large	0.6 mcg

Vitamin D

Vitamin D is also called the sunshine vitamin, since we make it when we are exposed to sunlight. However, we cannot make it in adequate amounts daily, so we really need to get it from our diet. Vitamin D is so important because it is what makes calcium work in our bodies. Without vitamin D, we can have problems with our bones. This is a common deficiency in individuals with celiac disease, since the small intestine damage leads to a decrease in its absorption—especially with steatorrhea (as is the case with vitamin A).

Even without gluten and digestive tract problems, most of us do not get enough vitamin D. Not many foods have adequate amounts, and with the increased use of sunscreen, vitamin D is produced in even smaller amounts. The best sources are fortified milk and cold water fish. Some other good sources of vitamin D are listed in the following table.

Fish, Dairy, Soy, Fruit	Serving size	Vitamin D (mcg)
Cod liver oil	1 tsp	11.3 mcg
Herring	3 oz	34.6 mcg
Salmon	3 oz	16.2 mcg
Trout	3 oz	12.7 mcg
Catfish	3 oz	10.6 mcg
Sardines	3 oz	10 mcg
Milk	1 cup	3.2 mcg
Soy milk, with added Ca, A, and D	1 cup	2.98 mcg
Orange juice, fortified with Ca and D	1 cup	3.55 mcg

Vitamin K

Vitamin K is like vitamins A and D in that it is fat-soluble. It is an important vitamin, since its job is to help your blood clot. It also works in the bone, so with a deficiency, bone strength is compromised. Some people with celiac disease will have symptoms of blood-clotting problems and will need to get vitamin K to resolve those issues. Vitamin K is found naturally in many foods, including dark green vegetables and all animal and plant foods.

Calcium

Calcium is a mineral that we need for many functions in the body. The most commonly known need is for bone strength. But it also contributes to proper function of muscle cell contraction and to nerve transmission. The body thinks that this is the most important function and will actually pull calcium from your bones, if there is not enough in the diet, to make sure there is enough for this work. So it is important to consume enough calcium to keep bones strong.

Because of the vitamin D deficiency that accompanies with celiac disease, calcium is usually also deficient—remember, vitamin D works to get calcium into your body. Once the intestinal villi return to normal, you should be absorbing calcium like the rest of us, but we all tend to have problems getting enough calcium (and depending how long it took for you to get diagnosed, you may have lost more calcium from your bones then an average person your age).

Calcium is found mainly in milk and dairy products, but can also be found in other foods.

Flours, Grains, Legumes, Seeds	Serving Size	Calcium (mg)
Soy flour	1 cup	251 mg
Corn flour (masa), white or yellow	1 cup	161 mg
Grains		
Cornmeal	1 cup	440 mg
Teff	1 cup	347 mg
Amaranth	1 cup	307 mg
Soybeans	1 cup	504 mg
Sesame seeds	1 oz	277 mg
Miso (Rice)	1 cup	157 mg
Sesame seed paste, tahini	2 Tbsp	127.8 mg
Navy beans	1 cup	126 mg
Great northern beans	1 cup	120 mg
Kidney beans	1 cup	117 mg
Protein, Vegetables, Fruits		
Sardines (with bone)	3 oz	321 mg
Salmon (with bone)	3 oz	233 mg
Mackerel	3 oz	203 mg

Protein, Vegetables, Fruits (Continued)	Serving Size	Calcium (mg)
Shrimp	3 oz	123 mg
Spinach, raw	1 cup	290 mg
Collards, cooked	½ cup	178.5 mg
Kale, raw	1 cup	137 mg
Turnip greens, raw	1 cup	105 mg
Broccoli rabe, cooked	½ cup	100 mg
Orange juice, calcium fortified	1 cup	500 mg

Dairy

	Serving Size	Calcium (mg)
Milk	1 cup	504 mg
Yogurt	1 cup	488 mg
Ricotta cheese	½ cup	335 mg
Romano cheese	1 oz	298 mg
Gruyere	1 oz	283 mg
Parmesan cheese	¼ cup	275 mg
Mozzarella	1 oz	269 mg
Cheddar	1 oz	253 mg
Provolone cheese	1 oz	212 mg
Monterey	1 oz	209 mg
Muenster	1 oz	201 mg
Gouda cheese	1 oz	196 mg
Colby cheese	1 oz	192 mg

Dairy (Continued)	Serving Size	Calcium (mg)
Roquefort cheese	1 oz	185 mg
Blue cheese	1 oz	148 mg
Feta cheese	1 oz	138 mg

Iron

Iron is also a mineral. It is very important in keeping oxygen in your blood. Without enough iron, you get anemia. Iron deficiency anemia is common in undiagnosed celiac disease. Once the intestine has healed and the iron deficiency corrected through supplements, it is important to continue to get enough iron. First, if you are a woman you lose iron monthly and your needs are greater. Second, iron (along with thiamin, riboflavin, niacin, and folate) is also part of the enrichment program, but as we've already discussed, that program doesn't quite cover a gluten-free diet.

Iron comes in two forms: heme and non-heme. The body absorbs heme iron—found in red meat, fish, and poultry—more easily. Non-heme iron—mainly found in vegetables, grains, eggs, and fruits—is not as easily absorbed, but we can increase absorption by increasing or decreasing the amounts of certain foods that we eat in meals that contain non-heme sources of iron.

Since non-heme iron can be better absorbed by changing what we eat (or don't eat) with it, we should start there.

- Eat red meat, poultry, or fish with a non-heme source of iron. This works because heme iron improves the absorption of non-heme iron. For example, you might have spinach with steak.

- Have a little vitamin C with your non-heme iron. This works because vitamin C helps the non-heme iron get into your body. For example, you could have your scrambled eggs with orange juice or have a mandarin orange and spinach salad. And in case you were wondering, vitamin C food sources are not only citrus fruits. You can also find vitamin C in kiwi, strawberries, cantaloupe, broccoli, tomatoes, potatoes, peppers, and cabbage.

- Avoid taking non-heme iron foods with coffee or tea, which contain tannins. Foods that contain tannins prevent the absorption of non-heme iron.
- Try to get more iron (heme or non-heme). Here is a short list of some foods that are a good source of iron:

Flours	Serving Size	Iron (mg)
Soy flour	1 cup	9.7 mg
Sorghum flour	1 cup	8.4 mg
Corn flour	1 cup	8.2 mg
Buckwheat flour	1 cup	4.9 mg
Chickpea flour	1 cup	4.5 mg
Sunflower seed flour	1 cup	4.2 mg
Rice flour, brown	1 cup	3.1 mg

Grains, Beans, Seeds	Serving Size	Iron (mg)
Amaranth	1 cup	14.7 mg
Teff	1 cup	14.7 mg
Rice, white, enriched	1 cup	9.8 mg
Quinoa	1 cup	7.8 mg
Millet	1 cup	6.0 mg
Corn, yellow or white	1 cup	4.5 mg
Buckwheat, groats (kasha)	1 cup	4.1 mg
Rice, wild	1 cup	3.1 mg
White beans	1 cup	21.1 mg
Kidney beans	1 cup	17.2 mg

Grains, Beans, Seeds (Continued)	Serving Size	Iron (mg)
Lima beans	1 cup	14.5 mg
Lentils	1 cup	13.4 mg
Chickpeas	1 cup	12.5 mg
Navy beans	1 cup	11.4 mg
Great northern beans	1 cup	10.0 mg
Pinto beans	1 cup	9.8 mg
Flaxseeds	1 oz	9.6 mg
Soybeans	1 cup	9.1 mg
Pumpkin seeds	¼ cup	5.3 mg
Sesame seeds	1 oz	4.1 mg

Protein, Vegetables

	Serving Size	Iron (mg)
Oysters	3 oz	10.2 mg
Mussels	3 oz	5.7 mg
Beef, all varieties	3 oz	3.3 mg
Lamb, all varieties	3 oz	2.3 mg
Turkey, dark meat	3 oz	2.1 mg
Turkey, white meat	3 oz	1.8 mg
Spinach, cooked	1 cup	6.4 mg
Tomatoes, sun-dried	1 cup	4.9 mg
Edamame, cooked	1 cup	3.5 mg
Asparagus, raw	1 cup	2.9 mg

Protein, Vegetables (Continued)	Serving Size	Iron (mg)
Kale, raw	1 cup	2.0 mg
Chard, Swiss, cooked	½ cup	2.0 mg
Peas, cooked	½ cup	1.9 mg
Fruits		
Raisins	1 cup	3.8 mg
Apricots, dried	1 cup	3.5 mg

Adding Extras: Fiber, Probiotics, and Omega-3 Fatty Acids

Fiber

Fiber is the part of food that we cannot digest. But just because we cannot digest it doesn't mean we don't need it. Fiber has many health benefits. It not only helps improve bowel function, but it also has been shown to decrease blood cholesterol (associated with heart disease) and improve blood sugar control (important when dealing with prediabetes or diabetes). Fiber may be helpful in preventing cancer, especially cancer of the intestinal tract. Certain kinds of fiber feed the "good" bacteria in your intestine, which also provides a world of health benefits (more on this shortly).

When you remove gluten from your diet, you automatically remove a lot of the fiber you may be consuming. With all the health benefits of fiber, you want to get your daily fiber requirement. Even without eliminating gluten, most people do not get enough fiber. So when you lose the gluten in your diet, you need to be diligent about getting your fiber needs met.

So how do you get that needed fiber without the gluten? Here are some tips:

- Consume whole fruits and vegetables instead of juices, since juice has all the fiber removed. While you're at it, don't remove the peel from those apples, pears, potatoes, or other edible peels—that's where much of the fiber is hiding.

- Add beans to many of your dishes. For example, enjoy chickpeas in salad, pinto beans in chili, lentils in soups, and kidney or pinto beans with rice.

- Add nuts and seeds to your meals. For example, enjoy almonds in your cream of rice, sesame seeds in your salad, pumpkin seeds on the tops of breads and muffins, and pecans in your cookies.

- Eat high-fiber snacks such as popcorn, dried fruits (like dried apricots or dried plums), and raw fruits and vegetables.

- Try to use some of the grains and flours that are higher in fiber in your cooking. Look at the chart below for a list of gluten-free foods that are good sources of fiber.

- If you are suffering from constipation and you have attempted to increase the fiber with the tips above, you may need a fiber supplement. Some of them are gluten-free, such as Benefiber® and Citrucel®.

- Last of all, remember to consume an adequate amount of water. This also helps the digestive tract move smoothly.

Flours, Grains	Serving Size	Fiber (g)
Carob flour	1 cup	41 g
Soy flour, defatted	1 cup	16 g
Sorghum flour	1 cup	12 g
Buckwheat flour, whole groat	1 cup	12 g
Corn flour (masa)	1 cup	11 g
Chickpea flour (besan)	1 cup	10 g
Peanut flour, defatted	1 cup	9 g
Potato flour	1 cup	9 g
Rice flour	1 cup	7 g
Arrowroot flour	1 cup	4 g

Flours, Grains (Continued)	Serving Size	Fiber (g)
Corn, bran, crude	1 cup	60 g
Rice bran, crude	1 cup	25 g
Buckwheat, groats (kasha)	1 cup	17 g
Cornmeal, whole grain	1 cup	9 g
Amaranth	1 cup	5 g
Quinoa	1 cup	5 g
Rice, brown	1 cup	4 g
Rice, wild	1 cup	3 g

Legumes

	Serving Size	Fiber (g)
Soybeans	1 cup	30 g
Small white beans	1 cup	19 g
Navy beans	1 cup	19 g
French beans	1 cup	17 g
Kidney beans	1 cup	16 g
Lentils	1 cup	16 g
Peas, split	1 cup	16 g
Pinto beans	1 cup	15 g
Black beans	1 cup	15 g
Miso (Rice)	1 cup	15 g
Lima beans	1 cup	13 g
Great northern beans	1 cup	12 g

Legumes (Continued)	Serving Size	Fiber (g)
Refried beans	1 cup	11 g
Fava beans	1 cup	9 g
Pink beans	1 cup	9 g

Nuts, Seeds, Fish, Vegetables

Coconut meat, dried	1 oz	5 g
Sesame seeds	1 oz	4 g
Almonds	1 oz	3 g
Flax seeds	3 Tb	9 g
Sunflower seeds	1 oz	3 g
Hazelnuts	1 oz	3 g
Pine nuts	1 oz	3 g
Pistachio nuts, dried roasted	1 oz	3 g
Pecans	1 oz	3 g
Peanut butter, chunky	2 Tbsp	3 g
Clams	3 oz	23.8 mg
Oysters	3 oz	10.2 mg
Mussels	3 oz	5.7 mg
Artichokes, cooked	1 medium	10 g
Squash, winter, cooked	1 cup	9 g
Parsnips, raw	1 cup	7 g
Peas, cooked	½ cup	4.5 g

Nuts, Seeds, Fish, Vegetables (Continued)	Serving Size	Fiber (g)
Edamame, cooked	½ cup	4 g
Mixed vegetables, without pasta	½ cup	4 g
Serrano pepper, raw	1 cup	4 g
Spinach, cooked	½ cup	4 g
Tomatoes, sun-dried	½ cup	3.4 g
Shitake mushrooms, dried	1 oz	3 g
Parsnips, cooked	½ cup	3 g
Brussels sprouts, cooked	½ cup	3 g
Broccoli, cooked	½ cup	3 g
Sweet potato in skin	½ cup	3 g
Okra, raw	1 cup	3 g
Yams, cooked	½ cup	2.5 g
Turnip greens, cooked	½ cup	2.5 g
Carrots, cooked	½ cup	2.5 g

Fruit

Passion fruit	1 cup	25 g
Elderberries	1 cup	10 g
Guava	1 cup	9 g
Raspberries	1 cup	8 g
Blackberries	1 cup	8 g
Figs, dried	½ cup	7.5 g

Fruit (Continue)	Serving Size	Fiber (g)
Prunes	½ cup	6 g
Blueberries	1 cup	6 g
Gooseberries	1 cup	6 g
Persimmon	1 medium	6 g
Banana	1 cup	6 g
Raisins	½ cup	5 g
Cranberries	1 cup	5 g
Prickly pear	1 cup	5 g
Pears, American versions	1 small	5 g
Plantains, cooked	1 cup	5 g
Apricots, dried	½ cup	4.5 g
Pears, Asian	1 medium	4 g
Carambola, starfruit	1 cup	4 g
Apple with skin	1 small	4 g
Oranges	1 cup sections	4 g
Tangerines	1 cup sections	4 g
Cranberries, dried	½ cup	3 g
Pomegranates	½ cup	3 g
Cherries	1 cup	3 g
Apricots	1 cup	3 g
Strawberries	1 cup	3 g
Mangos	1 cup	3 g

Fruit (*Continue*)	Serving Size	Fiber (g)
Papayas	1 cup	3 g
Peaches	1 large	3 g

Probiotics

Probiotics is the term health care professionals use to describe the "healthy" or "good" bacteria in the intestinal tract. These bacteria living in our small and large intestines do marvelous things. They consume some of the food that we cannot digest (fiber known as prebiotics) and produce something known as small chain fatty acids. These small chain fatty acids are then used by our gut cells for energy and repair. Also, we believe that these "good" bacteria fight off "bad" bacteria, helping prevent illness like stomach viruses.

When someone does not have enough probiotics in their gut, they are at risk for what is called permeable gut. Our intestinal tract has very special cells designed to allow small molecules of sugar, protein, and fat to enter our body and our bloodstream while preventing waste and pathogens from getting out. When the gut is not healthy, we develop larger "holes" or "gaps" that allow toxins into our body as well, where they can cause illness (like infections) or, as some believe, neurological and autoimmune problems. We will talk a little more about these types of illnesses in Chapter 15. For now, just understand that probiotics help our gut stay healthy and prevent it from becoming "leaky."

So how do you get those "good" bacteria into your body? There are many foods that you probably already eat that contain probiotics. For instance, yogurt is a good source of these "good bugs." Also, many manufacturers have recently begun adding probiotics to foods. Some of these are gluten-free, but some are not. Another good source of probiotics is supplements—but you will need to be careful to find probiotics that are gluten-free.

Gluten-free probiotic supplements include the following (although formulations change, so double-check these before starting to take them):

- Flora-Q Probiotic
- In-Liven

- Fast-Tract

- NuFerm Organic Whole Foods

- Innergy Biotic-Body Ecology Diet

Omega-3 Fatty Acids

We first learned about omega-3 fatty acids (their chemical makeup gives them their name) from studies into why the Eskimo population had such low heart disease rates. Research found that the Eskimos' diet was high in fish fat, which is high in omega-3 fatty acids. Some of these omega-3 fatty acids work in the body to reduce inflammation and therefore may provide health benefits such as reduced risk of cancer, heart disease, and rheumatoid arthritis (an autoimmune disease). Many studies are currently underway that look at the benefit of these fats on the brain and immune function—and, at the time of this writing, they look promising.

Omega-3 fatty acids come in many different forms. The first is what we call essential, meaning that we must get it in our diet. This one is known as alpha-linoleic acid (ALA) for short. The most beneficial forms are known as eicosapentanoic acid (EPA) and docosahexanoic acid (DHA). These forms can be made from ALA by our body, but unfortunately our body does not do this well. It seems that our body only converts 2–15 percent of ALA into EPA and only 2–5 percent into DHA. The percentage of conversion varies, and women seem to be better at converting than men, but at best it's a very small amount. Fish do a much better job of converting the algae they eat to EPA and DHA, which is why it's recommended that we consume fish two or more times a week.

Bearing in mind that only small amounts are converted, you can still get ALA in your diet. The best sources of ALA are flaxseeds, walnuts, pecans, and hazelnuts. You can also get eggs that are high in ALA omega-3 fatty acids from chickens who have been fed foods that increase the amount in the eggs. Oils that are high in omega-3 fatty acids are flaxseed oil and canola oil.

If you do not eat much fish and still want to make sure you get enough, consider a fish oil supplement. Supplements like cod liver oil or other fish oils will supply you with the EPA and DHA you need. Some people complain that the supplements cause "fish burps"; these can be reduced by refrigerating your supplement.

Using Gluten-Free Alternatives

Gluten-Free Products Are Everywhere

It wasn't very long ago that finding gluten-free foods other than those that are naturally gluten-free was next to impossible. And even if you could find it, it was very poor in quality, especially breads and desserts. In taste and consistency it was like eating cardboard. Thankfully, this is no longer the case. Gluten-free products have been getting better and better, and today they are the most rapidly increasing food category being manufactured.

In addition to the variety of choices, changes in food labeling laws are slowly making it easier to identify which foods are gluten-free and which are not. Gluten-free foods can now be found in restaurants and fast food establishments as well as in packaged foods. In addition, they are showing up in tasty bakery and dessert options and are working their way onto supermarket shelves.

What's Available

Gluten-free foods are everywhere, and thanks to the Internet you can now find

- Bread, bagels, pancakes, biscuits, coffee cake, waffles
- Pasta, pizza

- Cakes, cookies, pies

- Frozen meals, soups, casseroles

- Chain restaurants posting gluten-free menus online—many private restaurants offer gluten-free choices as well

The future holds much promise, especially since so many chefs are embracing gluten-free choices in their kitchens.

Where to Find Gluten-Free Items in Stores

Gluten-free foods are found in supermarkets in the health food and specialties aisle, as well as in the freezer case and mixed through-out the store. There are many foods that are gluten-free that do not indicate this on their packaging, so learning how to read labels will make it easier to identify more safe choices. There are also many gluten-free shopping guides now available, such as the *Gluten-Free Grocery Shopping Guide,* by Matison & Matison, which lists thousands of brand-name products that have already been checked for their gluten-free status.

Health food and specialty stores are the best place to find a large variety of gluten-free products. It is here that you may find more unusual or hard-to-find items. Since everyone has different taste buds, and one product may not appeal to everyone, it may be helpful to try some of the products before purchasing them. You can sample gluten-free foods at some of the many celiac fairs run throughout the country. Find out about events near you by checking with your local celiac organizations. To find a group in your area, go to www.csaceliacs.org.

Where to Find Gluten-Free Items on the Internet

The Internet now provides endless places to find gluten-free foods. Just going to some of the many gluten-free blogs or Web sites gives you a wonderful variety of products to try. At www.glutenfreehasslefree.com you can find a listing of many products for you to review. Also, listed below, you'll find some of the many companies that have great gluten-free choices.

Gluten-Free Grains are Available From

Aleia's
Pasta
www.aleias.com

AltiPlano Gold
Quinoa products
www.altiplanogold.com

Amazake, Grainaissance
Amazake and mochi
www.grainaissance.com

Amazing Grains
Montina and rice grass products
www.amazinggrains.com
www.montina.com

Anello's Pastries
Baked goods
www.anellospastries.com

Ancient Harvest Quinoa
Quinoa products
www.quinoa.net

Andean Dreams
Quinoa products
www.andeandream.com

Andrea's Fine Foods
Baked goods
www.andreasfinefoods.com

Arrowhead Mills
Grains
www.arrowheadmills.com

Aunt Gussie's Cookies
Cookies
www.auntgussies.com

Authentic Foods
Grains and almond meal
www.Authenticfoods.com

Azna Gluten-Free
Baked goods
www.aznaglutenfree.com

Bakery on Main
Bars and granola
www.bakeryonmain.com

Barbara's Bakery
Baked goods
www.barbarasbakery.com

Barkat
Breads, pastas, and desserts
www.glutenfree-foods.co.uk

Bio Nature
Pasta
www.bionature.com

The Birkett Mills
Grains and buckwheat products
www.thebirkettmills.com

Bittersweet Bakery
Baked goods
www.bittersweetgf.com

Bob's Red Mill
Grains, mixes, and cereals
www.bobsredmill.com

Breads From Anna
Cake and bread mixes
www.glutenevolution.com

BumbleBar Foods
Snack bars
www.bumblebar.com

Casa deFruta
Mesquite
www.casadefruta.com

Cause You're Special
Baking mixes
www.causeyourespecial.com

Gluten-free Grains (continued)

Celiac Specialties
Desserts and bakery products
www.celiacspecialtiesshop.com

Chebe Bread
Bread mixes
www.chebe.com

Cheecha Krackles
Potato snacks
www.cheecha.ca

Crave Bakery
Baked goods
www.cravebakery.com

Cream of The Crop
Buckwheat
www.alimentstrigone.com

Crunchmaster
Rice crackers
www.crunchmaster.com

Cybros
Baked goods
www.cybrosinc.com

Dale and Thomas
Popcorn and gourmet kettle corn
www.daleandthomas.com

De Boles
Pasta
www.deboles.com

Dietary Specialties
Bakery mixes
www.dietspec.com

Domata
Flours, consumer and foodservice sizes
www.domatalivingflour.com

Dowd & Rogers
Cake mixes
www.dowdandrogers.com

Enjoy Life Foods
Snack bars and bagels
www.enjoylifefoods.com

Ener-G Foods
Bread products
www.ener-g.com

Erewhon
Cereal
www.usmillsllc.com

Everybody Eats
Baked goods and fresh pasta
www.everybodyeats-inc.com

Expandex
Modified tapioca starch
www.expandexglutenfree.com

Farmer's Kitchen Café
Baked goods
www.farmerskitchencafe.com

Flying Apron Bakery
Baked goods
www.flyingapron.net

Food for Life Baking Company
Breads, corn, and rice tortillas
www.foodforlife.com

Foods by George
Baked goods, pasta, and pizza
www.foodsbygeorge.com

French Meadow Bakery
Baked goods
www.frenchmeadow.com

General Mills
Rice Chex (more products being developed)
www.generalmills.com

Get Healthy America
Gourmet foods
info@gethealthyamerica.com

Gluten-free Grains (continued)

GFN Foods, LLC
Mixes
www.gnffoods.com

Gibbs Wild Rice
Grains and wild rice
www.gibbswildrice.com

Gifts of Nature
Grains
www.giftsofnature.net

Gilberts Goodies
Allergy-friendly cookies and goodies
www.gilbertsgourmetgoodies.com

Gillian's Foods
Baked goods
www.gilliansfoods.com

Gluten-Free Bagel Company
Breads, bagels, and mixes
www.glutenfreebagelcompany.com

Gluten-Free Creations Bakery
Bakery
www.glutenfreecreations.com

Glutenfreeda Foods
Cookie dough
www.glutenfreedafoods.com

Gluten-Free Kneads
Cookie dough and flatbread
www.glutenfreekneads.com

Gluten-Free Mall
A variety of products
www.glutenfreemall.com

Gluten-Free Naturals
Cookie blends
www.gfnfoods.com

Gluten-Free Pantry
Mixes and snacks
www.glutenfree.com

Gluten Solutions
A variety of products and foods
www.glutensolutions.com

Glutino Food Group
Baked goods
www.glutino.com

GoGo Quinoa
Quinoa and amaranth products
www.quinoa.com

Good Eatz
Baked goods
www.goodeatz.org

Good Juju Bakery
Baked goods
www.goodjujubakery.com

The Grainless Baker
Baked goods
www.thegrainlessbaker.com

Haley's Corner Bakery
Baked goods
www.haleyscorner.com

Heaven Mills Bakery
Baked goods and matzah
www.heavenmillsbakery.com

Hoi-Grain
Snacks, sauces, and soups
www.conradricemill.com

1-2-3 Gluten-Free, Inc
www.123glutenfree.com

Gluten-Free Mall®
www.glutenfreemall.com

Gluten Solutions
www.glutensolutions.com

Island Gluten-Free Bakery
Baked goods
www.islandgfbakery.com

Gluten-free Grains (continued)

Jake Bakes
Baked goods
www.jakebakes.com

Jennies
Macaroons
www.macaroonking.com

Joan's GF Great Bakes
Bagels and pizza
www.gfgreatbakes.com

Jubilee Kafe
Baked goods
www.jubileekafe.com

Kathy's Creation
Baked goods
www.kathyscreationsbakery.com

Katz Gluten-Free
Kosher breads and bakery products
www.katzglutenfree.com

Kays Naturals
Cereals and snacks (protein-fortified)
www.kaysnaturals.com

Kingsmill Food
Baked goods
www.kingsmillfoods.com

Kinnikinnick Foods
Ready-to-eat breads and cakes
www.kinnikinnick.com

Kitchen Table Bakers
Cheese wafer crisps
www.kitchentablebakers.com

La Tortilla Factory
Teff tortillas
www.latortillafactory.com

Laurel's Sweet Treats
Bakery mixes
www.glutenfreemixes.com

The Little Aussie Bakery
Baked goods
www.thelittleaussiebakery.com

Little Bay Bakery
Baking mixes
www.littlebaybaking.com

Lundberg Family Farms
Rice products
www.lundberg.com

Lydias Organics
Natural sprouted grain, fruit, and
nut products
www.Lydiasorganics.com

**Madwoman Foods Bakeshop &
Foodery**
Baked goods
www.madwomanfoods.com

Maplegrove Gluten-free Foods
Potato pasta
www.perkysnaturalfoods.com

Manna From Anna
Prepared bread mixes
www.glutenevolution.com

Manishchewitz
Many kosher products
www.manischewitz.com

Mariposa Baking Company
Baked goods
www.mariposabaking.com

Mary's Gone Crackers
Crackers
www.marysgonecrackers.com

Miller's Gluten-Free
Bread
www.millersglutenfree.com

Minn-Dak Growers
Buckwheat products
www.minndak.com

Gluten-free Grains (continued)

Mochi
Brown rice puffs
www.grainaissance.com

Molly's Gluten-Free Bakery
Baked goods
www.mollysglutenfreebakery.com

Mr. Krispers
Chips
www.mrkrispers.com

Moose Lake Wild Rice
Grains and wild rice
www.Mooselakewildrice.com

Namaste Foods
Bakery mixes
www.namastefoods.com

Nana's Cookie Company
Cookie bars
www.nanasnatural.com

Nu-World Amaranth
Amaranth products
www.nuworldamaranth.com

Northern Quinoa Corporation
www.quinoa.com

Only Oats Farm Pure Foods
Oats
www.onlyoats.com

Outside the Breadbox
Baked goods
www.outsidethebreadbox.com

Pamela's Product
Bakery mixes
www.pamelasproducts.com

Pastariso
Pasta
www.maplegrovefoods.com

Perky's Natural Foods
Cereal
www.perkysnaturalfoods.com

Purefit Nutrition
Energy bars
www.purefit.com

The Really Great Food Company
Bakery mixes
www.reallygreatfood.com

Rice Expressions
Rice mixes
www.riceexpressions.com

Mr. Ritts
Baked goods
http://mrritts.com

Rose's Wheat-Free Bakery and Café
Baked goods
www.rosesbakery.com

The Ruby Range
Baked goods
www.therubyrange.com

Schar
A line of products
www.schar.com

The Sensitive Baker
Baked goods
www.thesensitivebaker.com

Shiloh Farms
Flours and sorghum
www.shilohfarms.com

The Silly Yak Bakery and Bread Barn
Baked goods
www.sillyyakbakery.com

Sinfully Gluten-Free
Baked goods
www.sinfullygf.com

Gluten-free Grains (continued)

Sunny Valley Wheat Free
Baked goods
www.sunnyvalleywheatfree.com

Sweet Christine's Gluten-Free Confections
Baked goods
www.sweetchristinesglutenfree .com

Sweet Escape Pastries, LLC.
Baked goods
www.sweetescpastries.com

Sweet Sin Bakery
Baked goods
www.glutenfreedesserts.com

Sylvan Border Farm
Whole-grain bakery mixes
www.sylvanborderfarm.com

The Teff Company
Teff products
www.teffco.com

The Sensitive Baker
Artisan breads
www.thesensitivebaker.com

Tinkyada
Brown rice pasta
www.ricepasta.com

Tom Sawyer
Flour blends and gums
www.glutenfreeflour.com

Twin Valley Mills, LLC
Grains and sorghum
www.twinvalleymills.com

Quinoa Corporation
Grains and quinoa products
www.quinoa.net

Nu-World Foods
Amaranth
www.nuworldamaranth.com

Van's International Foods
Waffles
www.wellnessfoods.ca

Whole Foods Market Gluten-Free Bakehouse
Baked goods
www.wholefoodsmarket.com

Gluten-Free Oats are Available From

Bob's Red Mill
www.bobsredmill.com

Cream Hill Estates
www.creamhillestates.com

Farm Pure Foods
www.onlyoats.com

Gluten-Free Oats
www.glutenfreeoats.com

Holly's Oatmeal
Porridge and oats
www.hollysoatmeal.com

Ready-Made Gluten-Free Foods are Available From

Allergaroo
Microwavable food
www.allergaroo.com

Alpine Aire Foods
Prepared meals
www.aa-foods.com

Amy's Kitchen
A wide variety of frozen meals
www.amyskitchen.com

Ready-Made Gluten-Free Foods (continued)

Annie's Homegrown
Meals
www.annies.com

Apetito
Textured meals
www.apetito.ca

Celinal Foods
Single-serve mixes and gluten-free starter kits
www.celinalfoods.com

GF Meals
Ready-to-cook meals
www.gfmeals.com

Gluten-Free Café
Frozen meals
www.myglutenfreecafe.com

Gluten-Free and Fabulous
Quinoa pasta and pizza
www.glutenfreefabulous.com

My Own Meals
Vacuum-sealed meals
www.myownmeals.com

Allergy-Free Gluten-Free Foods are Available From

Allergyfree Foods
www.allergyfreefoods.com

Allergaroo
Allergy-friendly foods
www.allergaroo.com

Arico Natural Foods
Gluten- and dairy-free foods
www.aricofoods.com

Cherrybrook Kitchen
gluten-, dairy-, and egg-free mixes
www.cherrybrookkitchen.com

Dr. Praeger's Sensible Foods
Fish sticks, pancakes, veggie burgers
www.drpraegers.com

Road End Organics
Gluten-, dairy-, egg-, and nut-free mixes and dips
www.edwardandsons.com

Gluten-Free Shakes are Available From

Boost Shakes
All products except for smoothies
1 (800) 247-7893
www.boost.com

Ensure Shakes
All products
1 (800) 986-8501
www.ensure.com

Glucerna Shakes
All products
1 (800) 227-5767
www.glucerna.com

Nutra Shakes
All products
1 (800) 654-3691
www.nutra-balance-products.com

Nutren Shakes
All products
1 (888) 240-2713
www.nestlenutritionstore.com

Gluten-Free Candy is Available From

Azure Chocolat
Kosher chocolate
www.azurechocolat.com

Candy Tree
Candy
www.healthflavors.com

Gluten-Free Broths and Asian Products are Available From

Annie Chun's
Asian foods
www.anniechun.com

Celinal Foods
Individual gluten-free packets
www.celinalfoods.com

Cuisine Sante
Broths
www.haco.ch

Eden Foods
Tamari
www.edenfoods.com

Kari-Out Company
Soy sauce
www.kariout.com

Kettle Cuisine
Frozen soups
www.kettlecuisine.com

Maplegrove Gluten-Free Foods
Broths
www.maplegrovefoods.com

Pacific Foods
Broths
www.PacificFoods.com

Premier Japan
Teriyaki and hoisin sauce
www.edwardandsons.com

San-J International
Tamari
www.san-j.com

Savory Choice
Broths
www.savorychoice.com

Simply Asia Foods
Asian noodles and sauces
www.simplyasia.net

Swiss Chalet
Broths and stocks
www.scff.com

Thai Kitchen
Many Asian products
www.thaikitchen.com

Gluten-Free Bars are Available From

Extend Bar
All products, including diabetic energy bar
www.extendbar.com

Larabar
Energy bar
www.larabar.com

Think Products
Bars
www.thinkproducts.com

Other Gluten-Free Products are Available From

Toaster Safety Bags
www.toastitbags.com

Prepared Gluten-Free Meals are Available From

AlpineAire Foods TyRy Inc
Rocklin CA
1 (800) 322-6325/(866)
322-6325
Fax (916) 624-1604
info@aa-foods.com
www.aa-foods.com

Amy's Kitchen
Petaluma, CA
1 (707) 578-7270
Fax (707) 578-7995
amy@amyskitchen.com
www.amyskitchen.com

Many frozen foods
Caesar's
Frozen meals
www.caesarspasta.com

Gluten-Free Beer is Available From

Anheuser-Busch (Redbridge)
www.anheuser-busch.com

Bard's Tale Beer (Dragon's Gold Gluten-Free Beer)
www.bardsbeer.com

BiAglut
www.biaglut.com/ITA/Prodotti/
Birra/default.htm

Fine Ale Club
www.ale4home.co.uk/fine_ale_
club.htm

Green's
www.glutenfreebeers.co.uk

LA Messagere
www.lesbieresnouvellefrance.com

Lakefront Brewery
www.lakefrontbrewery.com

Mongozo Beers
www.mongozo.org/engels/main.
php

Nick Stafford's Hambleton Ales
www.hambletonales.co.uk

O'Brien Brewing
www.gfbeer.com.au

Ramapo Valley Brewery
(Gluten-Free Honey Lager)
http://ramapovalleybrewery.com

Sprecher Brewery
www.sprecherbrewery.com/
index.php

Silly Yak
www.sillyyak.com.au/beer/faq.
html

Schlafly
www.schlafly.com

TIP
When drinking alcohol, remember that
All distilled alcohol (vodka, rum, gin, whiskey, scotch, etc.) is gluten-free.
All wine is gluten-free, unless a flavoring agent is added.
Most wine coolers contain gluten.
Most beers and ales are not gluten-free, because they are usually made from barley

Cooking Gluten-Free Dishes with Flair

Making Family Favorites Gluten-Free

We all have favorite foods that we have grown up with and enjoy. Learning how to make these favorites gluten-free can really make the difference in how you feel about following a gluten-free diet. There may be times when you are unable to find gluten-free foods that you can use as a substitute in a recipe, and you may need to change the recipe in order to make it work. In order to make things easier, start with simple versions of the recipes you want to change; later, you can work on making substitutions and more complicated changes as you become more experienced. The following examples demonstrate ways to modify recipes:

Original Green Bean Casserole: Casserole made with green beans, cream of mushroom soup, and dried onion rings.

Gluten-Free Modified Green Bean Casserole: In a casserole dish, combine green beans and gluten-free cream soup with sliced mushrooms. In place of the dried onion rings, sauté thin onion slices in olive oil until brown, crumble in gluten-free cereal or bread crumbs, add salt and pepper, and mix into green bean mixture and bake.

Original Chicken Cutlet Parmesan: Breaded and fried cutlets topped with mozzarella and tomato sauce and served with pasta.

Gluten-Free Modified Chicken Cutlet Parmesan: Toast gluten-free bread and process in food processor; add garlic, onion powder, Italian herbs, and parmesan cheese, and use breadcrumbs to bread the cutlets.

Proceed to make the recipe as above and serve with gluten-free brown rice or quinoa pasta and tomato sauce.

Original Butter Cookies: Made with butter, sugar, egg yolk, salt, baking powder, vanilla extract, and all-purpose flour.

Gluten-Free Modified Butter Cookies: Check baking powder to see if it is gluten-free, use an all-purpose gluten-free flour mixture (as found in Chapter 5), add a little extra gluten-free flour to achieve the same texture, and continue to finish the recipe as usual.

As you can see, if you are modifying recipes to make them gluten-free, you need to start by making small changes. On occasion, you will find a recipe that may require ingredients that are hard to find a gluten-free alternate for, such as puff pastry and phyllo dough. In these cases, you may have to modify the recipe a lot more to suit the ingredients you have available. More and more gluten-free products are on the horizon, so increasingly you will be able to find good substitutes for your ingredients; but, for now, we can work on the recipes with what is available in order to make the best possible alternatives. And I'd like to share with you some fabulous gluten-free recipes from my own collection.

The Gluten-Free Gourmet: Best Recipes

Breakfast

- Amaranth and Apricot Granola

- Pumpkin Pancakes/Waffles

- Blueberry Crumb Muffins

- Italian Frittata

- Pancakes with Cream Cheese Filling

Amaranth and Apricot Granola   Serves 6

This is great served on top of yogurt, as a cereal, or as a snack mix. It is easy to prepare, and any dried fruit or nuts can be substituted in this recipe.

Gluten-free cooking spray (or vegetable oil)
$1/3$ cup whole amaranth grain
2 cups gluten-free Rice Chex cereal

½ cup dried apricots, chopped
¼ cup dried cranberries
½ cup hazelnuts, chopped
½ cup sugar
3 Tb water
½ tsp cinnamon
¼ tsp nutmeg
1 tsp vanilla

1. Preheat oven to 325 degrees. Line a baking sheet with aluminum foil and spray with cooking spray.

2. Heat a small nonstick frying pan over medium-high heat until very hot. Pop the amaranth by adding 1 teaspoon at a time to the pan, cover and shake until grain pops. Pour out onto a plate and repeat with remaining amaranth.

3. In a large bowl, mix the popped amaranth with the Rice Chex, apricots, cranberries, and hazelnuts.

4. In a medium skillet, heat sugar, water, cinnamon, nutmeg, and vanilla to a boil. Boil for about 2 minutes, until sugar is dissolved.

5. Pour sugar mixture over amaranth in bowl. Stir gently to coat.

6. Spread mixture in a single layer on baking sheet. Bake in preheated oven for 15 minutes.

7. Remove from oven, cool slightly. Break granola apart to serve (about 1 cup per serving).

Nutritional information per serving: 247 calories, 3.6 grams protein, 47 grams carbohydrates, 7.5 grams fat, 3 grams fiber, 0 milligrams cholesterol, 89 milligrams sodium, 76 milligrams calcium, 3.6 milligrams iron.

Tips: The amaranth grain burns easily when popping. Be careful!

Pumpkin Pancakes/Waffles 6 (4-inch) pancakes (3 jumbo waffles)

Pumpkin pancakes are all the rage in the fall, but they are just as yummy as a special treat any time.

1 cup gluten-free all-purpose flour blend (below)
1 tsp baking powder

1 tsp salt
1 tsp cinnamon
¼ tsp nutmeg
⅛ tsp ginger
⅛ tsp cloves
2 Tb brown sugar
2 Tb granulated sugar
1 tsp xanthan gum
1 Tb butter, melted
1 egg, or 3 egg whites
2 Tb low-fat buttermilk (optional)
½ cup pumpkin purée
¾ cup skim milk
1 tsp vanilla extra
Gluten-free cooking spray

Gluten-Free Flour Blend

(*Makes 5¼ cups; store leftover in airtight canister.*)

1 cup sorghum ¾ cup brown rice flour
2 cups potato starch
1 cup tapioca starch
½ cup garbanzo bean flour

1. Mix dry ingredients together (1 cup gluten-free flour blend through xanthan gum).

2. Beat all wet ingredients together and pour into dry. Mix until just combined.

3. Spray a large skillet with cooking spray and heat until hot. Lower flame and pour in pancake batter to make 4-inch pancakes. (If making waffles, spray the waffle iron with cooking spray and follow manufacturer's directions for making waffles.)

4. Brown on both sides. Serve with maple syrup or jam. Looks great sprinkled with confectioner's sugar.

Nutritional information: 162 calories, 4.3 grams protein, 29.5 grams carbohydrates, 3.4 grams fat, 41 milligrams cholesterol, 487 milligrams sodium, 1.6 grams fiber, 96 milligrams calcium, 1.1 milligrams iron.

Tips: This is also delicious with sliced bananas and chocolate chips. To make without the pumpkin, omit the pumpkin, cinnamon, nutmeg, ginger, and cloves. Reduce the amount of milk to ½ cup. (Makes 2 jumbo waffles or four 4-inch pancakes.) If you like crisp waffles, leave in the waffle iron a few minutes longer.

Blueberry Crumb Muffins Serves 12

Light and delicious, the perfect breakfast. Freeze extras so you can take them out when you need them. Any berry can be used in this recipe.

½ cup white rice flour
½ cup brown rice flour
½ cup tapioca starch
½ cup sorghum flour
¼ cup granulated sugar
2 tsp baking powder
½ tsp baking soda
1 tsp xanthan gum
¼ tsp salt
1 tsp lemon zest
2 eggs
½ cup plain low-fat yogurt
1 cup low-fat 1% milk
4 Tb melted butter, divided in half
2 cups fresh or frozen blueberries
2 Tb brown sugar
¼ cup almond flour
¼ cup white rice flour
¼ tsp nutmeg

1. Preheat oven to 400 degrees. Line a 12-cup muffin tin with paper muffin cups.

2. Mix all dry ingredients (flour through lemon zest) in a large mixing bowl.

3. In a separate bowl, beat together eggs, yogurt, milk, and 2 tablespoons of the melted butter.

4. Make a well in the center of the dry ingredients. Pour in wet ingredients and stir until just combined.

5. Stir in blueberries. Divide batter evenly among the 12 prepared muffin cups.

6. In a small bowl, use a fork to mix together brown sugar, almond flour, white rice flour, nutmeg, and remaining 2 tablespoons of melted butter.

7. Sprinkle crumb mixture evenly over the 12 muffins.

8. Bake for 25 minutes or until a toothpick inserted in the middle comes out clean.

Nutritional information per serving: 209 calories, 4.6 grams protein, 36 grams carbohydrates, 6 grams fat, 47 milligrams cholesterol, 174 milligrams sodium, 72 milligrams calcium, <1 milligram iron.

Tips: These muffins are best served warm with butter or jelly. Freeze unused muffins so you can have delicious muffins whenever you want them.

Italian Frittata Florentine   Serves 4

Viva la Italy, this is rich delicious breakfast that tastes a lot like a crustless quiche. It is great served as a breakfast or a brunch treat.

Gluten-free cooking spray
1 medium onion, sliced thin
½ cup baby spinach
2 cups Egg Beaters
1 tsp gluten-free Dijon mustard
2 Tb 2% milk
½ tsp salt
¼ tsp pepper
2 Tb brown rice flour, or use a premade gluten-free flour blend like those sold by Bob's Red Mill
4 oz low-fat shredded Swiss cheese

1. Preheat oven to 350 degrees

2. Spray a medium skillet with cooking spray and sauté onion until light brown, stirring occasionally. Add baby spinach and sauté spinach until wilted and any additional liquid in the pan evaporates.

3. Spray a 10-inch casserole pan with cooking spray.

4. Whisk together Egg Beaters with Dijon mustard, 2% milk, salt, and pepper, and pour in casserole dish. Top with spinach mixture. Mix Swiss cheese with flour and sprinkle over the top.

5. Bake for 35–45 minutes until set through; cut into quarters and serve.

Nutritional information: 151 calories, 21.6 grams protein, 11.3 grams carbohydrates, 1.8 grams fat, 10.5 milligrams cholesterol, 499 milligrams sodium, 1 gram fiber, 360 milligrams calcium, 3.2 milligrams iron.

Tip: Egg whites or other egg substitute can be used in place of the Egg Beaters. Also, chopped cooked broccoli works well in place of the spinach, and low-fat cheddar in place of the Swiss.

Pancakes with Cream Cheese Filling   Serves 6

A bit like cheese blintzes, and terrific served with a side of sour cream.and strawberry jam.

Cream Cheese Filling

4 Tb light cream cheese
¾ cup 1% cottage cheese
1 Tb granulated sugar
1 cup skim milk
1 tsp vanilla extract
2 eggs
2 Tb butter, melted
1½ cups gluten-free flour blend (below, or prepurchased blend)
2 Tb sugar
2 tsp baking powder
1 tsp baking soda
½ tsp salt
½ tsp xanthan gum
Gluten-free cooking spray
1 Tb powdered sugar

Gluten-Free Flour Blend

(Makes 5¼ cups; reserve unused portion in an airtight container.)

1 cup sorghum

¾ cup brown rice flour
2 cups potato starch
1 cup tapioca starch
½ cup garbanzo bean flour
Optional fruit fillings: strawberries, blueberries, bananas, or all-fruit preserves.

1. Blend together cream cheese filling ingredients and set aside.

2. In a medium bowl, mix all remaining ingredients together (skim milk through butter).

3. In a large bowl, mix all dry ingredients together (gluten-free flour blend through xanthan gum) and set aside.

4. Fold wet ingredients into dry.

5. Heat a flat skillet and spray with cooking spray.

6. Drop batter by scant ¼ cupfuls onto hot griddle.

7. Brown pancakes on both sides.

8. Meanwhile, warm cream cheese filling in the microwave for about 30 seconds.

9. Fill each pancake with cream cheese filling and fruit if desired. Fold in half to serve. If using fruit preserves, spread pancake with preserves, then cream cheese filling, then fold.

10. Sprinkle pancakes with powdered sugar.

Nutritional information: 319 calories, 10.8 grams protein, 53.5 grams carbohydrates, 8.4 grams fat, 87.7 milligrams cholesterol, 596 milligrams sodium, 1 gram fiber, 132 milligrams calcium, 1.5 milligrams iron.

Tip: Cream cheese pancakes are yummy and a little like cheese blintzes. Ricotta cheese works well in place of cottage cheese in this recipe as well.

Breads

- Broccoli Cheese Calzones

- Mediterranean Pizza

- Potato Flat Bread

- Italian Pizza

- Hamburger Rolls

- Soft Pretzel Nuggets

- Basic Crêpes

- English Muffins

Broccoli and Cheese Calzones   Serves 4

Serve with tomato sauce, or wrap in aluminum foil and take with you as a great packed lunch choice to go.

1 package rapid-rise yeast
½ cup tapioca starch
⅓ cup chickpea flour
⅓ cup sorghum flour
1 tsp xanthan gum
½ tsp salt
1 tsp unflavored gelatin
1 tsp sugar
1 tsp garlic powder
¼ cup water
½ cup low-fat 1% milk
2 Tb olive oil
½ cup frozen, chopped broccoli, defrosted
½ cup part-skim ricotta cheese
½ cup part-skim mozzarella cheese
¼ tsp black pepper
1 tsp dried basil
1 egg white
1 Tb parmesan cheese

1. In a large bowl, sift together dry ingredients (yeast through garlic powder).

2. Heat water, milk, and olive oil in a small saucepan over medium heat until just simmering.

3. Add milk mixture to dry ingredients. Stir to combine. Dough should hold together. If too dry, add more milk; if too wet, add more white rice flour.

4. Put dough into a clean bowl that was sprayed with cooking spray; cover and let rest for 10 minutes.

5. Preheat oven to 400 degrees.

6. Mix broccoli, ricotta cheese, mozzarella cheese, black pepper, and basil together in a small bowl.

7. Divide dough into 4 equal-sized pieces. Press each piece into a 4-inch circle. Place about 2 tablespoons of broccoli mixture onto one half of each dough circle.

8. Fold dough in half and press with tines of a fork to seal edges. Brush each calzone with egg white and sprinkle with parmesan cheese.

9. Bake for 20 minutes, until crust is browned and filling is bubbly.

Nutritional information per serving: 316 calories, 16 grams protein, 37 grams carbohydrates, 13 grams fat, 20 milligrams cholesterol, 481 milligrams sodium, 3 grams fiber, 233 milligrams calcium, 2 grams iron.

Tips: Serve with a marinara sauce for dipping. Don't worry if the dough rips as you are trying to fill the calzones—just patch them back together and continue to wrap shut.

Mediterranean Pizza   Serves 2

This is so easy to prepare, and so full of flavor, that you'll be tempted to polish off the whole pizza yourself. You don't feel like you're missing anything when you make this delicious treat.

1 small individual gluten-free pizza dough (made to serve 2—Kinnikinnick pizza crusts, for example)
2 Tb prepared hummus
1 tomato, sliced
¼ tsp salt
¼ tsp oregano
1½ oz crumbled feta cheese

2 thin slices of red onion
2 Tb olives, chopped
1 tsp olive oil
¼ tsp garlic powder

1. Preheat oven to 350.

2. Cook pizza crust in oven on a cookie sheet that has been coated with aluminum foil until it starts to toast lightly.

3. Spread hummus on pizza crust and top with sliced tomato. Sprinkle with salt and oregano. Sprinkle with feta; top with onions, olives, olive oil, and garlic powder.

4. Turn oven up to broil and place pizza on a cookie sheet and cook for about 3 minutes, until cheese starts to melt.

5. Serve with a crisp green salad.

Nutritional information: 222 calories, 5.5 grams protein, 22.7 grams carbohydrates, 12.2 grams fat, 18.9 milligrams cholesterol, 750 milligrams sodium, 2.9 grams iron, 133 milligrams calcium, 1.3 milligrams iron.

Tip: This is delicious with any cheese or flavored bean dip—a real winner!

Potato Flat Bread   Serves 6

Potatoes have long been used throughout the world as a staple food. They are inexpensive and provide good flavor and can be used as an alternative in some traditional dishes.

2 russet potatoes
1 tsp salt
¼ stick butter or margarine, melted
1 egg
2 tsp sugar
½ cup gluten-free flour blend or brown rice flour
1 cup potato starch
2 tsp xanthan gum
2 Tb milk or buttermilk
Rice flour for rolling
Gluten-free cooking spray

Gluten-Free Flour Blend

(Makes 2¼ cups; reserve unused portion in an airtight container for future use.)

¾ cup sorghum flour
¾ cup potato starch or cornstarch
½ cup tapioca flour
¼ cup chickpea or almond flour

1. Boil potatoes until just cooked; cool and peel. (You can cut up the potatoes and cook them in the microwave in a small amount of water as well.)

2. Peel potatoes and process in a food processor with salt until smooth.

3. Meanwhile, in a large bowl, cream butter with egg and sugar; mix in potato mixture, then add gluten-free flour, potato starch, xanthan gum, and milk. Process together until smooth.

4. Work dough into ½-cup balls. If too sticky, add additional flour blend or potato starch.

5. On wax paper that has been dusted with rice flour, roll out each dough ball to make a ¼-inch-thick disk.

6. Spray skillet with cooking spray, then heat.

7. Cook each disk until brown and bubbling on each side.

Nutritional information: 237 calories, 3.8 grams protein, 47 grams carbohydrates, 4 grams fat, 35 milligrams cholesterol, 478 milligrams sodium, 2.2 grams fiber, 50.6 milligrams calcium, <1 milligram iron.

Tips: Great with dips or served as an open-face sandwich. Delicious when made with added seasoning such as garlic and onion powder. If made ahead of time and kept refrigerated, microwave for about 30 seconds before using.

Italian Pizza   Serves 10

This pizza is just fabulous—take care to follow the instructions for letting it rise, and you will have a pizza that tastes the way pizza should.

3½ cups all-purpose gluten-free flour blend (below)
¾ cup warm skim milk
¾ cup warm water
1 packet dry yeast (about 1 Tb)
2 tsp sugar
¼ cup olive oil
1¼ tsp salt
1 tsp xanthan gum
1 Tb cider vinegar
½ cup brown rice flour
4 Tb olive oil
2 Tb cornmeal
1 tsp dried oregano or Italian herb blend
2 cups tomato sauce
½ tsp garlic powder
½ tsp onion powder
1½ cups shredded mozzarella cheese
¼ cup parmesan cheese

Basic Gluten-Free Flour Blend

1 cup sorghum flour
1 cup potato starch
1 cup tapioca flour
½ cup chickpea flour or almond or corn flour

1. In a large bowl, mix 1 cup of flour blend with ¾ cup warm milk
    and ¼ cup warm water. Add yeast, sugar, ⅛ cup olive oil, and
    1 tsp salt. Mix together, cover with plastic wrap, and let sit for
    45 minutes.

2. Mix remaining flour with the remaining salt and xanthan gum.
    Mix together with yeasted mixture with ¼–½ cup warm water and
    cider vinegar for about 3–4 minutes, until the dough is a nice soft
    consistency that holds together but is not too wet.

3. Knead and form the dough into a ball; cover and let rest for about
    15 minutes. If too wet, add brown rice flour until a nice consis-
    tency.

4. Preheat oven to 450.

5. Drizzle a large flat pizza pan with 2 Tb olive oil and sprinkle with cornmeal.

6. Turn pizza dough out of bowl and shape and flatten, spreading out over pizza pan. Add brown rice flour if dough is too wet, and work it in as you fit the dough onto the pan, until the pan is completely covered with pizza dough (leave a thicker ridge around the edges). If the dough is too dry or crumbly, wet hands or a spatula and rub it across the top to smooth it out.

7. Sprinkle top of dough with remaining olive oil; sprinkle with oregano and let sit for about 20 minutes.

8. Place dough in the oven and precook for about 15 minutes

9. Top with tomato sauce, garlic, onion powder, mozzarella and parmesan cheese, and any other toppings you desire, and place it in the hot oven.

10. Bake for about 25–30 minutes, until crust is crispy. Makes 1 large or 2 medium-sized pies.

Nutritional information: 360 calories, 9.4 grams protein, 58 grams carbohydrates, 15.2 grams fat, 8.1 milligrams cholesterol, 551 milligrams sodium, 1.84 grams fiber, 154 milligrams calcium, 2.16 milligrams iron.

Tips: Add extra cheese or favorite toppings such as olives, shallots, and anchovies if so desired.

Hamburger Rolls   Serves 8

This recipe can be used to make either hamburger or hot dog rolls. Delicious fresh out of the oven, or toasted up on the barbeque.

¼ cup lukewarm water (105 degrees)
1 package rapid-rise yeast
½ cup mashed potatoes
¾ cup potato water
⅓ cup sugar
4 Tb butter
1 tsp salt
1½ cups brown rice flour
1 cup tapioca flour
1 cup quinoa or soy flour

½ cup dry milk powder
2 tsp xanthan gum
2 eggs
2 Tb sesame seeds

1. Combine water and yeast in a small bowl and let sit for 5 minutes.

2. Combine fresh hot mashed potatoes with potato water, sugar, butter, and salt. Whisk together until smooth. Let cool to lukewarm.

3. Combine flours with milk powder and xanthan gum.

4. Add 1 egg to potato mixture.

5. Mix yeast, water, 2 cups of flour mixture, and potato blend, mix until well-combined.

6. Stir in remaining flour to make a stiff dough.

7. Form dough into 8 round balls. Place on cookie sheet that has been lined with parchment paper. Flatten slightly.

8. Beat remaining egg. Brush on top of rolls and sprinkle with sesame seeds.

9. Let rise in a warm place for about 1 hour.

10. Bake at 400 degrees for 15–20 minutes, or until browned.

Nutritional information: 347 calories, 12 grams protein, 52 grams carbohydrates, 10.6 grams fat, 69 milligrams cholesterol, 418 milligrams sodium, 5 grams fiber, 150 milligrams calcium, 2.4 milligrams iron.

Tips: The oven is a good place for this dough to rise. Set oven at 175 degrees for 5 minutes. Turn off oven, put in hamburger rolls, and let rise for about 1 hour. To make potato water, boil potatoes in about 1½ cups of water until cooked. Mash potatoes and save water for potato water. Also, if you want a hot dog roll, shape each dough ball into a small log and follow the recipe as indicated for hamburger rolls.

Soft Pretzel Nuggets   Makes 36 Pieces

A nice treat for those late-night munchies, or for a party snack.

2 packages rapid-rise yeast
1 Tb brown sugar

1 tsp salt
2 Tb butter, melted
2¾ cups gluten-free flour blend
1 cup lukewarm water (105 degrees)
5 tsp baking soda
4 cups water
2 tsp kosher salt

Gluten-Free Flour Blend

(*Makes 4½ cups; reserve leftovers in an airtight container.*)

1½ cups sorghum flour
1½ cups potato starch
1 cup tapioca flour
½ cup chickpea flour

1. In a large bowl, combine yeast, sugar, salt, butter, and 1 cup flour mixture. Add water and stir until smooth and well-blended.

2. Add remaining flour and stir until mixed in and dough is stiff.

3. Spray a large cookie sheet with nonstick cooking spray, or line with parchment paper.

4. Break dough into 1½-inch pieces (nuggets) and place on cookie sheet.

5. Let sit, covered with a towel, for 1 hour.

6. Bring baking soda and water to a boil in a deep stainless steel pot.

7. Place pretzel nuggets a few at a time into the boiling water. Let boil for 1½ minutes. Remove with a slotted spoon, drain, and place on greased cookie sheet.

8. Preheat oven to 475 degrees.

9. Sprinkle with salt and bake for 9–10 minutes until golden brown.

Nutritional information (per pretzel): 52 calories, <1 gram protein, 10.5 grams carbohydrates, <1 gram fat, 1.7 milligrams cholesterol, 336 milligrams sodium, <1 gram fiber, 2.8 milligrams calcium, <1 milligram iron.

Tips: This dough falls apart easily, so it works best in nugget shape rather than traditional pretzel shape. These pretzels are best warm from the oven.

Basic Crêpes   **Serves 4**

Terrific filled with seafood or chicken and some shredded cheese. Works great as an appetizer entrée or as a dessert crêpe.

²/₃ cup sorghum flour
¹/₃ cup potato starch
2 eggs
1 cup low-fat milk
½ tsp salt
2 Tb butter, melted
Gluten-free cooking spray

1. In a large mixing bowl, whisk together flour, potato starch, and eggs. Add milk, and stir to combine.

2. Beat in salt and butter. Continue to mix until smooth.

3. Heat a medium size nonstick skillet over medium-high heat. Spray with cooking spray.

4. Pour ¼ cup batter onto a nonstick skillet pan. Tilt pan back and forth so that the batter coats the surface evenly.

5. Cook for about 1 minute, until the bottom starts to brown. Flip crêpe with spatula and cook the other side for about 30 seconds.

6. Remove to platter and cover to keep warm.

7. Fill as desired and serve.

Nutritional information: 272 calories, 8.8 grams protein, 40 grams carbohydrates, 9.8 grams fat, 124 milligrams cholesterol, 395 milligrams sodium, 2 grams fiber, 96.6 milligrams calcium, 1.8 milligrams iron.

Tips: Add a tablespoon of sugar to make a dessert crêpe.

English Muffins   **Makes 6**

Millet gives a nice texture and flavor to this English muffin—perfect toasted with jam and butter.

Gluten-free cooking spray
¼ cup gluten-free cornmeal
¾ cup millet flour
1 cup white rice flour

¼ cup potato starch
¼ cup tapioca starch
1 tsp cream of tartar
1 package rapid-rise yeast
½ cup dry milk powder
½ tsp salt
1 Tb sugar
1 cup lukewarm seltzer (105 degrees)
1 egg, beaten
2 Tb butter, melted

1. Grease 6 hamburger bun/muffin cups (available online, or see tip below) with cooking spray and dust lightly with cornmeal.

2. Mix all dry ingredients (flour through sugar) in a large bowl.

3. Mix seltzer, egg, and butter into the flour mixture. Stir until smooth and well-combined.

4. Pour into prepared cups. Let sit for 1 hour in a warm place, until doubled in size.

5. Preheat oven to 375 degrees.

6. Cook muffins for 15–20 minutes, or until a toothpick inserted into the middle comes out clean. (Muffins will not be browned.)

7. Let cool for 5 minutes in pan before removing. Cut in half and serve warm, or toast before eating.

Nutritional information: 265 calories, 6.6 grams protein, 47 grams carbohydrates, 5.7 grams fat, 46 milligrams cholesterol, 265 milligrams sodium, 2 grams fiber, 79 milligrams calcium, 1.5 milligrams iron.

Tips: If you do not have a hamburger muffin pan, 6-oz tuna cans that have been cleaned and had the label removed work just fine—or order an English muffin pan from a cooking supply company.

Appetizers

- Eggplant Dip

- Super Bean Dip

- Salmon Salad

- Chicken Satay

- Beets with Blue Cheese

- Albanian Meatballs (Quofte)

- Chicken Fingers with Apricot Sauce

- Hushpuppies

- Shrimp Scampi Wrapped in Bacon

- Grilled Stacked Eggplant and Mozzarella Tower

- Buffalo Chicken Wings

- Honey Soy Glazed Chicken Wings

Eggplant Dip   **Serves 8**

This is a terrific dip, delicious on gluten-free crackers, corn tortillas, or rice cakes, or served with a vegetable platter.

Gluten-free cooking spray
1 Tb olive oil
4 Tb garlic, minced
1 medium onion, finely chopped
2 green zucchini, cut into ½-inch pieces
1 green pepper, cut into ½-inch pieces
1 small eggplant, peeled and cut into ½-inch pieces
1 cup tomato sauce
1 tsp onion powder
½ tsp black pepper
1 tsp Italian seasoning
1 Tb sugar
1 Tb balsamic vinegar
2 Tb parmesan cheese

1. Spray skillet with cooking spray; add olive oil and sauté garlic, then add onion and sauté until translucent.

2. Add zucchini, green pepper, and eggplant; sauté until cooked through (add water if pan starts to dry out).

3. Add to pan 1 cup tomato sauce, onion powder, pepper, Italian seasoning, sugar, vinegar, and Parmesan cheese. Cover and simmer

for about 10–20 minutes (until vegetables are soft and tomato sauce is cooked down).

4. Refrigerate overnight to allow flavors to blend. Serve eggplant with gluten-free brown rice crackers.

Nutritional information: 67 calories, 2.3 grams protein, 11 grams carbohydrates, 2.3 grams fat, 1.1 milligrams cholesterol, 27 milligrams sodium, 3.5 grams fiber, 38 milligrams calcium, <1 milligram iron.

Tip: You can add more veggies to this dish and add extra garlic, onion powder, pepper, and Italian seasoning if you like. Hot sauce is also great added to this dip if you want it spicier—season to taste.

Super Bean Dip   Serves 8

This bean dip is high in fiber and loaded with flavor. Why not toast up a mini gluten-free pizza crust and spread bean dip on top and sprinkle with mozzarella cheese?

15 oz can chickpeas (garbanzo beans), drained
15 oz can kidney beans, drained
15 oz can black beans, drained
1 Tb garlic, minced
4–5 Tb lemon juice
1/3–1/2 cup water (for desired texture)
3 Tb tahini (sesame seed paste)
1 tsp cumin
1/2 tsp paprika
1 tsp salt
1 tsp pepper
1/2 cup parsley, chopped
1/2 cup green onions, chopped

1. Purée all ingredients together in a food processor.

2. Add extra water as needed to achieve desired texture.

3. Add additional spices to suit your taste.

4. Refrigerate until ready to use.

Nutritional information: 165 calories, 8.6 grams protein, 25 grams carbohydrates, 3.9 grams fat, 0 milligrams cholesterol, 506 milligrams sodium, 7.3 grams fiber, 56 milligrams calcium, 2.2 milligrams iron.

Tip: Most canned beans are gluten-free, but on occasion some companies have added gluten-containing products, so be sure to check your labels.

Salmon Salad   Serves 4

Serve this as part of an impressive salad platter, or rolled into a gluten-free wrap.

1 lb salmon fillets
2 Tb low-fat mayonnaise
2 Tb nonfat plain yogurt
1 tsp lemon juice
½ cup celery, chopped
1 Tb capers (optional)
1 tsp dried dill weed or 1 Tbsp fresh dill, chopped
1 tsp dried tarragon or 1 Tbsp fresh tarragon, chopped
¼ tsp black pepper
4 large lettuce leaves

1. Cook salmon fillets until just cooked (poach, grill, or broil) and cool to room temperature.

2. Mix remaining ingredients (except lettuce leaves) in a large bowl.

3. Flake salmon and stir into mixture.

4. Serve over lettuce leaves

Nutritional information per serving: 211 calories, 19.6 grams protein, 2.3 grams carbohydrates, 13 grams fat, 56.5 milligrams cholesterol, 190 milligrams sodium, <1 gram fiber, 46 milligrams calcium, <1 milligram iron.

Tips: Great served with other veggies such as sliced tomatoes, or roasted peppers. To check to make sure there are no bones in the salmon, run your hand across the top of the salmon to feel for bones, and use needlenosed pliers to pull out any you find.

Chicken Satay   Serves 4

This is an impressive appetizer that is sure to delight your guests. Serve as the perfect finger food, or as part of an appetizer platter.

1 lb chicken tenders, cleaned
½ cup coconut milk
1 tsp curry powder

1 tsp ginger
1 clove garlic, minced
Gluten-free cooking spray
2 Tb creamy peanut butter
2 Tb tahini (sesame seed paste)
1 Tb gluten-free soy sauce (such as La Choy, or San-J)
1 Tb brown sugar
½ cup (4 oz) gluten-free chicken broth
1 Tb lime juice
1 Tb red curry paste

1. Place chicken tenders, coconut milk, curry powder, ginger, and garlic in a 1-gallon zipper bag. Mix well and place in refrigerator to marinade for 1–2 hours.

2. Soak 4 wooden skewers in water for 30 minutes.

3. In a small saucepan, mix peanut butter, tahini, soy sauce, sugar, chicken broth, lime juice, and curry paste. Heat over low heat, stirring until smooth and well-combined.

4. Heat stove top grill pan or outdoor grill. Remove chicken from marinade.

5. Thread chicken onto skewers distributing chicken evenly.

6. Grill chicken for 3–5 minutes per side, until cooked through. Serve with peanut sauce.

Nutritional information per serving: 248 calories, 30 grams protein, 7 grams carbohydrates, 11 grams fiber, 66 milligrams cholesterol, 378 milligrams sodium, 34 milligrams calcium, 1.5 milligrams iron.

Tip: Use beef, pork, or shrimp in place of chicken.

Beets with Blue Cheese   Serves 4

This was inspired by the classic recipe often served in many top steak houses.

16 oz jar pickled beets, drained
4 oz bleu cheese
4 Tb gluten-free bread crumbs
4 cups mesculin greens, washed and dried
4 Tb shaved parmesan cheese

Dressing

2 Tb olive oil
2 Tb lemon juice
2 tsp sugar
Dash of salt
Dash of oregano
Dash of pepper
¼ cup white wine

1. Whisk together dressing ingredients.

2. Place beets on a cookie sheet and top with crumbling of bleu cheese and sprinkle with bread crumbs.

3. Turn oven to broil and place beets under broiler.

4. Arrange greens on 4 plates and top with dressing.

5. As soon as cheese starts to melt on the beets, remove from oven and arrange over greens.

6. Sprinkle with parmesan cheese and serve.

Nutritional information: 278 calories, 7.8 grams protein, 27 grams carbohydrates, 15.2 grams fat, 18.6 milligrams cholesterol, 785 milligrams sodium, 4.2 grams fiber, 204 milligrams calcium, 1 milligrams iron.

Tip: No time to make homemade dressing? Mix some gluten-free Italian dressing and squeeze in a little lemon juice.

Quofte (Albanian Meatballs)   Serves 8

These Mediterranean meatballs are lighter than the typical Italian meatballs. They can be served plain but are especially delicious with yogurt sauce.

1 lb ground beef sirloin
1 large Spanish onion, finely minced
1½ tsp dried mint
½ tsp pepper
1½ tsp salt
2 eggs
2 Tb water
¼ cup brown rice flour (or gluten-free flour blend)
½ cup additional brown rice flour (or gluten-free flour blend) for coating

Gluten-free cooking spray

1. Preheat oven to broil, and spray a baking sheet with cooking spray.

2. Mix meat, onion, spices, eggs, water, and ¼ cup flour together thoroughly. Mixture should be fairly wet; if not, add a little more water.

3. Shape meat into an oval shape with 2 teaspoons and roll in flour. It should resemble the shape of ⅓ of a cigar, a little bumpy.

4. Place meatballs on the prepared baking sheet.

5. Spray meatballs lightly with cooking spray and place in oven.

6. Broil until brown on both sides.

7. Serve with garlic yogurt sauce (see sauces).

Nutritional information: 174 calories, 15.6 grams protein, 13.4 grams carbohydrates, 6 grams fat, 84 milligrams cholesterol, 506 milligrams sodium, 1 gram fiber, 19 milligrams calcium, 1.8 milligrams iron.

Tip: Traditionally these meatballs are made with a higher-fat meat and deep-fried. This recipe cuts down the fat and calories. I find these just as delicious as the traditional version. Other meats can be mixed with these meatballs. Dried currants and nuts make a nice addition as well.

Chicken Fingers with Apricot Sauce   Serves 4

Both kids and adults will love these delicious, easy-to-make chicken fingers. They can be served with any sauce.

16 oz skinless boneless chicken breast
2 Tb gluten-free cornmeal
2 Tb seasoned gluten-free breadcrumbs
2 Tb crushed pecans
2 tsp garlic powder
1 tsp onion powder
8 egg whites
Gluten-free cooking spray
4 Tb apricot preserves

2 Tb gluten-free light mayonnaise
1 dash of gluten-free hot sauce (optional)

1. Preheat oven to 350.

2. Clean and pound chicken cutlets. Cut into chicken fingers 3–4 inches long and 2–3 inches wide.

3. Toss cornmeal, breadcrumbs, pecans, garlic powder, and onion powder together in a medium bowl.

4. Dip chicken in egg whites and then coat in cornmeal mixture.

5. Spray baking sheet with cooking spray, put coated chicken on baking sheet and spray top with cooking spray.

6. Cook until brown on one side; turn, spray again with cooking spray, and bake until just cooked through and crispy and brown on the outside.

7. Mix together apricot preserves, light mayo, and hot sauce and serve with chicken fingers.

Nutritional information: 280 calories, 34.5 grams protein, 21 grams carbohydrates, 6.7 grams fat, 68 milligrams cholesterol, 247 milligrams sodium, <1 gram fiber, 29 milligrams calcium, 1.3 milligrams iron.

Tip: If gluten-free breadcrumbs are not available, toast 1 slice of gluten-free bread and process in a food processor with ¼ tsp Italian seasoning and ¼ tsp salt and a dash of pepper

Hushpuppies   Serves 12

Put these in a basket, sprinkle with powdered sugar, and watch them disappear.

1 cup buttermilk
1 egg
2 cups gluten-free cornmeal
½ cup gluten-free flour blend (store-bought, or see blends in Chapter 5)
¼ cup frozen corn kernels, defrosted
4 Tb granulated sugar
1 tsp salt
½ tsp gluten-free baking soda
½ tsp gluten-free baking powder

1 tsp xanthan gum
Corn oil for frying
4 Tb powered sugar (for garnish)

1. Beat together buttermilk and egg.

2. Combine egg mixture with all other ingredients except corn oil and powdered sugar, and stir to combine.

3. In a fryer, heat corn oil until hot.

4. Spoon a few tablespoons of cornmeal mixture at a time into the hot oil.

5. Fry until golden. Remove from oil with slotted spoon and drain on paper towels.

6. Sprinkle with powdered sugar and serve warm.

Nutritional information: 165 calories, 3.5 grams protein, 38.6 grams carbohydrates, 2 grams fat, 18 milligrams cholesterol, 290 milligrams sodium, <1 gram fiber, 39 milligrams calcium, <1 milligram iron.

Tip: For spicier hushpuppies, add cayenne pepper and skip the powdered sugar.

Shrimp Scampi Wrapped in Bacon   Serves 4

This classic recipe never goes out of style.

12 oz jumbo shrimp, shells removed
6 pieces of gluten-free bacon
Olive or canola oil gluten-free cooking spray
2 Tb butter or margarine
2 Tb garlic, minced
½ tsp salt
1 Tb lemon juice
¼ cup white wine
2 Tb parmesan cheese

1. Preheat oven to 350 degrees.

2. Lightly cook bacon in microwave until just cooked, but still soft.

3. Cut each piece of bacon in half and wrap around shrimp, secure with a toothpick.

4. Spray a cooking sheet with cooking spray, and place shrimp on the sheet.

5. Mix together butter, garlic, salt, lemon juice, and wine and heat in microwave, just to melt butter.

6. Pour mixture over shrimp on baking sheet and cook until shrimp are just cooked (pink).

7. Sprinkle with parmesan cheese and serve.

Nutritional information: 220 calories, 21.4 grams protein, 2.2 grams carbohydrates, 12.4 grams fat, 158 milligrams cholesterol, 714 milligrams sodium, <1 gram fiber, 77 milligrams calcium, 2.1 milligrams iron.

Tip: Scallops or chicken can be used in this recipe in place of the shrimp as well. Garnish with chopped scallions and lemon wedges.

Grilled Stacked Eggplant and Mozzarella Tower   Serves 6

This makes an impressive appetizer, layered and served on individual plates.

1 large eggplant peeled and sliced into ½-inch round slices
2 Tb garlic, minced
½ tsp salt
½ tsp pepper
2 Tb olive oil
6 slices gluten-free bread
2 Tb olive oil
1 tsp garlic powder
2 Tb parmesan cheese
2 roasted red peppers sliced
2 tomatoes, sliced thin
6 oz fresh mozzarella, sliced thin (if you are following a low-fat diet, substitute skim mozzarella)
4 Tb fresh basil, finely chopped

1. Mix eggplant slices with garlic, salt, pepper, and 2 Tb olive oil, and then grill in a George Foreman–type countertop grill until just cooked.

2. Meanwhile, preheat your oven to broil, and toast all 6 pieces of bread.

3. Using a coffee cup or a muffin cutter, cut a circle in the middle of each piece of toast, brush the top of each round with olive oil, sprinkle with garlic powder and parmesan cheese, and broil on a baking sheet until cheese melts.

4. Layer garlic crouton, eggplant, roasted peppers, tomatoes, and mozzarella on 6 small plates.

5. Garnish with fresh chopped basil and serve.

Nutritional information: 257 calories, 8.5 grams protein, 22 grams carbohydrates, 15.6 grams fat, 24 milligrams cholesterol, 483 milligrams sodium, 2.6 grams fiber, 222 milligrams calcium, 1.5 milligrams iron.

Tip: This recipe works well without the garlic crouton, if desired. It is best prepared with fresh roasted peppers. To roast peppers, preheat your oven to 450, place aluminum foil on a baking sheet and cook peppers until they just start to blacken. Take out of the oven and wait until peppers cool, peel, and pop out seeds. Can be made ahead and kept in the refrigerator in a glass jar for a few days.

Buffalo Chicken Wings   Serves 16

Settle down with a crowd of friends to watch the football game and polish off a bucket of chicken wings—add hot sauce to taste.

5 lbs chicken wings, separated into winglet and drumlet
½ cup brown rice flour
1 tsp salt
½ tsp pepper
½ cup vegetable oil
6 Tb lite butter
1 Tb hot sauce or to taste
½ cup gluten-free bleu cheese salad dressing
8 celery stalks, sliced long, then quartered

1. Mix together brown rice flour, salt, and pepper.

2. Wash and dry chicken wings, and dredge into flour mixture.

3. Heat vegetable oil in a saucepan and fry wings in hot vegetable oil until golden; discard remaining oil.

4. In a small saucepan, melt butter and mix with hot sauce.

5. Preheat oven to broil.

6. Toss wings with butter mixture, and place on a cookie sheet that has been covered with aluminum foil.

7. Cook under the broiler until the wings are crispy.

8. Serve with bleu cheese dressing and celery sticks.

Nutritional information: 422 calories, 25 grams protein, 4.7 grams carbohydrates, 34 grams fat, 125 milligrams cholesterol, 370 milligrams sodium, <1 gram fiber, 18.4 milligrams calcium, 1.77 milligrams iron.

Tip: To make your own bleu cheese dressing, in a food processor combine 4 oz bleu cheese, 1 cup light mayonnaise, ½ cup light gluten-free sour cream (such as Friendship), 2 Tb lemon juice, ½ tsp garlic powder, 1 Tb grated onion, and salt and pepper to taste.

Honey-Soy Glazed Chicken Wings   Serves 8

This Chinese favorite is cooked until the chicken practically falls off the bone.

2 lbs chicken wings
4 Tb vegetable oil
⅓ cup light gluten-free soy sauce (such as La Choy or San-J)
4 Tb honey
2 Tb sherry
1 tsp garlic, minced
½ tsp fresh ginger, minced
2 stalks scallions chopped
1 Tb brown sugar
1 Tb vinegar
4 Tb scallions, chopped

1. Separate each wing into 2 pieces.

2. In a large skillet, heat oil and stir fry chicken wings in small batches until lightly browned.

3. Drain on paper towels.

4. Mix together all remaining ingredients (except the scallions) and heat in a medium-sized sauté pan.

5. Cook chicken wings in sauce mixture for about 30 minutes, until chicken is soft.

6. Garnish with additional chopped scallions if desired.

Nutritional information: 358 calories, 21.7 grams protein, 11 grams carbohydrates, 25 grams fat, 87 milligrams cholesterol, 610.8 milligrams sodium, <1 gram fiber, 27 milligrams calcium, 1.6 milligrams iron.

Tip: Gluten-free tamari works well in this recipe as an alternate to the soy sauce.

Soups, Sandwiches, and Salads

- Cranberry-Quinoa Salad
- French Onion Soup
- Beef Stew
- Swiss Chard and White Bean Soup
- Crispy Chopped Chicken Salad
- Pear, Gorgonzola Cheese, and Walnut Mixed Green Salad
- Sautéed Spinach Salad
- Butternut Squash and Apple Soup

Cranberry-Quinoa Salad   Serves 6

This tasty salad is great as a side or, tossed with slices of grilled chicken, as an entrée.

1 cup whole quinoa, rinsed 2–3 times
2 cups gluten-free chicken or vegetable broth (such as Pacific)
2 tsp olive oil
1 medium yellow onion, chopped
½ cup frozen peas, defrosted and drained
¼ cup dried cranberries
¼ cup walnuts, chopped
2 Tb fresh parsley, roughly chopped

1. Cook quinoa in gluten-free broth for 15–20 minutes, or until cooked.

2. In separate skillet, heat oil; then, add onion and cook until soft.

3. Add cooked onion and peas, dried cranberries, walnuts, and parsley to cooked quinoa.

4. Can be served hot or cold.

Nutritional information: 197 calories, 6.6 grams protein, 29 grams carbohydrates, 6.6 grams fat, 0 milligrams cholesterol, 166 milligrams sodium, 4.2 grams fiber, 35 milligrams calcium, 1.9 milligrams iron.

Tip: Unless you buy pre-rinsed quinoa, it is important to rinse it several times to remove the bitter outer coating. Quinoa is cooked when a little tail pops out of each grain.

French Onion Soup   Serves 4

This rich, flavorful soup can stand alone as a meal. If you want to make it really decadent, sprinkle extra shredded cheese on top of the soup before broiling.

2 Tb vegetable oil
1 Tb unsalted butter
2 sweet onions (such as Vidalia), thinly sliced
1 Tb cornstarch
1 tsp dried thyme leaves
1 qt (32 oz) gluten-free beef stock (such as Kitchen Basics)
4 slices gluten-free bread
2 tsp olive oil
4 tsp shredded parmesan cheese

1. Place vegetable oil and butter in a large (4-qt) saucepan and heat over medium heat until butter is melted.

2. Add onions and cook for 10–15 minutes until softened and golden brown.

3. Stir in cornstarch and thyme until well blended with onions.

4. Add beef stock and bring to a boil. Reduce heat and simmer for 20 minutes.

5. Preheat broiler.

6. Using a cookie cutter, cut a 2-inch round circle from the center of each slice of bread.

7. Brush with olive oil and sprinkle with cheese.

8. Place bread under broiler for 2–3 minutes until cheese is melted.

9. Pour soup into 4 bowls and top with bread croutons and serve.

Nutritional information: 289 calories, 4 grams protein, 26.4 grams carbohydrates, 18 grams fat, 16 milligrams cholesterol, 797 milligrams sodium, 1.8 grams fiber, 84 milligrams calcium, 1.6 milligrams iron.

Tip: Swiss or provolone cheese works great in this recipe when melted over the top of the soup.

Beef Stew   **Serves 10**

Beef stew is a satisfying standalone meal. Serve with toasted gluten-free English muffins to soak up the extra juices.

1½ lbs beef chunks for stew
2 Tb gluten-free rice flour
Gluten-free cooking spray
3 Tb garlic, minced
1 medium onion, chopped
2 tsp Italian seasoning
1 tsp salt
1 tsp pepper
1 cup baby carrots
6 small potatoes cut into 2-inch pieces
8 oz button mushrooms
1 large can crushed tomatoes
10 oz package frozen green beans
48 oz low-sodium gluten-free beef broth (such as Pacific)

1. Toss beef with rice flour.

2. Spray a large pot with cooking spray and sauté beef in batches until browned.

3. Set beef on the side. To the pot add a few tablespoons water, garlic and onion, and cook until onion is translucent.

4. Add Italian seasoning, salt, pepper, baby carrots, potatoes, mushrooms, tomatoes, and green beans and heat for about 10 minutes.

5. Add beef, broth, and 2 cups of water and simmer for about 1½–2 hours, until beef is soft and veggies are cooked.

Nutritional information: 220 calories, 21.5 grams protein, 21.8 grams carbohydrates, 6 grams fat, 33 milligrams cholesterol, 432 milligrams sodium, 3.7 grams fiber, 66.3 milligrams calcium, 3.3 milligrams iron.

Tip: If stew gets too thick when cooking, add some water as needed. Any kind of leftover veggies work well added to the beef stew.

Swiss Chard and White Bean Soup   Serves 6

This classic Italian favorite is easy to make and delicious. If you like it really garlicky, add extra garlic to taste.

2 Tb olive oil
2 large onions, chopped into medium-sized pieces
1 cup carrots, chopped
4 stalks celery, chopped
4 Tb garlic, chopped
1 large bunch fresh Swiss chard, thoroughly washed and chopped into medium pieces
48 oz low-sodium gluten-free chicken broth (such as Pacific)
½ tsp salt
1 tsp pepper
2 Tb fresh oregano, finely minced
1 19 oz can white beans (cannelloni beans) drained and rinsed
2 tsp sugar
1 Tb balsamic vinegar
4 Tb parmesan cheese

1. Heat olive oil and sauté onion, carrots, celery, and chopped garlic until the onions start to brown.

2. Add Swiss chard; heat until wilted.

3. Add chicken broth salt, pepper, oregano, beans, sugar, and balsamic vinegar.

4. Cook 40 minutes until all flavors are incorporated and the Swiss chard is soft.

5. Sprinkle with Parmesan cheese and serve.

Nutritional information: 208 calories, 12.9 grams protein, 27.9 grams carbohydrates, 7 grams fat, 2.9 milligrams cholesterol, 485 milligrams sodium, 6.5 grams fiber, 134.6 milligrams calcium, 2.6 milligrams iron.

Tip: Escarole works nicely in this recipe in place of the Swiss chard.

Crispy Chicken Chopped Salad   Serves 4

This is an amazing salad—when you are making it, be sure to make extra breaded chicken breasts, which are great for quick meals.

12 oz skinless, boneless chicken breast
1 egg, beaten
¼ cup seasoned gluten-free breadcrumbs (see tip)
Gluten-free cooking spray
6 cups romaine lettuce, chopped
2 oz bleu cheese crumbled
1 apple, peeled and chopped
1 cup tomato, chopped
1 cup cucumber, chopped
1 cup red pepper, chopped
1 cup carrots, chopped

1. Clean chicken breasts and pound until 1 inch thick (if you get thin chicken breasts, you can skip this step).

2. Preheat oven to 350 degrees.

3. Dip chicken in egg and then breadcrumbs.

4. Spray a baking sheet with cooking spray and place chicken on it, then spray the top of chicken lightly with cooking spray.

5. Bake chicken until it starts to brown on one side, then turn, spray top again with cooking spray, and bake until golden brown and cooked through.

6. Slice chicken into 2-inch pieces. Mix in large bowl with all other ingredients and serve with favorite gluten-free salad dressing or balsamic vinegar.

Nutritional information: 251 calories, 26.8 grams protein, 18.7 grams carbohydrates, 8.1 grams fat, 112.8 milligrams cholesterol, 328 milligrams sodium, 5.5 grams fiber, 152 milligrams calcium, 2.3 milligrams iron.

Tips: Grilled chicken or shrimp can be used in place of the crispy chicken as well. To make seasoned gluten-free breadcrumbs, process gluten-free bread in a food processor until you have crumbs; mix with a little garlic, onion powder, and Italian seasoning.

Pear, Gorgonzola, and Walnut Mixed Green Salad   Serves 6

Serve this salad at the beginning of a holiday meal for an impressive start.

2 pears, sliced, cored, and sectioned into ¼-inch pieces
2 Tb lemon juice
Gluten-free cooking spray
¼ cup walnuts, chopped
2 Tb sugar
½ tsp cinnamon
3 oz gorgonzola cheese crumbled
6 cups mixed greens, chopped
1 cup cherry tomatoes
1 cup shredded carrots
1 cup, sliced and peeled cucumbers
¾ cup gluten-free, fat-free Italian dressing (as needed)

1. Toss pears with lemon juice until ready to combine with salad.

2. Spray a skillet with cooking spray and heat. Give the nuts a quick spray with cooking spray and heat about 2 minutes. Add sugar and cinnamon, remove from heat, and set aside to cool.

3. Drain pears.

4. Combine all ingredients and serve.

Nutritional information: 167 calories, 5.5 grams protein, 22.2 grams carbohydrates, 7.7 grams fat, 22 milligrams cholesterol, 516 milligrams sodium, 4.2 grams fiber, 120 milligrams calcium, <1 milligram iron.

Tip: Try using mandarin orange sections or cranberries in place of the pears for delicious alternatives.

Sautéed Spinach Salad   Serves 4

This show-stopping recipe is always a hit.

1 slice white gluten-free bread, crust removed and cut into 1-inch pieces

Gluten-free cooking spray
⅛ tsp garlic and onion powder
1 red pepper
5 scallions, chopped
1 cup mushrooms, sliced
2 tomatoes, cut into small wedges
½ cup cucumber, peeled, sliced, and cut into half-moons
4 Tb gluten-free, fat-free balsamic salad dressing
2 Tb balsamic vinegar
1 7-oz bag baby spinach
4 oz drained mandarin oranges
1½ Tb parmesan cheese

1. Preheat oven to 450 degrees.

2. Spray a baking sheet with cooking spray and place bread cubes on it; sprinkle with garlic and onion powder.

3. Bake until light brown and set aside.

4. Place red pepper in 450 degree oven on a pan covered with aluminum foil and bake until black on the outside about 30 minutes (taking care not to burn).

5. Set red pepper aside to cool, then peel and remove seeds and skin. Cut into 1-inch strips.

6. Spray sauté pan with cooking spray and heat pan.

7. Sauté scallions in sauté pan about 4 minutes.

8. Add mushrooms to pan and sauté until they start to soften.

9. Add tomatoes, cucumber, and roasted pepper with salad dressing and vinegar and heat for several minutes until well-combined.

10. Add baby spinach and heat about 1–2 minutes (do not wilt spinach).

11. Toss everything together in a large salad bowl with Mandarin oranges and top with parmesan cheese, then with gluten-free croutons.

Nutritional information: 71.6 calories, 3.8 grams protein, 12.3 grams carbohydrates, 1.2 grams fat, 1.5 milligrams cholesterol, 249 milligrams sodium, 2.7 grams fiber, 70 milligrams calcium, 1 milligrams iron.

Tip: This is a real crowd-pleasing salad, great with an Italian meal of gluten-free pasta and meat sauce.

Butternut Squash and Apple Soup   Serves 8

All I can say is: creamy, sweet, satisfying, delicious.

3 Tb butter
1 onion, minced
½ tsp nutmeg
1 tsp fresh ginger, chopped
1 tsp cinnamon
1 Tb garlic, chopped
2 apples, peeled, cored, and chopped
½ cup apple juice
5 cups low sodium gluten-free chicken stock (such as Pacific blend)
2 lbs butternut squash, peeled, seeded, and cut into 1-inch cubes
1 tsp salt
1 tsp pepper
½ cup fat-free half-and-half
1 cup light sour cream (such as Friendship)

1. Melt butter in large pot over a medium heat and sauté onion until it starts to brown.

2. Add nutmeg, ginger, cinnamon, garlic, apples, apple juice, chicken stock, and squash. Bring to a boil.

3. Lower heat to a simmer and cook uncovered about 30–45 minutes, until apple and squash are tender.

4. Purée in small batches in a blender until smooth, and return to pot. Add salt and pepper.

5. Fold in ½ cup fat-free half-and-half.

6. Serve with sour cream garnish.

Nutritional information: 191 calories, 5.8 grams protein, 27.3 grams carbohydrates, 8.2 grams fat, 20.6 milligrams cholesterol, 411.6 milligrams sodium, 3.7 grams fiber, 123.6 milligrams calcium, 1.4 milligrams iron.

Tip: You can use acorn squash or pumpkin in place of the butternut squash in this recipe if so desired.

Entrées

- Beer Battered Shrimp
- Roasted Chicken Breast with Caramelized Onions
- Veggie Stir Fry
- Shrimp Teriyaki
- Chicken Cutlet Francese
- Lasagna
- Pasta
- Crescent Ravioli
- Chicken Enchilada
- Grouper Piccata
- Walnut-Crusted Chicken Breast in Mustard Sauce
- Parmesan Gnocchi
- Chicken Vegetable Curry with Mango Chutney
- Chicken- and Spinach-Stuffed Crepes
- Pierogis with Potato Cheese Filling
- Chili
- Chicken Cutlet Parmesan

Beer-Battered Shrimp   Serves 4

These shrimp are best deep-fried, the gluten-free beer gives them a light crispy coating.

1 lb large raw shrimp (shells removed except tail)
1 egg separated (room temperature)
½ Tb olive oil
½ cup gluten-free flour blend
1 tsp xanthan gum
½ tsp salt
½ cup gluten-free beer

Corn oil for frying
Gluten-free cocktail or tartar sauce

Gluten-Free Flour Blend

(Makes 5¼ cups; store leftover blend in an airtight container as a gluten-free all-purpose flour.)

1 cup sorghum
¾ cup brown rice flour
2 cups potato starch
1 cup tapioca starch
½ cup garbanzo bean flour

1. Mix together egg yolk, olive oil, gluten-free flour, xanthan gum, salt, and gluten-free beer until smooth.

2. Beat egg white until stiff peaks form and fold into batter.

3. Spray a non-stick skillet and heat until hot.

4. Dip shrimp one at a time in batter and place in skillet; use a teaspoon to put a little extra batter on top.

5. Heat corn oil in a fryer or a medium pot and fry shrimp until golden brown; remove shrimp with a slotted spoon, and drain on paper towels.

6. Keep shrimp warm until all are cooked; serve with gluten-free cocktail sauce or tartar sauce.

Nutritional information: 271 calories, 26 grams protein, 19.6 grams carbohydrates, 8.7 grams fat, 225 milligrams cholesterol, 496 milligrams sodium, 1 gram fiber, 95 milligrams calcium, 3.4 milligrams iron.

Tips: Make sure you use a fryer dedicated to gluten-free frying. If you prefer not to fry shrimp, you can spray a skillet with cooking spray and cook shrimp on both sides until golden. They will be a little flat in shape but still delicious. This batter also works well for onion rings.

Roasted Chicken Breasts with Caramelized Onions   Serves 4

A real family favorite, this is great with any sides on any occasion.

16 oz (4 4-oz) bone-in chicken breasts with skin
½ tsp salt

½ tsp pepper
Gluten-free cooking spray
4 yellow or white onions
1 Tb olive oil
1 Tb butter
2 Tb sugar
1 Tb red wine vinegar

1. Preheat oven to 375 degrees. Place chicken on baking sheet and season with salt and pepper. Bake for 40–45 minutes or until chicken is cooked.

2. Peel and thinly slice onions.

3. In large skillet, heat olive oil and butter over medium-high heat. Add onions and stir to coat. Reduce heat to medium, and cook onions for 8–10 minutes, stirring frequently; if pan is too dry, add a little water.

4. Stir in sugar. Continue to cook for 15–20 minutes, until golden brown in color, stirring occasionally.

5. Remove from heat; stir in vinegar.

6. Remove skin from chicken and serve covered with onions.

Nutritional information: 327 calories, 25 grams protein, 20 grams carbohydrates, 11 grams fat, 90 milligrams cholesterol, 395 milligrams sodium, 3 grams fiber, 81.2 milligrams calcium, 1.8 milligrams iron.

Tip: If you use sweet onions, such as Vidalia, you do not need to add any sugar.

Veggie Stir Fry   Serves 4

Restaurant stir fries include gluten from soy sauce, but you can make a gluten-free version at home. This recipe can be prepared with chicken, pork, or beef and served over brown rice as a complete meal.

¼ cup (2 oz) gluten-free vegetable or chicken broth (such as Kitchen Creations)
2 Tb gluten-free soy sauce (such as La Choy or San-J)
1 tsp cornstarch
1 tsp brown sugar

½ tsp fresh ginger, chopped
¼ tsp red pepper flakes
2 tsp vegetable oil
1 cup sugar snap peas
2 cups bok choy, washed and cut into small pieces
1 cup carrots, sliced
1 cup mushrooms, sliced
4 green onions, sliced
1 red pepper, sliced
1 clove garlic, minced
½ cup water chestnuts, drained

1. Whisk together broth, soy sauce, cornstarch, brown sugar, ginger, and red pepper flakes in a small bowl and set aside.

2. Heat oil in a large wok or skillet. Add vegetables (peas through red pepper).

3. Stir fry vegetables 1–4 minutes, until vegetables start to soften. Add garlic and water chestnuts and continue to cook for 1 more minute.

4. Add sauce and sauté for 1–2 minutes, until sauce thickens.

Nutritional information: 96 calories, 4 grams protein, 15 gram carbohydrates, 3 grams fat, <1 milligram cholesterol, 430 milligrams sodium, 4.4 grams fiber, 80.5 milligrams calcium, 1 milligram iron.

Tip: Use any combination of vegetables you wish.

Shrimp Teriyaki   **Serves 4**

The teriyaki sauce in this recipe is perfect for salmon, beef, chicken, or scallops.

16 oz raw shrimp, cleaned and shelled
2 tsp garlic, minced
½ tsp onion powder
¼ cup low sodium gluten-free soy sauce (such as San-J)
2 Tb honey
1 Tb white vinegar
½ tsp dried ginger
½ tsp sesame oil
4 scallions, chopped
¼ cup red pepper, chopped

1. Preheat oven to 350.

2. Mix together minced garlic, onion powder, gluten-free soy sauce, honey, vinegar, ginger, and sesame oil; pour over shrimp in an oven-safe casserole dish.

3. Arrange scallions, and chopped red pepper over the top of shrimp. Bake about 15 minutes, until shrimp are pink, and serve.

4. Great with brown rice or quinoa and steamed broccoli.

Nutritional information: 184 calories, 25 grams protein, 14 grams carbohydrates, 26 grams fat, 172 milligrams cholesterol, 699 milligrams sodium, <1 gram fiber, 75 milligrams calcium, 3.1 milligrams iron.

Tip: This recipe works well with salmon or tuna steaks.

Chicken Francese   Serves 4

This dish is so easy to prepare that you'll want to make it over and over again.

1 lb boneless, skinless chicken breasts, cleaned and sliced thin or pounded
Gluten-free cooking spray
1 Tb garlic, minced
2 scallions, chopped
2 eggs, lightly beaten
½ cup brown rice or chickpea flour
2 Tb butter or olive oil
1 cup mushrooms, sliced
½ tsp salt
½ tsp pepper
1 tsp Italian seasoning
½ cup white wine
½ Tb lemon juice
2 Tb scallions, chopped (for garnish)

1. Spray a skillet with cooking spray. Sauté garlic and scallions for a few minutes.

2. Dip chicken in egg, then flour.

3. Add chicken to pan and brown on both sides. Add butter, mushrooms, salt, pepper, Italian seasoning, white wine, and lemon

juice to the pan and continue cooking until chicken is cooked through, mushrooms are soft, and sauce thickens.

4. If needed, add a little extra white wine.

5. Garnish with scallions and serve.

Nutritional information: 295 calories, 31.8 grams protein, 17.7 grams carbohydrates, 10.3 grams fat, 186.7 milligrams cholesterol, 445 milligrams sodium, 1.5 grams fiber, 41.2 milligrams calcium, 2 milligrams iron.

Tip: Egg substitutes can be used in place of whole eggs if so desired.

Lasagna   Serves 16

This is perfect for when you have company and want a one-dish meal that you can serve to everyone. For a smaller lasagna, cut this recipe in half.

Gluten-free lasagna noodles (2 [10-oz] boxes gluten-free lasagna noodles)
2 Tb olive oil
3 Tb garlic, minced
2 large onions, chopped
2½ lbs ground sirloin
3 tsp Italian seasoning
1 tsp salt
1 tsp pepper
3 qts marinara sauce
3 cups part-skim ricotta cheese
⅓ cup parmesan cheese
1½ lbs shredded skim mozzarella

1. Cook lasagna noodles until just cooked.

2. In a large pot, heat olive oil; sauté garlic 2 minutes.

3. Add onions to oil mixture and sauté until onions start to brown; add a little water to pan if needed to keep onions from sticking.

4. Add sirloin to the pot and sauté until brown; then add Italian seasoning, salt, and pepper.

5. Preheat oven to 350 degrees.

6. Pour some sauce over the bottom of a lasagna pan. Cover with 3 lasagna noodles, pour ½ meat mixture, some sauce, and 1½ cups ricotta cheese spread across, 5 Tb parmesan cheese, and ½ lb mozzarella cheese.

7. Start again with another layer, then finish with another layer of noodles, sauce, Parmesan, and mozzarella cheese. Reserve about 2 cups of the sauce to serve on the side.

8. Place the lasagna pan on top of a baking sheet.

9. Cover with aluminum foil and bake for about 30–45 minutes, until cheese is bubbling.

Nutritional information: 626 calories, 38 grams protein, 66.7 grams carbohydrates, 21.5 grams fat, 90.6 milligrams cholesterol, 1172 milligrams sodium, 5.9 grams fiber, 531 milligrams calcium, 3.5 milligrams iron.

Nutritional information (reduced-fat version): 505 calories, 37 grams protein, 66 grams carbohydrates, 8 grams fat, 56 milligrams cholesterol, 1171 milligrams sodium, 5.9 grams fiber, 452 milligrams calcium, 2 milligrams iron.

Tips: To reduce the fat in this recipe, use fat-free ricotta and fat-free mozzarella cheese and reduce the mozzarella to only 1 lb; you can also use white meat ground turkey in place of the sirloin. Note that although lasagna can be made ahead and frozen until you are ready to use, 2 days' defrosting in the refrigerator will be required prior to baking.

Pasta   **Serves 16**

If you want to make delicious homemade gluten-free pasta or lasagna noodles, this recipe is a sure winner.

1 cup sorghum flour
½ cup brown rice flour
1½ cup tapioca flour
1⅓ cup potato starch
⅔ cup cornstarch
6 tsp xanthan gum
4 eggs, beaten
4 Tb olive oil

2 tsp salt

²/₃ cup water

Brown rice flour (about ½ cup, for rolling)

1. In a large bowl, combine dry ingredients except for extra brown rice flour for rolling.

2. Add eggs and oil to the dry ingredients and blend in (by hand or with a food processor).

3. Work in water a little at a time, until the dough has a nice consistency. Cover dough until ready to use.

4. Sprinkle some rice flour on parchment paper.

5. Break off tennis-ball-size pieces of dough and roll into oval logs.

6. Press dough into parchment paper, sprinkle the top with rice flour, and roll out into a ⅛-inch thick and 6-inch wide rectangular noodle.

7. Trim off edges so it makes a clean-looking rectangle and cover with a damp dish cloth.

8. Leave as a lasagna noodle or cut into desired pasta shape.

9. Boil a large pot of water with ½ tsp salt and 1 Tb olive oil.

10. Add pasta noodles and cook until desired doneness is achieved (undercook a little for al dente pasta).

11. Rinse noodles under cool water in a colander before using.

Nutritional information: 217 calories, 40.4 grams carbohydrates, 3.3 grams protein, 5 grams fat, 52.8 milligrams cholesterol, 336 milligrams sodium, 2.3 grams fiber, 55 milligrams calcium, 1.8 milligrams iron.

Tips: This pasta recipe can be used to make tortellini, ravioli, or any favorite noodle. To make noodles, cut into ¼-inch strips. To make tortellini, roll into marble-sized balls and flatten into half-dollar-size disks, fill with ricotta cheese, fold in half and seal shut by pinching ends together (refrigerate or freeze until ready to use). For ravioli, lay the long pieces of rolled pasta over a ravioli pan; fill with desired filling, top with another piece of pasta, and cut using the top of the ravioli pan.

Crescent-Shaped Ravioli   Serves 6

This pasta recipe gives a nice texture to all those recipes that call for a pasta with a little more chew that holds up to many sauces.

2 eggs
4 Tb olive oil
2 tsp salt
⅓ cup water
¾ cup brown rice flour
½ cup tapioca flour
½ cup potato starch
¼ cup cornstarch
3 tsp xanthan gum
Brown rice flour (for dusting)
1 cup part skim ricotta
¼ cup parmesan cheese
1 tsp Italian seasoning
2 eggs, beaten

1. Beat together 2 eggs, ⅓ cup water, and 3 Tb olive oil.

2. In a bowl combine brown rice flour, tapioca flour, potato starch, cornstarch, xanthan gum, and 1 tsp salt.

3. Either by hand or in a food processor, work in wet ingredients until they become a well-incorporated dough; add extra rice flour if needed.

4. Mix together skim ricotta, parmesan, Italian seasoning, and remaining eggs.

5. On parchment paper dusted with brown rice flour, take tennis-ball-size balls of dough and roll to about 1/8 inch thick. Use a biscuit cutter to cut small round circles. Roll again so the surface of each circle is doubled in size.

6. Use a tablespoon to portion out 1 spoon of ricotta filling to fill each circle, then fold in half and shut by crimping the edges with a fork.

7. Boil a large pot of water. Add 1 tsp of salt and 1 Tb of olive oil. Add ravioli and cook for about 10 minutes until desired texture is achieved.

8. Rinse in a colander with warm water.

9. Serve with favorite pasta sauce.

Nutritional information: 346.7 calories, 10.5 grams protein, 44.7 grams carbohydrates, 14 grams fat, 121.4 milligrams cholesterol, 562 milligrams sodium, 2.6 grams fiber, 221 milligrams calcium, 2 milligrams iron.

Tip: You can mix a variety of fillings in these ravioli—try folding in some spinach with the cheese filling, or some sun-dried tomatoes.

Chicken Enchiladas   Serves 4

This delicious Spanish dish goes great with rice and beans and is easy on your budget as well.

2 whole bone-in chicken breasts with skin
¼ tsp black pepper
2 Tb vegetable oil
2 Tb water
2 Tb cornstarch
2 Tb chili powder
1 (8 oz) can tomato sauce
1½ cups water
½ tsp cumin
½ tsp garlic powder
Gluten-free cooking spray
½ cup onions, chopped
½ cup low-fat cream cheese
1 can (4 ounces) diced green chili peppers
8 gluten-free corn tortillas, warmed until they are just starting to soften
½ cup shredded monterey jack cheese

1. Sprinkle chicken with black pepper and bake at 375 degrees for 40–45 minutes, until cooked through. Remove, and set aside to cool slightly.

2. Remove skin and bone from chicken. Using 2 forks, shred chicken and set aside.

3. Heat oil in a medium saucepan over medium-high heat. Add cornstarch and chili powder. Decrease heat to medium and cook for 3–4 minutes until light brown, stirring constantly.

4. Stir in tomato sauce, water, cumin, and garlic powder. Continue to cook for 5–10 minutes, until slightly thickened. Add additional water if sauce is too thick.

5. Spray a large nonstick skillet with cooking spray and heat over medium-high heat.

6. Add onions and cook for 3–4 minutes, until softened. Add cream cheese and chili peppers. Stir to combine. Continue to cook until cream cheese starts to melt. Add chicken and 1 cup of the enchilada sauce. Stir to combine. Remove from heat.

7. Preheat oven to 350 degrees. Spray a 9 × 13-inch pan with cooking spray.

8. Spread ¼ cup enchilada sauce on bottom of pan.

9. Divide filling among 8 tortillas. Roll up and place seam-side down in pan.

10. Cover with remaining sauce and sprinkle with cheese.

11. Bake for 25 minutes, until hot and bubbly.

Nutritional information per serving: 450 calories, 29 grams protein, 38 grams carbohydrates, 20 grams fat, 78 milligrams cholesterol, 575 milligrams sodium, 6 grams fiber, 216 milligrams calcium, 3 milligrams fiber.

Tips: Serve with shredded lettuce and tomatoes.

Grouper Piccata   Serves 2

Grouper is a delicious fish, especially when served with the capers, olives, and tomato sauce.

8 oz grouper
2 Tb brown rice flour
1 Tb olive oil
1 Tb butter
4 Tb white wine
1 Tb capers
1 tomato, chopped
¼ cup black olives, sliced
2 Tb lemon juice

1. Dredge fish in brown rice flour.

2. Heat olive oil in a skillet over medium-high heat

3. Place fish in skillet and brown fish slowly on both sides. Remove from pan and set aside.

4. To pan, add butter, wine, capers, tomatoes, and olives, heating until the mixture begins to simmer.

5. Add fish back to the pan with the sauce, and heat until cooked through.

6. Add lemon juice and serve.

Nutritional information: 309 calories, 23.6 grams protein, 13.5 grams carbohydrates, 15.9 grams fat, 57.2 milligrams cholesterol, 379 milligrams sodium, 1.9 gram fiber, 37 milligrams calcium, 2 milligrams iron.

Tip: Any fish works well in this recipe, including catfish, cod, orange roughy, flounder, and tilapia.

Walnut-Crusted Chicken Breasts with Mustard Sauce   Serves 4

This fabulous chicken dish can be served plain but is great with any sauce. The walnut coating makes a great cutlet.

1 lb (4 [4-oz]) boneless, skinless chicken breasts
Gluten-free cooking spray
¼ cup crushed walnuts
4 Tb gluten-free cornmeal
½ tsp salt
1 tsp garlic powder
1 tsp onion powder
1 tsp paprika
½ tsp pepper
¼ tsp cinnamon
¼ tsp nutmeg
1 egg, beaten

Mustard Sauce

1 Tb olive oil
1 shallot, chopped
1 tsp garlic, chopped
2 Tb brown mustard

1 Tb wine vinegar
½ tsp oregano
4 Tb fat-free half-and-half

1. Preheat oven to 350 degrees.

2. Mix walnuts and all spices together.

3. Lightly toast walnut spice mixture in sauté pan about 2–3 minutes, then remove from heat.

4. Dip chicken breasts in egg, then coat chicken breasts in walnut spice mixture.

5. Spray cooking spray in a large skillet over medium heat.

6. Brown chicken on both sides and cook through.

7. To make sauce, heat olive oil in a sauté pan over medium heat. Add shallots and garlic and sauté about 5 minutes, until softened.

8. Add mustard, vinegar, and oregano, and heat for several minutes.

9. Add fat-free half-and-half and heat through.

10. Serve chicken with mustard sauce over the top.

Nutritional information: 268 calories, 30.4 grams protein, 12.3 grams carbohydrates, 9.4 grams fat, 119.3 milligrams cholesterol, 585.3 milligrams sodium, 2.1 grams fiber, 48.6 milligrams calcium, 1.8 milligrams iron.

Tip: Shrimp or pork loin can be used in this recipe in place of the chicken breasts.

Parmesan Gnocchi   Serves 4

These gnocchi taste just like the classic version. Serve with vodka sauce and fresh peas or with olive oil and Parmesan cheese, as below.

2 large russet potatoes
2 eggs
2 tsp salt
2 cups gluten-free flour blend
1 tsp xanthan gum
2 Tb olive oil
¼ cup parmesan cheese

1. Bake potatoes; cool and peel skin.

2. Mash potatoes in a food processor, adding eggs, salt, flour blend, and xanthan gum; process until smooth.

3. Boil a large pot of water.

4. Take out dough in baseball-sized pieces, one at a time, and roll into a log of cigar thickness. Cut into ½-inch pieces; add extra flour blend if too sticky. Keep the rest of the dough covered with plastic wrap.

5. Cook gnocchi in small batches, taking care not to overcrowd the pot. Cook for about 8 minutes; then remove with a slotted spoon, place in a colander, and rinse with warm water.

6. When gnocchi are done, drizzle with olive oil and sprinkle with parmesan cheese.

Gluten-Free Flour Blend

(Makes 2¼ cups; store leftover blend in an airtight container as a gluten-free all-purpose flour.)

¾ cup sorghum flour
¾ cup potato starch or cornstarch
½ cup tapioca flour
¼ cup chickpea, almond, or corn flour

Nutritional information: 481 calories, 11.8 grams protein, 84 grams carbohydrates, 12.3 grams fat, 110 milligrams cholesterol, 1301 milligrams sodium, 2.7 grams fiber, 111 milligrams calcium, 2.7 milligrams iron.

Tip: Gnocchi is also delicious with tomato, pink, or pesto sauce, or with roasted garlic and olive oil as well.

Chicken Vegetable Curry with Mango Chutney　　　　Serves 4

Bursting with the flavors of curry and sweet potatoes, you will want to make this savory dish time and time again.

½ lb boneless, skinless chicken breast
2 Tb vegetable oil
1 small yellow onion, chopped
2 cloves garlic, minced
1 tsp fresh ginger, minced

½ tsp ground cumin
½ tsp turmeric
½ tsp cinnamon
1 Tb curry powder
½ tsp salt
2 tomatoes, chopped
2 cups gluten-free low sodium chicken broth
1 medium sweet potato, peeled and cut into ½-inch cubes
1 medium russet potato, peeled and cut into ½-inch cubes
½ cup plain nonfat yogurt
1 tsp garam masala
2 cups frozen cauliflower, defrosted

1. Cut chicken into bite-sized pieces. Heat oil in a large nonstick skillet. Add chicken and cook until browned.

2. Remove chicken from pan. Add onion, garlic and ginger. Sauté for 2–3 minutes, until softened.

3. Add cumin, turmeric, cinnamon, curry, and salt, and stir for 1–2 minutes, until curry becomes fragrant—be careful not to burn.

4. Add tomatoes, broth, chicken, and potatoes, then cover and simmer over low heat for about 45 minutes, until chicken is cooked and potatoes are tender.

5. Stir in yogurt, garam masala, and cauliflower, then cook for about 5 more minutes, until heated through.

6. Serve with mango chutney (see sauces and seasoning section) and brown rice.

Nutritional information: 266 calories, 21 grams protein, 27 grams carbohydrates, 9 grams fat, 33.5 milligrams cholesterol, 430 milligrams sodium, 5.2 grams fiber, 139.5 milligrams calcium, 2.7 milligrams iron.

Tips: Garam masala is an aromatic North Indian spice blend that can be used in everything from flat breads to soups.

Chicken- and Spinach-Stuffed Crêpes   Serves 4

The crêpes in this recipe can be stuffed with any filling and served for any occasion, from breakfast to appetizers to desserts. A simple recipe that yields amazing results.

1 Tb vegetable oil

1 shallot, finely chopped

12 oz boneless, skinless chicken breast tenders, cut into bite-sized pieces

2 cups fresh spinach, chopped

1 Tb butter

2 Tb cornstarch

1 cup milk

¾ cup gluten-free, low-sodium chicken broth (such as Pacific)

¼ tsp salt

¼ tsp white pepper

1/8 tsp nutmeg

A basic crêpes recipe follows the recipe for this chicken filling.

1. Heat vegetable oil in a large nonstick skillet over medium-high heat. Add shallot and cook for 2–3 minutes, until softened.

2. Add chicken and continue to cook until chicken is cooked through. Add spinach and remove from heat.

3. In a medium saucepan, melt butter. Stir in cornstarch until smooth.

4. Add milk, chicken broth, salt, pepper and nutmeg. Whisk until smooth. Bring to a boil, stirring constantly, until sauce starts to thicken. Remove from heat.

5. Return chicken to medium heat. Stir in 1 cup of the sauce. Remove from heat.

6. Use filling for crêpes. Spoon remaining sauce over the crêpes to serve (basic crêpe recipe follows).

Basic Gluten-Free Crêpes   **Serves 4**

⅔ cup sorghum flour

⅓ cup potato starch

2 eggs

1 cup low-fat milk

½ tsp salt

2 Tb butter, melted

Gluten-free cooking spray

1. In a large mixing bowl, whisk together sorghum flour, potato starch, and eggs. Add milk, and stir to combine.

2. Beat in salt and butter. Continue to mix until smooth.

3. Heat a medium nonstick skillet over medium-high heat. Spray with cooking spray.

4. Pour ¼ cup of batter onto pan. Tilt pan back and forth so that the batter coats the surface evenly.

5. Cook for about 1 minute, until the bottom starts to brown. Flip crepe with spatula and cook the other side for about 30 seconds.

6. Remove to platter and cover to keep warm.

Nutritional information for Chicken and Spinach Crepes: 515 calories, 35 grams protein, 52 grams carbohydrates, 20 grams fat, 188 milligrams cholesterol, 760 milligrams sodium, 5.6 grams fiber, 324 milligrams calcium, 4.5 milligrams iron.

Tips: Asparagus would also work well in this dish.

Nutritional information for Crepes: 272 calories, 8.8 grams protein, 40 grams carbohydrates, 9.8 grams fat, 124 milligrams cholesterol, 395 milligrams sodium, 2 grams fiber, 96.6 milligrams calcium, 1.8 milligrams iron.

Tips: Add a tablespoon of sugar to make a dessert crepe

Pierogis with Potato Cheese Filling   Serves 8

Serve with melted butter and sautéed onions, with sour cream on the side.

Filling
2 Tb vegetable oil
1 cup onion, finely chopped
2 cups hot mashed potatoes
1 cup sharp cheddar cheese, shredded

Dough
2 cups gluten-free flour blend
2 tsp xanthan gum

½ tsp salt
3 Tb vegetable oil
2 eggs
⅓ cup plain seltzer water

Brown rice flour (for rolling)

1. Heat oil in a medium skillet. Add onions and sauté for 3–4 minutes until softened.

2. Mix onions and cheese with mashed potatoes. Stir to combine and make sure cheese melts. Set aside to cool.

3. In a large bowl, combine the flour blend, xanthan gum, and salt. Make a well in center.

4. In a separate bowl, combine vegetable oil, eggs and seltzer. Pour into well in flour mixture. Stir to combine and form a stiff dough. Add extra flour blend if too wet.

5. Cut dough into 4 pieces. Roll out the first ball about ¼ inch thick, using additional brown rice flour for dusting. Using a biscuit cutter, cut out individual pierogi. Repeat with remaining 3 dough pieces.

6. Take each individual circle and roll out until double in size.

7. Take 1 teaspoon of filling and place on one half of each circle. Fold over, and wet edges and press edges together with fork tines.

8. Place pierogis on 2 large cookie sheets and freeze for 1–2 hours before cooking.

9. Bring large pot of water to boil. Cook pierogi in batches of 10. Boil for 6–8 minutes, until they rise to the top. Cook for an additional 1–2 minutes. Remove with a slotted spoon and serve immediately.

Gluten-Free Flour Blend

¾ cup brown rice flour
½ cup tapioca flour
½ cup potato starch
¼ cup cornstarch

Nutritional information: 364 calories, 9.2 grams protein, 45.6 grams carbohydrates, 17 grams fat, 68 milligrams cholesterol, 368 milligrams sodium, 2.7 grams fiber, 155.6 milligrams calcium, 1.7 milligrams iron.

Tips: Pierogi can be cooked and frozen. To serve, defrost and sauté in butter or drop into boiling water for 3–4 minutes.

Chili   Serves 8

This chili is great as a main course and can also be stuffed into a pepper, a potato, or a corn tortilla with melted cheddar.

2 Tb olive oil
3 Tb garlic, chopped
1 large onion, chopped
2 green or red peppers, chopped
1 lb sirloin, chopped
½ tsp cumin
1 tsp paprika
¼ tsp pepper
¼ tsp chili powder
1 tsp oregano
½ tsp cinnamon
2 Tb brown sugar
1 Tb balsamic vinegar
2 15.5-oz cans cooked kidney beans
28 oz can crushed tomatoes
½ can water

Hot sauce to taste

1. Heat olive oil. Sauté garlic, onions, and peppers.

2. Add beef, seasonings, and balsamic vinegar.

3. Add beans, tomatoes, and water, then cook at least ½ hour for all flavors to merge.

4. Add hot sauce and additional seasoning to taste.

Nutritional information: 285 calories, 19.4 grams protein, 31.7 grams carbohydrates, 9.8 grams fat, 36.8 milligrams cholesterol, 455.8 milligrams sodium, 9.1 grams fiber, 87.2 milligrams calcium, 4.3 milligrams iron.

Tips: Any kind of bean can be used in this recipe; you can easily use ground chicken or turkey in place of the beef.

Chicken Cutlet Parmesan   Serves 4

This same basic recipe can be used to make shrimp parmesan, veal parmesan, or eggplant parmesan.

Gluten-free cooking spray
1 cup gluten-free breadcrumbs
1 tsp garlic powder
1 tsp onion powder
½ tsp oregano
1/8 tsp pepper
½ tsp salt
3 Tb parmesan cheese
1 egg
1 lb boneless, skinless chicken breasts
1 cup marinara sauce
½ tsp garlic powder
1 cup shredded mozzarella

1. Spray a cookie sheet with cooking spray

2. Mix breadcrumbs, garlic powder, onion powder, oregano, pepper, salt, and 2 Tb parmesan cheese.

3. Beat egg, then dip chicken in egg and then in breadcrumb mixture. Coat on both sides.

4. Place chicken on cookie sheet and spray the top with cooking spray.

5. Set oven to broil and cook chicken until brown on both sides.

6. Pour ⅓ sauce in casserole dish. Top with chicken, then with rest of the sauce, 1 Tb Parmesan cheese, and mozzarella cheese.

7. Turn oven to 350 degrees and bake chicken for about 20 minutes until bubbling and the cheese is melted.

Nutritional information: 401.4 calories, 38.6 grams protein, 24.7 grams carbohydrates, 15.9 grams fat, 138 milligrams cholesterol, 986 milligrams sodium, 4 grams fiber, 324.6 milligrams calcium, 2.2 milligrams iron.

Tip: If gluten-free breadcrumbs are not available, crush 1½ cups of gluten-free cornflakes as a substitute.

Sides

- Black Beans and Rice

- Red Potatoes and Bacon

- Steamed Broccoli in Garlic Sauce

- Quinoa with Sautéed Onions and Lima Beans

- Wild Rice and Pecan Pilaf

- Escarole and White Beans

- Spicy Sweet Potato Fries

- Stuffed Tomatoes

- Kasha Varnishkes

- Cranberry Quinoa Salad

Black Beans and Rice   Serves 4

This is a great Spanish side dish that works well with almost any entrée.

1 cup brown rice
2 cups (16 oz) water or gluten-free (such as Pacific)
½ tsp salt
1 tsp olive oil
1 small red onion, finely chopped
¾ cup gluten-free salsa
16 oz can black beans, drained and rinsed
1 Tb lime juice
¼ cup cilantro, roughly chopped
Guacamole, sour cream, cheese, if desired

1. Cook brown rice in salted water or gluten-free broth for 45– 50 minutes until cooked through.

2. Heat oil in bottom of a skillet. Add red onion, and cook 2–3 minutes. Add salsa, black beans, and lime juice and heat through.

3. Combine black bean salsa mixture with cooked brown rice. Before serving, toss in cilantro. If desired, top with guacamole, sour cream, and cheese.

Nutritional information per serving: 283 calories, 10 grams protein, 56 grams carbohydrates, 2.6 grams fat, 0 milligrams cholesterol, 762 milligrams sodium, 7.2 grams fiber, 64.8 milligrams calcium, 2.2 milligrams iron.

Tip: If you like it spicy, add hot sauce, extra salsa, and cilantro.

Red Potatoes and Bacon   Serves 4

Serve this with roasted chicken and steamed vegetables for a satisfying and delicious meal.

1½ lbs red potatoes
2 tsp olive oil
½ tsp dried thyme leaves
½ tsp dried parsley
¼ tsp salt
⅛ tsp black pepper
4 slices turkey bacon, diced

1. Fill a large pot with water and add potatoes. Bring to a boil and cook for 5– 6 minutes, until just fork tender.

2. Drain and cool slightly.

3. Preheat oven to 400 degrees.

4. Cut potatoes into ½-inch cubes and place in a 2-qt baking dish.

5. Add oil, thyme, parsley, salt, and pepper. Toss until potatoes are coated.

6. Top with bacon.

7. Bake for 40 minutes, until bacon is crisp and potatoes are browned. Add a little water if the pan is too dry.

Nutritional information: 212 calories, 8 grams protein, 34 grams carbohydrates, 5 grams fat, 15 milligrams cholesterol, 326 milligrams sodium, 4 grams fiber, 37.3 milligrams calcium, 2.1 milligrams iron.

Tip: Using the red potatoes gives this dish a nice look—I like the small red potatoes because they taste so sweet.

Steamed Broccoli in Garlic Sauce   Serves 4

Steaming the broccoli saves a lot of calories over sautéing.

1 medium head garlic
½ tsp olive oil
1 Tb butter
1 Tb cornstarch
½ cup fat-free milk
½ cup gluten-free chicken broth (such as Kitchen Basics)
¼ tsp salt
⅛ tsp pepper
2 cups broccoli florets
½ cup water

1. Preheat oven to 400 degrees. Slice off top of garlic head: drizzle with olive oil and wrap in foil. Bake for 45–50 minutes, until very soft. Cool.

2. Melt butter in small saucepan over medium heat. Stir in cornstarch, until well blended.

3. Using a wire whisk, add milk and broth. Bring to a boil, stirring constantly until thickened. Reduce heat.

4. Remove the garlic cloves from the skin and stir into the sauce. Remove from heat and season with salt and pepper.

5. In a large skillet, place broccoli and water. Cover and cook for 5– 6 minutes until tender.

6. Drain broccoli. Serve with sauce.

Nutritional information: 74 calories, 3 grams protein, 7.5 grams carbohydrates, 4 grams fat, 11 milligrams cholesterol, 243 milligrams sodium, 1.2 grams fiber, 67 milligrams calcium, <1 milligram iron.

Tip: This garlic sauce is nice on any vegetable, such as asparagus, spinach, zucchini, and yellow squash.

Quinoa with Sautéed Onions and Lima Beans   Serves 4

This recipe is high in protein and fiber and loaded with flavor.

2 tsp vegetable oil
½ cup diced onion

1 tsp turmeric

½ tsp ground coriander

¼ tsp ground cinnamon

¼ tsp allspice

1 cup quinoa (if not pre-rinsed, rinse 2–3 times)

2 cups (16 oz) gluten-free vegetable broth, such as Kitchen Basics

1 cup precooked lima beans

1. Heat oil in a large saucepan over medium-high heat. Add onions and sauté for 3–4 minutes until softened.

2. Add spices and quinoa and stir to coat.

3. Add broth and bring to a boil. Reduce heat and simmer for 10–15 minutes.

4. Stir in lima beans and continue to simmer for another 5–10 minutes, until quinoa is tender and liquid is absorbed.

Nutritional information: 259 calories, 9.4 grams protein, 44.5 grams carbohydrates, 5 grams fat, 0 milligrams cholesterol, 261 milligrams sodium, 6 grams fiber, 51 milligrams calcium, 3.6 milligrams iron.

Tips: Millet and brown rice work nicely in this recipe as well. If you use brown rice, a little additional liquid may be needed in the recipe.

Wild Rice and Pecan Pilaf   Serves 4

Wild rice and pecans add a nutty texture to this wonderful rice dish.

1 cup wild rice, uncooked

1 Tb butter or olive oil

½ cup red onions, chopped

4 Tb raisins

2 cups gluten-free chicken broth (such as Pacific)

4 Tb pecans, coarsely chopped

1. In saucepan toast rice for about 2–4 minutes, then add butter, onions, and raisins. Heat for about 5 minutes, until onions are translucent.

2. Add chicken broth and bring to boil. Stir, lower heat, and cover.

3. Cook for about 45–50 minutes until rice is done.

4. Fold in pecans and serve.

Nutritional information per serving: 270 calories, 9.5 grams protein, 40.4 grams carbohydrates, 8.9 grams fat, 7.6 milligrams cholesterol, 413 milligrams sodium, 3.8 grams fiber, 28 milligrams calcium, 1.4 milligrams iron.

Tip: Wild rice is much denser than regular rice. If too chewy, add some water or broth and cook a little longer.

Escarole and White Beans   Serves 4

This Italian classic is a perfect side to your gluten-free pasta dinner.

1 head of escarole, washed, drained and chopped
½ cup (4 oz) gluten-free chicken broth (such as Pacific)
1 Tb olive oil
½ head fresh garlic, chopped
½ large onion, chopped
15.5 oz can white navy beans, drained
½ tsp salt
½ tsp pepper
1 Tb balsamic vinegar
1 tsp sugar
1 Tb lemon juice

1. In a large pot, cook escarole in chicken broth until cooked (if broth evaporates, add additional broth or water).

2. Place olive oil in skillet over medium heat. Sauté garlic and onions for about 5 minutes, until softened.

3. Add beans, salt, pepper, and balsamic vinegar to garlic and onions.

4. Add sugar and lemon to cooked escarole.

5. Add escarole and broth to bean mixture and cook for about 10 minutes, then serve.

Nutritional information: 127 calories, 7.7 grams protein, 21.5 grams carbohydrates, 4.1 grams fat, 0 milligrams cholesterol, 590 milligrams sodium, 7.2 grams fiber, 91 milligrams calcium, 1.9 milligrams iron.

Tip: To peel garlic: cut head in half, microwave in small bowl with a little water about 30 seconds, peel off cloves and chop.

Spicy Baked Sweet Potato Fries   Serves 4

These potatoes are so easy to make and are truly a treat. Baking these fries saves a lot of fat over traditional deep-fried fries.

2 medium sweet potatoes, cut into thin French fries
1 tsp onion powder
1 tsp garlic powder
2 tsp paprika
1 tsp salt
½ tsp cinnamon
½ tsp pepper
Gluten-free cooking spray

1. Preheat oven to 375 degrees.

2. Mix all spices together in a large bowl.

3. Toss sweet potatoes with the spices.

4. Spray a cookie sheet with cooking spray and place sweet potato mixture on tray.

5. Spray tops of sweet potato fries with cooking spray.

6. Bake until crisp on the outside and cooked through, turning frequently, and spraying again with cooking spray if too dry. Should be cooked in about 35–40 minutes.

Nutrition Information: 64.5 calories, 1.4 grams protein, 15 grams carbohydrates, <1 gram fat, 0 milligrams cholesterol, 618 milligrams sodium, 2.7 grams fiber, 28.2 milligrams calcium, <1 milligram iron.

Tip: Other spices can work well in this recipe, too. If you like your sweet potato fries plain, skip the spices and proceed from step 4 on. If you want, you can fry the potatoes, but baking this way reduces the fat drastically. Many gluten-free foods are often very high in fat, so it helps to cut back when you can.

Stuffed Tomatoes   Serves 2

This recipe is perfect for barbeques, or served up with a steak, chicken, or hamburger.

2 large tomatoes
1 Tb olive or canola oil

1 small onion, chopped
2 Tb garlic, chopped
1 tsp Italian seasoning
1 Tb capers
½ tsp salt
¼ tsp pepper
½ cup seasoned gluten-free breadcrumbs (see cooking tips)
2 Tb parmesan cheese
¼ cup white wine

1. Preheat oven to 350 degrees.

2. Cut off top of tomato; remove pulp and place in small bowl.

3. Heat a medium skillet and add oil.

4. Sauté onion in skillet until translucent; add garlic and sauté 2–3 minutes.

5. Add tomato pulp, Italian seasoning, capers, salt, pepper, and gluten-free breadcrumbs and heat a few minutes.

6. Stuff mixture into tomatoes, place in casserole dish, and sprinkle with parmesan cheese.

7. Pour wine into casserole dish.

8. Bake for about 25 minutes, until tomatoes start to soften.

Nutritional information: 257 calories, 5 grams protein, 25.9 grams carbohydrates, 13 grams fat, 4.4 milligrams cholesterol, 894 milligrams sodium, 4.7 grams fiber, 130 milligrams calcium, 1.1 milligrams iron.

Tip: If gluten-free bread crumbs are not available, toast gluten-free bread and put through a food processor with some Italian seasoning, garlic, onion powder, and a little salt.

Kasha Varnishkes   Serves 8

This is a terrific side dish that can be served just as easily with scrambled eggs as with a piece of chicken or steak.

6 oz spiral brown rice or quinoa pasta
3 Tb olive oil

1 Tb garlic, minced

1 large Spanish onion, chopped into ½-inch pieces

2 cups mushrooms, sliced

1½ tsp salt

½ tsp pepper

1 cup whole kasha (buckwheat groats)

1 egg beaten

2 cups gluten-free chicken broth (Pacific)

1. Cook and drain pasta.

2. While pasta is cooking, heat olive oil in a skillet over medium heat and sauté garlic and onion.

3. When onion is starting to brown, add about 2 Tb water, mushrooms, salt, and pepper. Cover and continue to cook until mushrooms are soft.

4. Drain pasta and place in a large bowl. Stir in onion and mushroom mixture.

5. In a separate medium pot, put on a high heat and add buckwheat groats. When hot, add egg and keep stirring until egg is absorbed and buckwheat groats are separated from each other. Add chicken broth, lower heat, and cover. Cook about 10–15 minutes, until liquid is absorbed.

6. Toss buckwheat with pasta and mushrooms and serve.

Nutritional information: 227.3 calories, 6.9 grams protein, 35.7 grams carbohydrates, 6.8 grams fat, 26.4 milligrams cholesterol, 648.8 milligrams sodium, 2.7 grams fiber, 16.1 milligrams calcium, 1.7 milligrams iron.

Tip: To reheat leftovers place in a casserole dish, add a little additional gluten-free chicken broth, cover, and bake at 300 degrees until hot.

Cranberry-Quinoa Salad   Serves 6

This is a perfect recipe just like what you would buy in a gourmet store, only at a much lower cost.

1 cup quinoa, (if not pre-rinsed, rinse 3 times)

2 cups gluten-free chicken or vegetable broth or water

2 tsp olive oil
1 medium yellow onion, chopped
½ cup frozen peas, defrosted and drained
¼ cup dried cranberries
¼ cup walnuts, chopped
2 Tb fresh parsley, roughly chopped

1. Cook quinoa in gluten-free broth for 15–20 minutes, until cooked.

2. In separate skillet, heat oil, then add onion and cook until soft.

3. Add cooked onion and peas, dried cranberries, walnuts, and parsley to cooked quinoa. Can be served hot or cold.

Nutritional information: 196.7 calories, 6.6 grams protein, 28.9 grams carbohydrates, 6.6 grams fat, 0 milligrams cholesterol, 166.4 milligrams sodium, 4.2 grams fiber, 34.7 milligrams calcium, 1.9 milligrams iron.

Tip: Cooked millet or amaranth can be used in place of the quinoa, and raisins, currants, or apricots can be used in place of the cranberries.

Sauces and Seasonings

- Mango Chutney

- Yogurt Sauce

- Salsa

- Steak Sauce

- Barbeque Sauce

- Cream Sauce

Mango Chutney   Serves 4

This is great addition to many dishes. Papaya or peaches work well in place of the mango in this recipe.

1 (12-oz) bag frozen mango, or 2 cups cubed fresh mango
¼ cup golden raisins
½ cup cider vinegar
½ cup brown sugar

1 Tb garlic, minced
1 tsp fresh ginger, minced
¼ tsp cayenne pepper
¼ tsp black pepper
½ tsp salt

1. In a large skillet, bring all of the ingredients to a boil over medium heat.

2. Reduce heat to low and simmer, uncovered, for about 30 minutes, stirring constantly.

3. Remove from heat and cool before serving.

Nutritional information: 161.6 calories, <1 gram protein, 40.6 grams carbohydrates, <1 gram fat, 0 milligrams cholesterol, 300 milligrams sodium, 2 grams fiber, 33 milligrams calcium, <1 milligram iron.

Tips: This chutney can be stored in the refrigerator for up to a week.

Yogurt Sauce   Serves 4

A terrific Middle Eastern sauce that is great with so many dishes.

2 Tb olive oil
½ tsp sugar
2 cups nonfat plain yogurt
1 tsp garlic powder
½ tsp salt
2 scallions, chopped, or ½ tsp onion powder
4 Tb lemon juice
½ cucumber, chopped (optional)
1 tsp dried mint

1. Mix all ingredients together.

2. Refrigerate until ready to use.

Nutritional information: 81.5 calories, 7.5 grams protein, 12.5 grams carbohydrates, <1 gram fat, 2.4 milligrams cholesterol, 242 milligrams sodium, <1 gram fiber, 256.7 milligrams calcium, <1 milligram iron.

Tip: Add extra garlic and lemon to taste. Great served with kabobs.

Salsa   Serves 4

Salsa can be made from vegetables, fruits and a variety of spices and seasoning agents. It is the perfect addition to almost any meal.

2 cups plum tomatoes, seeds and juice removed and chopped coarsely
½ jalapeno pepper, minced finely
½ cup red onions, finely chopped
½ cup cilantro, finely chopped
½ tsp salt
¼ tsp pepper

1. Combine all ingredients; chill until ready to serve.

Nutritional information: 25.5 calories, 1 gram protein, 5.6 grams carbohydrates, <1 gram fat, 0 milligrams cholesterol, 297 milligrams sodium, 1.5 grams fiber, 15.8 milligrams calcium, <1 milligram iron.

Tip: Salsa is great with chips or as a topping for fish or chicken. Try adding corn, chopped vegetables, fruits, and different spices to salsa to create your own signature variety.

Steak Sauce   Serves 8

This sweet, savory steak sauce is a terrific addition to almost any meal.

¼ cup olive oil
⅓ cup gluten-free soy sauce (such as La Choy or San-J)
3 Tb brown sugar
3 Tb gluten-free Worcestershire sauce
2 Tb garlic, minced
½ tsp onion powder
½ tsp pepper

1. Whisk all the ingredients together; refrigerate until ready to use.

Nutritional information: 86.3 calories, <1 gram protein, 5.7 grams carbohydrates, 6.7 gram fat, 0 milligrams cholesterol, 750 milligrams sodium, <1 gram fiber, 7.5 milligrams calcium, <1 milligram iron.

Tip: This steak sauce is perfect as a topping choice for any barbeque.

Barbecue Sauce   **Serves 12**

Barbecue sauce is easy to make and delicious for using on your grilled recipes. Add your favorite spices until you get a flavor that is perfect for you.

2 Tb olive oil
½ small red onion, chopped
1 Tb garlic, minced
½ cup apricot preserves
½ cup catsup
1 Tb molasses
1 Tb vinegar
1 tsp gluten-free hot sauce (more, if you like it hot)
2 Tb gluten-free Worcestershire sauce
⅛ tsp ground celery seeds
½ tsp salt
¼ tsp pepper

1. Heat olive oil and sauté onion until translucent. Add garlic and sauté for about 2–3 minutes more.

2. Add all other ingredients; simmer for about 5 minutes.

3. Taste and add extra seasoning if desired.

4. Refrigerate until ready to use.

Nutritional information: 73.3 calories, <1 gram protein, 13.7 grams carbohydrates, 2.3 grams fat, 0 milligrams cholesterol, 257.5 milligrams sodium, <1 gram fiber, 11.1 milligrams calcium, <1 milligram iron.

Tip: Any kind of preserves can be used in place of the apricot.

Cream Sauce   **Serves 4**

This is great to use as a base for a cream soup, or with any recipe that originally calls for a cream sauce.

2 Tb butter
2 Tb rice flour
1 cup half-and-half
½ tsp salt
⅛ tsp pepper

1. Melt butter in a sauce pan and stir in rice flour, stirring until it is a thick paste.

2. Slowly add half-and-half a little at a time, stirring until all half-and-half is added and the sauce begins to thicken and is smooth.

3. Add salt and pepper, heat for an additional 2–3 minutes, and serve.

Nutritional information: 147 calories, 2.2 grams protein, 6.4 grams carbohydrates, 12.7 grams fat, 37.4 milligrams cholesterol, 356.6 milligrams sodium, <1 gram fiber, 65.8 milligrams calcium, <1 milligram iron.

Tips: Add an egg yolk and shredded parmesan cheese and heat and stir until thickened for a terrific Alfredo sauce. To make a cheese sauce, substitute milk for the half-and-half and add some shredded cheddar cheese. Stir over a low heat until the cheese is melted.

Desserts

- Double Chocolate Chip Cookies
- Apple-Almond Tart
- Italian Ricotta Pie
- Apple Cranberry Crumb Pie
- Strawberry Shortcake
- Chocolate Lava Cakes
- Cheesecake Bars
- Pumpkin Pie
- Linzer Tarts
- Cream Cheese Butter Cookies
- Chocolate Chip Coconut Meringue Cookies
- Oatmeal Butterscotch Cookies
- Moist and Delicious Carrot Cake

Double Chocolate Chip Cookies   **Makes 48 Servings**

The ultimate chocolate chip cookie—no one would ever know they are gluten-free!

2¼ cups gluten-free flour blend
½ cup brown rice flour
2 tsp gluten-free baking soda
1 tsp gluten-free baking powder
1 tsp salt
2 tsp xanthan gum
2 sticks of butter
¾ cup white sugar
¾ cup brown sugar
2 eggs, slightly beaten
1 tsp vanilla extract
12 oz gluten-free semi sweet chocolate chips
6 oz gluten-free semi sweet chocolate chunks
Gluten-free cooking spray

Gluten-Free Flour Blend

(Makes 4½ cups; store leftover blend in an airtight container as a gluten-free all-purpose flour.)

1½ cups sorghum flour
1½ cups potato starch or cornstarch
1 cup tapioca flour
½ cup chickpea or almond flour

1. Preheat oven to 350 degrees.

2. Combine all dry ingredients except sugar and chips.

3. Cream butter, then add sugar and beat until well-combined.

4. Add eggs and vanilla extract to the butter mixture and mix well.

5. Mix flour mixture into creamed mixture; if too wet, add a little extra flour blend or brown rice flour. Dough should be moist but hold together well.

6. Add ¾ of the chips, reserving the rest of the chips and chocolate chunks for topping. (See tips below for baking.)

7. Use a tablespoon scoop to place cookies on the baking sheet—spray scoop with cooking spray to keep the dough from sticking. Scoops that have a handle that pushes out the dough work best.

8. Only spoon 3 cookies across on each row on the baking sheet, or they may spread into each other.

9. Top cookies with reserved chocolate chips and chunks, pushing in a little.

10. Bake cookies until they are just starting to brown but still a little light in the middle. Remove from oven, let sit for about 1–2 minutes, and remove from baking sheet to cool on aluminum foil or rack.

Nutritional information: 140 calories, 1.5 grams protein, 19.7 grams carbohydrates, 7.2 grams fat, 19 milligrams cholesterol, 141 milligrams sodium, <1 grams fiber, 13.6 milligrams calcium, <1 milligram iron.

Tips: Baking flour blends should be mixed and kept in containers, handy when all-purpose flour is called for in recipes. Also, note that nuts are also a great addition to these cookies. This recipe makes a soft, puffy cookie. If you like a crispy, flatter cookie, use a little less flour.

Apple Almond Tart   Serves 12

This decadent tart was adapted from a classic French tart often offered among dessert options at fine restaurants.

Crust

1¼ cups all-purpose gluten-free flour blend (see below)
1 tsp xanthan gum
¼ tsp salt
5 Tb cold, unsalted butter, cut into little pieces
1 egg yolk
3–4 Tb ice water
½ Tb unsalted butter, softened
9-inch tart pan

Gluten-Free Flour Blend

(Makes approximately 3 cups; store leftover blend in an airtight container as a gluten-free all-purpose flour.)

1 cup sorghum flour
1 cup potato starch
⅔ cup tapioca flour
¼ cup almond flour

Filling

1 cup slivered almonds (or almond meal)
½ cup dark brown sugar
¼ cup gluten-free flour blend
½ tsp salt
1 tsp ground cinnamon
6 Tb unsalted butter, softened
2 eggs
2 Tb dark rum
3 golden delicious apples, cored, peeled, halved, and thinly sliced
½ cup dark brown sugar

1. Preheat oven to 400 degrees.

2. By hand or in a food processor, blend together the flour blend, xanthan gum, salt, and 5 Tb butter until mixture resembles small peas.

3. Work in egg and ice water until the dough begins to hold together nicely (add more ice water if needed).

4. Wrap dough in plastic wrap and place in freezer for about 15 minutes.

5. On parchment paper, sprinkle a little of the leftover flour blend and then flatten out the dough. Sprinkle out the flour blend and then carefully roll out the dough until large enough to cover the inside of a tart pan.

6. Butter tart pan inside with ½ Tb butter.

7. Flip the dough into the tart pan and press into pan to fix nicely, reserving any pieces of extra dough for patching.

8. Bake tart dough for about 10–15 minutes, until it is dry to the touch and light brown.

9. If the crust has cracked at all, use leftover dough to patch insides. If no dough is left over, combine a little gluten-free flour with softened butter and spread over the crack.

10. Set crust aside.

11. In a food processor, pulse slivered almonds until they are chopped fine, and place them in a large bowl. (If using almond meal, skip this step.)

12. To the almonds add ½ cup brown sugar, ¼ cup gluten-free flour blend, ½ tsp salt and ½ tsp cinnamon and mix together.

13. Beat into the almond mixture 4 Tb of the soft butter, until well blended.

14. Blend 2 eggs and rum into this mixture.

15. Spread creamed mixture into the baked shell.

16. Arrange the apples over the top of the tart in a flower design.

17. Melt remaining butter, pour over top of apples, sprinkle with brown sugar and remaining cinnamon.

18. Bake for about 1 hour, until apples are golden.

19. Let cool for about ½ hour, until set; carefully remove from tart pan and place on a platter.

Nutritional information per serving: 308 calories, 4.7 grams protein, 35 grams carbohydrates, 17 grams fat, 82 milligrams cholesterol, 170 milligrams sodium, 2.4 grams fiber, 56.8 milligrams calcium, 1.1 milligrams iron.

Tip: This tart is yummy made with pears or peaches as well.

Italian Ricotta Pie   Serves 12

Don't be surprised when everyone cuts into this delicious treat.

Crust

1⅔ cup gluten-free flour blend (see below)
2 Tb sugar
½ tsp salt
½ tsp gluten-free baking powder
1 tsp xanthan gum
½ cup butter
2 eggs

Filling

15 oz part-skim ricotta cheese
1 cup sugar
1 Tb gluten-free flour blend
½ tsp grated lemon peel
Dash of salt
4 eggs
2 tsp vanilla extract
⅓ cup gluten-free semi sweet chocolate chips
1 tsp orange extract
½ tsp cinnamon
Dash of nutmeg
9-inch pie pan

Gluten-Free Flour Blend

(Makes approximately 4½ cups; store leftover blend in an airtight container as a gluten-free all-purpose flour.)

1½ cups sorghum flour
1½ cups potato starch or cornstarch
1 cup tapioca flour
½ cup chickpea, almond, or corn flour

1. Combine gluten-free flour blend, sugar, salt, baking powder, and xanthan gum with butter; mix together with a fork or a food processor until the mixture resembles small crumbs.

2. Add eggs and work mixture until it holds together as a ball.

3. Wrap dough in plastic wrap and place in freezer for about 20 minutes.

4. Remove dough from freezer and place on parchment paper that has been dusted lightly with gluten-free flour, pressing dough down into a circle.

5. Sprinkle top of dough with gluten-free flour blend and carefully roll out into a large disk that will cover the inside of a pie pan.

6. Flip dough into pie pan and press into any cracks to make sure crust covers all areas of pie pan. Crimp edges.

7. Preheat oven to 350 degrees.

8. In a large bowl, mix together ricotta, sugar, flour, lemon peel, and salt.

9. In a small bowl, beat eggs for about 3 minutes and fold into ricotta mixture.

10. Add all remaining ingredients and pour into prepared crust.

11. Bake for about 1 hour until just set; turn off oven, and let sit in warm oven another 15 minutes before removing and cooling.

Nutritional information: 334 calories, 8.9 grams protein, 43 grams carbohydrates, 14.8 grams fat, 137 milligrams cholesterol, 280 milligrams sodium, <1 gram fiber, 130 milligrams calcium, 1.3 milligrams iron.

Tip: This delicious pie freezes beautifully and can be cut and defrosted one piece at a time. Using a porcelain pie pan gives it a nice presentation.

Apple Cranberry Crumb Pie   Serves 8

This pie can be made with many fruit fillings and is always perfect, especially topped with vanilla ice cream.

Crust

¼ cup potato starch
¼ cup tapioca starch
½ cup white rice flour
2 tsp granulated sugar
½ tsp xanthan gum
½ tsp gluten-free baking powder
½ sp salt
6 Tb unsalted cold butter
⅓ cup cold water
1 tsp cider vinegar

1. Sift all dry ingredients (flour through salt) into a large mixing bowl.

2. Add butter and use a pastry cutter or fork to work butter into the dry ingredients until they are well incorporated and mixture looks crumbly.

3. Mix together water and vinegar. Stir into the flour. The dough should be soft but hold together when squeezed. Wrap in plastic wrap and refrigerate while making filling.

Filling

3 large green apples
½ cup fresh cranberries
1 Tb lemon juice
2 Tb cornstarch
½ cup granulated sugar
1¼ tsp ground cinnamon
2 Tb unsalted butter, melted
¼ cup almond flour, finely ground
¼ cup white rice flour
2 Tb brown sugar

1. Peel and thinly slice the apples. Place in a medium mixing bowl. Add cranberries and lemon juice and stir gently to mix.

2. Add cornstarch, sugar, and 1 teaspoon of cinnamon. Stir until combined.

3. Mix butter, almond and rice flour, brown sugar, and remaining ¼ teaspoon cinnamon in a small bowl with a fork until mixed and crumbly.

4. Preheat oven to 375 degrees.

5. Remove crust from refrigerator and plastic wrap. Place between 2 sheets of waxed paper and roll out into a 9-inch circle (use a little flour blend if dough is sticking to the wax paper).

6. Remove one sheet of waxed paper and invert crust into a 9-inch pie plate. Remove second sheet of waxed paper so pie crust fits nicely into the pan. Trim and crimp edges of the crust to make decorative border.

7. Pour apple mixture into crust. Sprinkle with crumb topping.

8. Bake for 40 minutes. If pie browns too quickly, cover with aluminum foil.

Nutritional information per serving: 286 calories, 1.6 grams protein, 44 grams carbohydrates, 12.5 grams fat, 32 milligrams cholesterol, 96 milligrams sodium, 2.5 grams fiber, 29 milligrams calcium, <1 milligram iron.

Tips: Use any kind of berry in this pie: blueberry, raspberry—the sky's the limit! Handle the crust as little as possible so that it will stay flaky.

Strawberry Shortcake   Serves 4

In the spring and summer, when seasonally ripe berries are everywhere, this cake is a sure hit.

Gluten-free cooking spray
½ cup brown rice flour
½ cup white rice flour
¼ cup tapioca starch
2 tsp gluten-free baking powder
½ tsp gluten-free baking soda
3 Tb sugar
¾ cup low-fat buttermilk
1 Tb raw turbinado sugar (white granulated sugar can be used)
2 cups strawberries, sliced
⅓ cup gluten-free whipped cream

1. Preheat oven to 425 degrees. Coat a cookie sheet with cooking spray.

2. In a large mixing bowl, mix brown rice flour, white rice flour, tapioca starch, baking powder, baking soda, and 2 tablespoons of sugar together in a large mixing bowl.

3. Add buttermilk; stir to combine.

4. Using two spoons, drop batter onto cookie sheet in 4 equal portions. Sprinkle with raw sugar.

5. Bake in preheated oven for 15 minutes, until golden brown.

6. Mix sliced strawberries with remaining 1 tablespoon sugar.

7. When biscuits have cooled, slice in half. Top one half with ½ cup strawberries and 1 tablespoon whipped cream; place other half of biscuit on top and serve.

Nutritional information per serving: 283 calories, 4.7 grams protein, 58 grams carbohydrates, 4.2 grams fat, 12 milligrams cholesterol, 330 milligrams sodium, 2.8 grams fiber, 113 milligrams calcium, <1 milligram iron.

Tips: Turbinado sugar or sugar in the raw is pure cane sugar; it is coarser and contains natural molasses.

Chocolate Lava Cakes   Serves 6

This gooey chocolate cake is just perfect for the chocoholic in you.

Gluten-free cooking spray
3 oz gluten-free semi sweet chocolate
3 oz gluten-free bittersweet chocolate
3 Tb unsalted butter
4 egg yolks
5 Tb sugar
1 tsp vanilla extract
2 egg whites (room temperature)
½ tsp cream of tartar
1 Tb confectioner's sugar

1. Preheat oven to 425 degrees. Coat the inside of 6 ¾-cup oven-safe custard cups with cooking spray. Place custard cups on a cookie sheet.

2. Combine chocolates and butter in top of a double boiler. Heat over simmering water until chocolate is melted, stirring frequently. Remove from heat and cool for 10 minutes (or microwave chocolate to melt it).

3. In a large bowl, beat egg yolks and sugar with an electric beater about 2 minutes, until thick and light in color. Fold in vanilla and chocolate.

4. Beat egg whites and cream of tartar in a separate clean bowl, until stiff peaks form. Gently fold into the chocolate mixture.

5. Divide batter evenly among 6 custard cups. Bake in preheated oven about 10 minutes, until cakes are puffed but still soft in the center.

6. Transfer cookie sheet to a rack. Let cool 1 minute.

7. Using a small knife, cut around sides of cakes to loosen. Remove cakes to a serving dish. Sprinkle with confectioner's sugar and serve.

Nutritional information per serving: 274 calories, 4 grams protein, 24 grams carbohydrates, 18 grams fat, 154 milligrams cholesterol, 24 milligrams sodium, 2 grams fiber, 28 milligrams calcium, 1.6 milligrams iron.

Tip: Serve with fresh raspberries or blueberries.

Cheesecake Bars   **Makes 36 Servings (Serving Size 1 Bar)**

These delicious bars are like miniature cheesecakes, perfect for an afternoon treat.

¾ cup crushed gluten-free graham crackers (such as Kinnikinnick gluten-free)
½ cup gluten-free flour blend (below)
½ cup walnuts, chopped fine
¼ cup sugar
½ cup butter melted
8 oz cream cheese
⅓ cup sugar
1 egg
1 Tb lemon juice
½ tsp grated lemon peel

Gluten-Free Flour Blend

(*Makes 4½ cups; store leftover blend in an airtight container as a gluten-free all-purpose flour.*)

1½ cups sorghum flour
1½ cups potato starch or cornstarch
1 cup tapioca flour
½ cup chickpea or almond flour

1. Preheat oven to 350 degrees.

2. Stir together first four ingredients, except 2 Tb of the graham cracker crumbs. Add melted butter and combine.

3. Press into a 9 × 9-inch square nonstick baking pan.

4. Bake in a 350 degree oven for 12 minutes.

5. Cream together cream cheese and ⅓ cup sugar.

6. Add egg, lemon juice, and lemon peel; mix well.

7. Pour over baked layer, sprinkle with remaining gluten-free graham cracker crumbs, and bake for an additional 20–25 minutes.

8. Cool and cut into bars.

Nutritional information: 85 calories, 1.1 grams protein, 7 grams carbohydrates, 6 grams fat, 13.7 milligrams cholesterol, 54 milligrams sodium, <1 grams fiber, 7.8 milligrams calcium, <1 milligram iron.

Tip: If you prefer a taste besides lemon, why not use orange peel and orange juice in place of the lemon?

Pumpkin Pie   Serves 8

There is no need for you to pass on the pumpkin pie on Thanksgiving—this recipe is a sure hit.

9-inch Pie Crust

1⅔ cups gluten-free flour blend (following the filling)
2 Tb sugar
½ tsp salt
½ tsp baking powder
1 tsp xanthan gum
½ cup butter
2 eggs

1. Combine gluten-free flour blend, sugar, salt, baking powder, and xantham gum.

2. Work butter into the dry mixture with a fork or a food processor until the mixture resembles small crumbs.

3. Add eggs, and work mixture until it holds together as a ball.

4. Wrap in plastic wrap and place in freezer for about 20 minutes.

5. Remove dough from freezer and place on parchment paper that has been dusted lightly with gluten-free flour; press dough down into a circle.

6. Sprinkle top of dough with gluten-free flour blend and carefully roll out into a large disk that will fit into a pie pan.

7. Flip dough into pie pan and press into any cracks to make sure crust covers all sections of the pie pan.

8. Crimp edges to make a nice pie edge.

Filling

¾ cup dark brown sugar
1 tsp cinnamon
½ tsp salt
½ tsp ground ginger
¼ tsp ground cloves
2 eggs
1 tsp vanilla extract
15 oz pumpkin purée
12 oz evaporated milk

Gluten-Free Flour Blend

(Makes 4½ cups; store leftover blend in an airtight container as a gluten-free all-purpose flour.)

1½ cups sorghum flour
1½ cups potato starch or cornstarch
1 cup tapioca flour
½ cup chickpea, corn, almond, or hazelnut flour

1. Preheat oven to 425 degrees.

2. In a small bowl, mix together brown sugar, cinnamon, salt, ginger, and cloves.

3. In a large bowl, beat eggs, vanilla, pumpkin, and add into spice mixture. Fold in evaporated milk.

4. Pour pumpkin mixture into pie crust and bake for 15 minutes. Lower temperature to 350 degrees and bake for an additional 50 minutes, until knife inserted in the center comes out clean.

5. Refrigerate until ready to serve.

6. Top with gluten-free whipped cream if desired.

Nutritional information per serving: 256 calories, 4.5 grams protein, 33.5 grams carbohydrates, 10 grams fat, 92 milligrams cholesterol, 302 milligrams sodium, 1.6 grams fiber, 120 milligrams calcium, 1.4 milligrams iron.

Tip: If you want to use homemade pumpkin purée, cut a small pumpkin in half and remove the seeds; place pumpkin halves cut-side down on a baking sheet and bake at 350 degrees until pumpkin is soft and can be pierced with a fork. Scoop out pumpkin flesh; purée and strain. Refrigerate until ready to use.

Linzer Tarts   45 (3-inch) tarts

These tarts are actually easier to roll than those made from gluten-containing flour. They are so light and delicious, you'll want to have them every day.

4 sticks unsalted butter
1½ cups sugar
4 egg yolks
2 tsp vanilla extract
6½–7 cups all-purpose gluten-free flour blend
1½ cups almond flour
1 tsp salt
2 tsp xanthan gum
½ cup rice flour
½ cup powdered sugar
30 oz red raspberry preserves

Gluten-Free Flour Blend

(Makes 6¾ cups; store leftover blend in an airtight container as a gluten-free all-purpose flour.)

2¼ cups sorghum flour
2¼ cups potato starch or cornstarch
1½ cups tapioca flour
¾ cup almond or hazelnut flour (nut flours give the best taste) or chickpea or corn flour

1. In a large bowl, beat butter until creamy. Then cream sugar into butter, add egg yolks and vanilla, and blend together.

2. Combine 6½ cups all-purpose gluten-free flour blend with almond flour, salt, and xanthan gum. When well-combined, dough should be easy to shape with hands but not wet or sticky. If the dough is too wet, add gluten-free all-purpose blend until you get the right consistency. Dough should be a little softer than Play-Doh.

3. Preheat oven to 350 degrees.

4. On a work surface, spread a large piece of waxed paper and sprinkle with rice flour. Take a softball-sized piece of dough and shape into a ball; then flatten it out and flip so both sides have some rice flour on them.

5. Take a rolling pin and roll out to about ⅓-inch thick. If dough is too sticky, add a little more rice flour.

6. Take a cookie cutter about 3 inches across and cut out dough. You will need to cut 2 pieces for each tart. Take a smaller cookie cutter and cut a small design in the center of one of the cookies. I like to save the cutaway shapes to make smaller cookies (otherwise, just reincorporate it into the dough).

7. Bake the cookies for about 9–10 minutes, until cookies are set and just starting to turn golden in color.

8. Remove from tray with a spatula, and place on aluminum foil to cool. Sprinkle with powdered sugar.

9. When cookies are cool, spread about 1 Tb of preserves on each uncut cookie, and spread. Top with a cookie with a design cut out, and arrange cookies on a platter. Serve 1 tart per person.

Nutritional information per serving: 257 calories, 2.3 grams protein, 42 grams carbohydrates, 9.7 grams fat, 40.3 milligrams cholesterol, 59 milligrams sodium, <1 gram fiber, 12.8 milligrams calcium, <1 milligram iron.

Tip: If you would like to just make smaller cookies without the cutout in the center, halve the recipe and cut 2 small cookies for each jam-filled cookie. Cookies can be kept in an airtight container for weeks or can be stored in the freezer and defrosted when ready to use. Dough can also be made ahead of time, then wrapped in plastic and refrigerated or frozen until ready to use.

Cream Cheese Butter Cookies   Makes 48 Servings

These cookies are simple to make and the perfect ultimate buttery cookie to dip into coffee. These cookies have been adapted from my mother-in-law Helen's famous cream cheese cookies.

1 cup (2 sticks) unsalted butter or margarine
3-oz package cream cheese, softened

1 cup granulated sugar
1 egg yolk
1 tsp vanilla extract
3½ cups all-purpose gluten-free blend
1 tsp salt
2 tsp xanthan gum
¼ cup powdered sugar

Gluten-Free Flour Blend

(Makes 5 cups; store leftover blend in an airtight container as a gluten-free all-purpose flour.)

1½ cups sorghum flour
½ cup rice flour
1½ cups potato starch or cornstarch
1 cup tapioca flour
½ cup chickpea, corn, almond, or hazelnut flour (nut flours give the best taste)

1. Preheat oven to 350 degrees.

2. In a large bowl, cream together butter and cream cheese; add sugar and blend until smooth.

3. Add egg yolk and vanilla to butter mixture and mix to combine.

4. In a small bowl, combine flour blend, salt and xanthan gum.

5. Combine wet and dry ingredients until a nice dough forms.

6. Shape cookies into small balls and make a thumbprint in the center.

7. Place cookies on a cookie sheet and bake for 10–12 minutes, until they are just hinting at light gold.

8. Remove from cookie sheet and place on aluminum foil or rack to cool.

9. Sprinkle with powdered sugar; store in airtight container until ready to use.

Nutritional information per serving: 102.7 calories, <1 gram protein, 14.7 grams carbohydrates, 4.8 grams fat, 16.5 milligrams cholesterol, 58 milligrams sodium, <1 gram fiber, 9 milligrams calcium, <1 milligram iron.

Tip: Cookies can be kept in an airtight container for weeks or can be stored in the freezer and defrosted when ready to use. Dough can also be made ahead of time and wrapped in plastic and refrigerated or frozen until ready to use.

Chocolate Chip Coconut Meringue Cookies   Serves 8

These delicious cookies just melt in your mouth.

2 egg whites (room temperature)
¼ tsp salt
⅛ tsp cream of tartar
⅔ cup granulated sugar
¼ cup cocoa powder
⅓ cup mini gluten-free chocolate chips
2 Tb dried cranberries
¼ cup shredded coconut
¼ cup walnuts, chopped
Gluten-free cooking spray

1. Preheat oven to 300 degrees.

2. In a mixer, beat egg whites with salt and cream of tartar until they start to peak.

3. Blend in sugar and cocoa powder 1 tablespoon at a time, until well-combined and stiff peaks are formed.

4. Fold in chocolate chips, cranberries, coconut, and walnuts.

5. Spray cookie sheet with cooking spray and cover with parchment paper.

6. Drop batter by teaspoon onto parchment paper.

7. Bake for 30–40 minutes, until cookies are crisp.

8. Wait until cool before trying to remove from cookie sheet.

Nutritional information: 147 calories, 2.4 grams protein, 24.4 grams carbohydrates, 5.6 grams fat, 0 milligrams cholesterol, 88 milligrams sodium, 3.8 grams fiber, 9.1 milligrams calcium, <1 milligram iron.

Tip: Why not try dried blueberries, cherries, or chopped pecans in this recipe? Everything tastes great in a meringue. Let your imagination go wild!

Spicy Oatmeal Butterscotch Cookies   Makes 36 Cookies

These cookies make you feel like you are at a country picnic.

1 cup butter, softened
1 cup brown sugar
½ cup white granulated sugar
2 eggs
1 tsp vanilla extract
1¾ cups gluten-free flour blend
1 tsp gluten-free baking soda
¼ tsp xanthan gum
½ tsp salt
2 tsp cinnamon
2½ cups gluten-free rolled oats
1 cup gluten-free butterscotch chips
½ cup sweetened coconut

Gluten-Free Flour Blend

(*Makes 4½ cups; store leftover blend in an airtight container as a gluten-free all-purpose flour.*)

1½ cups sorghum flour
1½ cups potato starch
1 cup tapioca flour
½ cup almond flour

1. Preheat oven to 350 degrees. Line a cookie sheet with parchment paper.

2. In a large bowl, cream butter; then add brown and white sugar and beat until light and fluffy.

3. Add eggs and vanilla. Continue to beat until smooth.

4. Combine the gluten-free flour blend, gluten-free baking soda, xanthan gum, salt, and cinnamon. Stir into the sugar mixture.

5. Stir in the gluten-free oats, chips, and coconut.

6. Drop by rounded teaspoons onto prepared cookie sheet.

7. Bake for 10–12 minutes, until light and golden. Do not overbake. Let them cool for 1–2 minutes on cookie sheet. Set on aluminum foil or wire rack to cool completely.

8. Store in an airtight container or freeze until ready to use.

Nutritional information (per cookie): 165 calories, 1.6 grams protein, 21.6 grams carbohydrates, 8 grams fat, 25 milligrams cholesterol, 119 milligrams sodium, <1 grams fiber, 9.7 milligrams calcium, <1 milligrams iron.

Tips: Use chocolate chips or dried fruit in place of butterscotch chips if desired.

Moist and Delicious Carrot Cake   Serves 16

Everyone loves this carrot cake. Cut it into squares, and it's a perfect dessert to go.

Gluten-free cooking spray
2 cups gluten-free flour blend
2 tsp gluten-free baking soda
1 tsp gluten-free baking powder
2 tsp cinnamon
½ tsp xanthan gum
½ tsp salt
½ tsp allspice
2 cups white granulated sugar
¾ cup vegetable oil
2 Tb ground flaxseed
3 eggs
1 tsp vanilla extract
½ cup walnuts, chopped
1 (8-oz) can crushed pineapple
1½ cups finely grated carrot

Gluten-Free Flour Blend

(Makes 4½ cups; store leftover blend in an airtight container as a gluten-free all-purpose flour.)

1½ cups sorghum flour
1½ cups potato starch

1 cup tapioca flour
½ cup almond flour

Cream Cheese Frosting

1 (8-oz) package light cream cheese
1 lb confectioner's sugar
2 Tb butter, softened

1. Preheat oven to 350 degrees. Spray 2 9-inch round cake pans with cooking spray.

2. Sift together flour, baking soda, baking powder, cinnamon, xanthan gum, salt, and allspice.

3. In a large bowl, beat sugar, oil, and flaxseed until well blended. Add the eggs, one at a time, beating well after each addition. Stir in the vanilla.

4. Stir flour mixture into wet ingredients until just blended. Do not overmix.

5. Fold in walnuts, pineapple, and carrots. Pour batter into prepared pans.

6. Bake for 30–35 minutes or until toothpick inserted in middle comes out clean. Remove from oven and cool cake.

7. While cake is cooling, prepare frosting by beating together frosting ingredients until light and creamy.

8. Cover cake with frosting and serve.

Nutritional information: 448 calories, 4.3 grams protein, 75 grams carbohydrates, 15.9 grams fat, 51.4 milligrams cholesterol, 322 milligrams sodium, 1.2 grams fiber, 44 milligrams calcium, 1 milligrams iron.

Tips: For a festive touch, sprinkle cake with toasted coconut or finely ground walnuts.

Creating Your Own Gluten-Free Recipes

Learning how to create gluten-free recipes allows you to easily prepare delicious, healthy meals every day. It also can save you a lot of money! Recipe development can be as simple or gourmet as you want it to be. Even if you haven't been much of a cook before, you'll find that taking it one step at a time will bring very satisfying results.

So How Do You Get Started?

Step 1: Pick up a basic all-purpose cookbook (I suggest one of the classics, such as *Fannie Farmer*, *The Joy of Cooking*, or *Good Housekeeping*). Any of these will give you a leg up in regard to basic techniques, cooking times, and so forth. You'll also find inspirations for combining different ingredients. Although typical cookbooks will include gluten-containing ingredients, the cooking methods will help you as you develop your own gluten-free recipes. Carol Fenster's book *1000 Gluten-Free Meals*, is a great gluten-free addition to your cooking library that provides 1,000 gluten-free versions of classic recipes. Having a basic all-purpose cookbook and Carol's book can give you a lot of options and tips to choose from. As you get comfortable, you may want to add to this basic library other books on different types of cuisine.

Step Two: Make a list of your favorite foods, whether you know how to make them or not. Add to your list other types of recipes you'd like to learn to prepare.

Step Three: For your first attempts, start with simple recipes so that you will be able to be successful from the beginning. You can build up to more challenging dishes from there.

Example

You love chicken and fruit, and you're looking to develop a recipe that includes both. You picked up some chicken thighs and pineapple at the supermarket, and you're ready to get started. Open your all-purpose cookbook to check cooking times and temperatures for the chicken. Decide which seasonings appeal to you, and be sure you have these on hand. Let's say that for the chicken you decide to use olive oil, garlic, onion powder, salt, and pepper. In addition, you have found a recipe for fruit salsa in your cookbook that you can alter a little, using your pineapple in place of the other fruit suggestions. Your dish will be "Baked Chicken with Pineapple Salsa," and on the side you've decided to serve rice and steamed broccoli. So the recipe would go as follows:

Baked Chicken with Pineapple Salsa   Serves 4

3 chicken thighs
1 Tb olive oil
¼ tsp garlic powder
¼ tsp onion powder
1/8 tsp pepper
¼ tsp salt

Pineapple Salsa   Serves 4

1 cup fresh pineapple, chopped
½ cup red onion, chopped
1 small jalapeno pepper, chopped
¼ tsp salt
Dash of pepper
½ cup cilantro, chopped
1 Tb olive oil
Juice of one lime

1. Preheat oven to 350 degrees.

2. In a casserole dish place chicken, drizzle with olive oil, sprinkle with garlic, onion powder, salt, and pepper.

3. Roast chicken for about 30 minutes, until chicken is cooked through and golden brown.

4. While chicken is cooking, prepare salsa by combining all salsa ingredients in a medium bowl.

5. Serve salsa over baked chicken with a side of rice and steamed broccoli.

These development techniques can be used for almost any recipe. Gluten-free baking can be a bit trickier, so it is best to take already-tested and successful gluten-free baking recipes and use them as your base. Pick gluten-free flour blends like those found in Chapter 5 to ensure a happy result.

If you bravely choose to develop your own gluten-free flour blends, it is important to understand how to combine flours in order to achieve the best results. Gluten-free flours generally produce denser breads, so adding a lighter starch to the blend can be helpful to obtain a desirable texture. Starches such as tapioca or potato starch work well when incorporated into the gluten-free flour blend to lighten things up. For improving texture, 1–2 tsp xanthan gum or expandex (usually about 1 tsp to every 2–3 cups of gluten-free flour blend) should be added to provide a better rise in your final product. Sometimes you'll need to adjust the amount of flour or modify the rising time of a recipe to get better results. Bread recipes work best when they include higher-protein selections (such as bean flours, eggs, milk, and cheese) that help provide an even better overall texture.

Dessert recipes usually work very well using the gluten-free flour combinations, but cakes usually require a little extra starch in the flour blend. The trick is starting with some basic skills, picking your favorite foods, and—above all—being creative and having fun.

Dining Out without Gluten

Tips for Stress-Free Dining Out

Dining out is supposed to be an enjoyable experience. For the gluten-free diner, it is also one of the greatest challenges; after all, this is when you have the least control over the food preparation and the least access to food labels for review. Because food is the basis of most social and business interactions, this is more than a little nuisance, and it is difficult to avoid. In order to make dining out easier for you, it is essential to have an understanding of how restaurants work.

Restaurants are usually busy places, and asking for special requests can be difficult or uncomfortable, especially when the staff is in a rush and have little time to listen to your questions. Some establishments don't make any provisions for those with special needs, and specific menus do not allow for any alterations or substitutes without tacking on an extra charge for each change or addition.

The fact is that most restaurants are truly afraid of people with food allergies or intolerances; the last thing that they want is for someone to get sick in their establishment. They would rather just give you plain unseasoned foods than take a chance of giving you a food that may be unsafe. Sometimes they may be so uncomfortable or overwhelmed by the restrictions that apply to creating a gluten-free dish that they may even make you feel unwelcome.

Of course, all you are looking for is a delicious, safe meal. When placing your order, you are not looking to draw a lot of attention to yourself or to make a scene. You just want them to listen to your requests and bring back something amazing from the kitchen. Of course, this is less likely to happen in restaurants that have cooks with little experience and establishments that use mostly prepared broths, soups, sauces, and gravies.

In order to make sure you have a pleasant dining experience, try to call restaurants (or look them up online) prior to your visit and get a copy of their menu. When you call, ask to speak to the manager and be sure to call off-hours (for example, the middle of the afternoon, after the lunch rush and before dinner service); when they are not busy, and they will be able to talk to you without being rushed. Selecting your meal will always be easier if you have identified gluten-free foods prior to your arrival at the restaurant. A night out is supposed to be fun, and it shouldn't feel like a chore. Some restaurants are clearly more amenable to special requests than others, so try to choose those whenever you can. It's win–win when you give your business to establishments that make you feel most welcome.

It's a given that, at times, your restaurant experience will be rocky— be patient. And when you have a great meal, show the chef and wait staff that you appreciate it by thanking them and tipping generously. The following list offers many suggestions to make it easier for you when ordering gluten-free choices.

SIMPLE TIPS WHEN DINING OUT

- Check with local celiac support groups for restaurant suggestions.
- Select restaurants that have gluten-free menus; there are many listed in the resource section at the end of this book.
- Review the restaurant's menu ahead of time.
- Call ahead and speak to the manager or chef to find out whether they can provide you with safe and delicious selections. Call in the middle of the afternoon, when they are more likely to be slow and can answer all your questions.

- Try to avoid restaurants that may have a higher risk of cross-contamination, such as those who prepare bakery items in the same area where other foods are being made.
- It takes more care for a restaurant to prevent cross-contamination, so try to dine out when the restaurant is less busy, either early or late in the evening.
- Bring a copy of the gluten-free dining sheets found in this chapter, making it easier for the chef to provide you with safe selections.
- Explain to the server that you will become ill if particular care is not taken with your food.
- Send back food that has been contaminated with gluten, breadcrumbs, croutons, etc. Let them know that removing or scraping off the problem food will not be enough to keep you from getting sick.

A Look Inside a Restaurant Kitchen

Even when a restaurant is trying to accommodate special requests, they may have equipment and space constraints that make it difficult to provide the level of safety you need.

First, some kitchens are very small, and all foods may be prepared within the same area. It may be impossible to separate pots and utensils, or even to find a separate safe counter area in order to prepare your food. On busy nights, chefs will be racing around so fast that the risk of cross-contamination will be huge. Even when they are trying to offer food choices that are not contaminated with gluten, it is easy to make a mistake.

Evaluate your restaurant choices carefully, and when it appears that space may be an issue during the food preparation, it is better to dine out during slow times when it is easier for the chef to keep your food isolated from gluten-containing ingredients and utensils that have been used in prepping unsafe foods.

Also, take into consideration the equipment used to prepare the food; a restaurant that cooks foods in individual sauté pans has more control over each dish served. Nevertheless, with a restaurant that uses premarinated meats and sauces, preparing everything on the same grill, with the same tongs, it is difficult to impossible for them to accommodate those who have food intolerances or allergy issues.

Chain restaurants often have specific operating procedures for every recipe, often using premixed seasoning blends and preprepped foods, so it could be difficult for them to make many adjustments to their selections. Try calling their corporate offices prior to your visit for additional support. In addition, when you visit a chain restaurant that has a gluten-free menu and find when you arrive that the wait staff is uninformed about it, you should treat this restaurant just like one that doesn't have a gluten-free menu. After all, the menu can only be safe if those serving you are aware of cross-contamination issues.

Safe Choices to Order

Even if a restaurant has a gluten-free menu and knowledgeable staff, asking questions is necessary. Often larger establishments have high staff turnovers, and they may not adequately train everyone equally in terms of their gluten-free offerings. In these types of situations, a mistake can be made. Double-check when each course is served, asking about toppings, sauces, sides, and garnishes to make sure something wasn't mistakenly added to your food. You may feel a little uncomfortable about doing this, but remember: you are out for an enjoyable experience, and you don't want to get sick.

D's Dieting Dilemmas

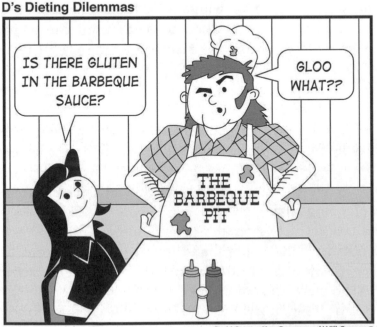

By M Brown Ken Brown and Will Cypser ©

Because wheat, flour, bread, and soy sauce are where most gluten is lurking, it is sometimes easier to just say that you are allergic to wheat, flour, bread, and soy sauce than to explain all the details about the gluten-free diet. Remember that in restaurants barley is most commonly found in salad dressings and in desserts as malt, and rye is mostly found in bakery goods, so avoiding these items can make it possible to meet your needs without overwhelming the kitchen.

If you say, "I can't eat wheat, flour, bread, and soy sauce," and your waiter replies, "Do you mean gluten?" you know immediately that you are ahead of the game.

In general, when ordering from a typical menu, try to avoid pre-pared sauces, dressings, or broths that are not made completely from scratch. In Chapter 5, you'll find some ways to dress up foods when there are no safe seasonings and sauces available at the restaurant. Generally, safe foods will include salads, plain veggies, meat, pork, chicken, and fish. Using the dining-out cards found in this chapter will help the chef understand what you can or can't eat. Sometimes just providing the information to the restaurant is enough for them to prepare many safe options for you. When you feel you are in an establishment that really isn't going to take your requests seriously, stick to plain food and jazz it up yourself.

The Gluten-Free Traveler

When traveling for business, it's likely you'll take part in meetings, group meals, or even buffets at which choices may be limited. In these cases, it is best to research ahead of time. If flying, call the airline and see whether they can provide gluten-free meals on long flights. Because most airlines now offer very few food options, always carry snacks with you. Even if the airline has promised you a gluten-free meal, you'll want to carry gluten-free snacks just in case. Good travel choices include gluten-free bars, trail mix, cereals, and individual cheese sticks. If you are taking a road trip, carry a cooler with salads, fresh fruit, gluten-free cereal, gluten-free wraps, and cold cuts. If possible, try to book a hotel that has a mini kitchen so you can stock up on favorites, making it easier to put together gluten-free meals. If a hotel with a mini kitchen is not available, ask if you can get a small refrigerator in your room. Let the hotel staff know it is for medical reasons—they will be more likely to accommodate you. For a list of dining and travel resources, see Chapter 15.

D's Dieting Dilemmas

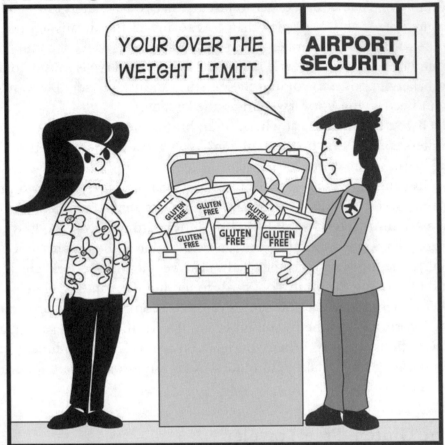

By M Brown Ken Brown and Will Cypser ©

Find out what restaurant choices will be available in your hotel, and research gluten-free restaurants in the area. To find gluten-free restaurants in the United States, go to www.glutenfreerestaurants.org or contact the local celiac support groups.

For business meetings, see if you can order special meals for your meetings prior to arrival. If you are unable to make any requests ahead of time and find that you are in an environment where you do not feel comfortable asking a lot of questions, request that your food be prepared as plain as possible, without sauces or marinades, and spice it up with some of the suggestions in Chapter 5.

If travel is for pleasure, you'll likely have more flexibility. You might look into gluten-free tour groups—several are listed in the resource section at the end of this book. If traveling with a traditional tour group or cruise, I recommend that you not book your trip unless they can guarantee a gluten-free menu will be available at all your meals. This doesn't means a buffet, or a preselected dinner, but a gluten-free menu. Some groups will say that the tour director will accommodate you, but this can mean anything from you getting a great meal to having the same choice over and over, to having no choice at all every time you dine out. Part of the enjoyment of traveling is sampling foods, especially in other countries. If you are paying the same money as everyone else, you should be taken care of properly.

In order to make it easier when traveling abroad, I have put together a listing of international celiac organizations that can help you find gluten-free choices wherever you go. It is delightful to discover that there are many gluten-free restaurants throughout the world.

International Celiac Organizations

Argentina: www.celiac.org.ar
Australia: (Coeliac Society of South Australia): www.coeliac.org.au
Australia: (The Coeliac Society of NSW): www.nswcoeliac.org.au
Australia: (The Queensland Coeliac Society): www.qld.coeliac.org.au
Austria: www.zoeliakie.or.at
Belgium: www.coeliakie.be; www.vcv.coeliakie.be
Bermuda: +1 441 232 0264
Brazil: www.acelbra.org.br
Canada: www.celiac.ca
French Canada: www.fqmc.org
Chile: www.coacel.cl
Croatia: www.celiac.inet.hr
Czech Republic: www.coeliac.cz
Denmark: www.coeliaki.dk
Finland: www.keliakia.org
France: www.afdiag.org
Germany: www.dzg-online.de
Greece: www.koiliokaki.com
Hungary: www.coeliac.hu
Ireland: www.coeliac.ie
Israel: www.celiac.org.il
Italy: www.celiachia.it
Luxemburg: www.alig.lu

Mexico: www.celiacosdemexico.com

Netherlands: www.coeliakievereniging.nl

New Zealand: www.coeliac.co.nz

Norway: www.ncf.no

Pakistan: www.celiac.com.pk

Portugal: www.celiacos.org.pt

Poland: www.celiakia.org.pl

Russia: www.celiac.spb.ru

Slovenia: www.drustvo-celiakija.si

Spain: www.celiacos.org

Spain: (S.M.A.P. Celiacs de Catalunya): www.celiacscatalunya.org

Sweden: www.celiaki.se

Switzerland: www.zoeliakie.ch; www.coeliakie.ch; www.celiachia.ch

United Kingdom: www.coeliac.co.uk

Uruguay: www.acelu.org

When Dining Out

In general, unless a restaurant has a gluten-free menu,

Avoid

- Anything that could be thickened with flour

- Breaded foods

- Casseroles

- Cream sauces

- Creamed soups

- Croutons

- Flour-coated food

- Gravies

- Imitation seafood

- Soups that have base added (unless the stock is 100 percent home-made)

Question

- Fried food (unless from a dedicated fryer)
- Marinades and basting agents
- Salad dressings
- Sauces

Safe

- 100 percent dairy
- Fresh fruits and vegetables
- Meat, chicken, and fish (except self-basting or marinated)
- Vegetable oils and added fat
- Wine, herbs, and pure spices such as garlic and onion powder

Gluten-Free Cards for Easier Dining Out

In order to help chefs understand more about what is safe for you to eat, I have created the following dining-out sheets in 14 different languages. They include lists of safe and unsafe food choices that are specific to each country. They can be copied directly from this book or downloaded and printed from http://glutenfreehasslefree.com/facts/living/cards.asp. Some establishments will be more willing than others to explore gluten-free choices with you, so there are two types of dining-out sheets available. One is simple and to the point and should be used in busy restaurants when you just want them to understand some of the basics about gluten-free eating. The second sheet is for those restaurants that are willing to put more effort into providing you with a special meal. These detailed dining sheets provide different foods that are specific to that culture and are provided in both English and the native language. These cards can also help you to identify safe food choices for each cuisine, making it easier to select gluten-free selections when traveling.

Gluten-Free Meal Card   English

To the Chef:
　　I am on a medically required diet and need special assistance with my meal. I cannot eat wheat and gluten (gluten is found in wheat, rye, and barley) . Even the smallest amount of gluten can make me sick, and therefore I must avoid any food, sauce, or garnish containing gluten and any of its byproducts, including wheat flour, oats, breadcrumbs, soy sauce, bouillon cubes and purchased stocks, teriyaki sauce, commercial seasoning blends, marinades, and sauces (unless they are labeled gluten-free) .I can safely eat fruits, vegetables, rice, quinoa, buckwheat, amaranth, corn, potatoes, peas, legumes, millet, chicken, red meats, fish, eggs, dairy products, fats and oils, distilled vinegars, and homemade stocks and gravies, as long as they are not cooked with wheat flour, breadcrumbs, or sauce.
　　Please prepare my food in a way that avoids cross-contamination with wheat. Use fresh water separate oil, pots, pans, and utensils. If you are not sure about an ingredient that the food contains, please let me know and I may be able to give you more information.
　　Thank you for helping me to have a safe and pleasant dining experience.

Gluten-Free Meal Card   English

To the Chef:

I am on a medically required diet and need to know how my food is prepared. I cannot eat wheat and gluten (gluten is found in wheat, rye, and barley). Even the smallest amount of gluten can make me sick, and therefore I must avoid any food, sauce, or garnish containing gluten and any of its by products. If you are not sure if a menu item, recipe, or ingredient contains gluten, please let me know and I may be able to give you more information.

Foods that I can safely eat include:
- Beef, fish, lamb, pork, duck, goose and other poultry, rabbit, seafood, tofu and most soy products (except soy sauce made with wheat)
- Eggs
- 100% natural dairy products
- Fruits and juices, vegetables, including canned tomato products
- All beans, legumes, nuts, including peanut butter and nut butters
- Amaranth, buckwheat, corn, millet, certified gluten-free oats, potatoes, rice, quinoa, sorghum, and teff
- Homemade stocks and broths (without added wheat)
- Butter, margarine, and vegetable oils
- Pure spices and herbs, distilled vinegars that do not contain malt, wheat-free soy sauce
- Distilled alcohol, wine

Foods that I cannot safely eat (unless they have been checked to be gluten-free) include:
- Some luncheon and processed meats, self-basting poultry, artificial bacon bits, imitation crab meat
- Seasoning blends, modified wheat starch, soy sauce, teriyaki sauce, hydrolyzed vegetable protein, Worcestershire sauce
- Bouillon cubes, canned stocks and broth, packaged soup and soup bases, gravies, cream sauces, and some marinades
- Salad dressings and sauces that include malt or any gluten-containing byproduct
- Barley, bread, bulgur, couscous, orzo, pasta, rye, semolina, spelt, stuffing, tabouli, wheat, wheat germ
- Beer

If a label says that a food product was made on equipment that processes wheat, rye, or barley, I cannot eat it. If the label lists malt or barley, I cannot eat it.

In the preparation of my food:

Please prepare my food in a safe way to avoid cross-contamination with wheat, rye, and barley. Use fresh water and separate oil, pots, pans, colanders, and utensils.

Thank you for preparing my meal in a creative way that includes safe foods so I can have a wonderful dining experience.

Gluten-Free Meal Card   Arabic

To the chef:

I am on a medically required diet and need special assistance with my meal. I cannot eat wheat and gluten (gluten is found in wheat, rye and barley). Even the smallest amount of gluten can make me sick and therefore I must avoid any food, sauce or garnish containing gluten and any of its byproducts including wheat flour, oats, breadcrumbs, soy sauce, bouillon cubes and purchased stocks, teriyaki sauce, commercial seasoning blends, marinades and sauces (unless they are labeled gluten free).

I can safely eat fruits, vegetables, rice, quinoa, buckwheat, amaranth, corn, potatoes, peas, legumes, millet, sorghum and nuts, chicken, red meats, fish, eggs, dairy products, fats and oils, distilled vinegars, and homemade stocks and gravies, as long as they are not cooked with wheat flour, breadcrumbs or sauce.

Please prepare my food in a way that avoids cross contamination with wheat. Use fresh water, separate oil, pots, pans and utensils. If you are not sure about an ingredient that the food contains, please let me know and I may be able to give you more information.

Thank you for helping me to have a safe and pleasant dining experience.

Arabic

إلى رئيس الطهاة:

انا أتّبع نظام غذائيه ُوصى عليه طبياً و أحتاج مساعدة خاصة في وجباتي. أنا محظور عن تناول منتجات القمح والغلوتين (الغلوتين هي مادة بروتينية توجد في الدقيق و الشعير) حتى اقل آمية من الغلوتين تضرّني صحياً و لذلك يجب علىَّ تجنُّب أي طعام أو مرقة أو توابل تحتوي على هذه المادة أو أياً من منتجاتها مثل دقيق الخبز أوالبليلة أوالشعير أوفتات الخبز أوصلصة الصويا أومكعبات مرقة الدجاج أوخلطة التوابل أومرق نقع قطع اللحم أو الخل (إلا إذا آان مطبوع عليها علامةخالي من الغلوتين) أستطيع أآل الفواآه والخضروات والأرز وحبة الحنطة والذرة والبطاطس والبازلاء والبقوليات والسرغوم والمكسرات والدواجن واللحوم والسمك والبيض ومنتجات الألبان والمواد الدهنية والزيوت ومرقة اللحم والشربة المنزلية طالما تم طبخها بدون دقيق أوفتات الخبز أوالصلصة. أرجوإعداد طعامي بما لا يدع مجالاً لخلط أي نوع من الدقيق. أرجوإستعمال ماء نقي وزيوت نقية وأدوات وأوعية معقمة. إن لم تكن متيقناً من محتويات أي من مقادير الطعام أرجو أن تُخبرني فبإستطاعتي إعطاءك معلومات أآثر.
شكرآ لمساعدتي على تناول طعام صحِّي وشهي.

Gluten Free Meal Card   Arabic

To the Chef:

I am on a medically required diet and need to know how my food is prepared. I cannot eat wheat and gluten (gluten is found in wheat, rye and barley). Even the smallest amount of gluten can make me sick, and therefore I must avoid any food, sauce, or garnish containing gluten, and any of its byproducts. If you are not sure if a menu item, recipe or ingredient contains gluten, please let me know and I may be able to give you more information.

Foods that I can safely eat include:

- Beef, fish, lamb, pork, poultry, seafood, tofu and most soy products
- Eggs
- Dairy products, yogurt
- Fruits and juices, baba ganoush, all vegetables including cabbage, eggplant, okra, zucchini, and canned tomato products
- All beans, chick peas, legumes, lentils, seeds and nuts including: peanut butter, nut butters, hummus, tahini
- Potatoes, rice
- Homemade stocks and broths (without added wheat)
- Butter, margarine, olives, olive, sesame and vegetable oil
- Pure spices and herbs, distilled vinegars that do not contain malt, wheat free soy sauce
- Distilled alcohol, wine

Foods that I cannot safely eat (unless they have been checked to be gluten free) include:

- Any meat or seafood that has been dusted or dredged in wheat flour or basted with wheat flour based marinades, ground meat patties (kafta), meat pastries (sambousik)
- Bread, bulgur, cracked wheat, couscous, egg noodles, falafel made with wheat flour, pancakes, pastries such as baklava, pita, porridge made with wheat, semolina and anything made with semolina such as easter cakes
- Seasoning blends, modified wheat starch, soy sauce, teriyaki sauce, hydrolyzed vegetable protein, Worcestershire sauce
- Bouillon cubes, canned stocks and broth, packaged soup and soup bases, gravies, cream sauces and some marinades
- Salad dressings, and sauces that include malt or any gluten containing byproduct
- Beer

If a label says that a food product was made on equipment that processes wheat, rye or barley, I cannot eat it. If the label says malt or barley, I cannot eat it.

In the Preparation of my Food:

Please prepare my food in a safe way to avoid cross contamination with wheat, rye, and barley. Use fresh water, separate oil, pots, pans, colanders and utensils.

Thank you for preparing my meal in a creative way that includes safe foods so I can have a wonderful dining experience.

بطاقة الوجبة الخالية من الغلوتين   **Arabic**

إلى رئيس الطهاة:

انا اُتّبع نظام غذائي مُوصى عليه طبياً وأرغب في معرفة طريقة إعداد طعامي. انا محظور عن تناول منتجات القمح والغلوتين (الغلوتين هي مادة بروتينية توجد في الدقيق و الشعير) حتى أقل آمية من الغلوتين تضرّني صحياً و لذلك يجب علىَّ تجنُّب أي طعام أو مرقة أو توابل تحتوي على هذه المادة أو أياً من منتجاتها. إن لم تكن متيقناً من إحتواء أياً مما في قائمة الطعام أوبوصفة الطهي أوالمقادير على مادة الغلوتين، أرجوأن تُخبرني فبإستطاعتي إعطاءك معلومات آأثر.

الغذاء الآمن المسموح تناوله:

- اللحوم، الاسماك، الضأن، لحم الخنزير، الدواجن، الوجبات البحرية ومعظم منتجات الصويا.
- البيض
- منتجات الالبان والزبادي اللبنة
- الفوآلة والعصير، آل الخضروات مثل الكرنب والباذنجان والبامية والقرع ومعلبات الطماطم، بابا غنوج، آل الخضروات مثل الكرنب والباذنجان والبامية والقرع ومعلبات الطماطم
- آل أنواع البقوليات مثل الفول والبازلاء والعدس واللّب والمكسّرات آاللوز وزبدة الفول السوداني والحمُص و الطحينة
- البطاطس والارز
- المرقة المنزلية (بدون إضافة لمنتجات القمح)
- السمن، الزبدة، زيت الزيتون والسمسم وزيت الخضروات
- التوابل والاعشاب النقية والخل الخالي من الشعيرالمنقوع وصلصة الصويا الخلية من الشعير
- النبيذ والمشروبات الكحولية المرشحة

الغذاء المحظور تناوله (إلا إذا آان عليه علامة خالي من الغلوتين) يشمل:

- أي من اللحوم أوالوجبات البحرية المغمّسة أوالمرشوشة أو المطعَّمة بدقيق القمح أو المغمّسة بماء النقع المخلوط بدقيق القمح أوالكُفتة أوالسمبوآة
- الخبز بأنواعه وحبوب القمح والكُسكس والشعرية والفلافل المحتوية على الدقيق والفطائر والحلويات آالبقلاوة والجلاش والكُنافة والعصيدة المصنوعة بالقمح والسميد والسميد لباب الدقيق وأي شئ مصنوع بلباب الدقيق مثل آعك العيد
- عصارات النكهة ونشاة الدقيق المعالج وصلصة الصويا وصلصة الدواجن وبروتينات الخضروات المحللة بالماء والصلصة الحريفة بالخل والتوابل
- مكعبات المرقة والشربة والمرقة المعلبة أوالمحفوظة أوالمر آزة وصلصة مرقة اللحم وصلصة القشدة وبعض أنواع مرقة الغموس
- مزيج توابل السلطة أو المرقة المحتوية على الشعير النابت أو أي من منتجات الغلوتين
- البيرة

لا أستطيع تناول أي عبوة إذا آانت علامة المعلب تشير أن المُنتج مصنوع بأدوات مستعملة في إعداد دقيق الخبز أو البليلة ولا أستطيع تناول أى عبوة تحتوي على الشعير النابت أو البليلة

عند إعداد طعامي:

أرجوإعداد طعامي بما لايدع مجال لخلط أي نوع من الدقيق أوالقمح أو البليلة. أرجو إستعمال ماء نقي وزيوت مرشحة وأدوات ومصافي مُعقَّمة.

شكراً جزيلاً على إعداد وجبتي بطريقة مبتكرة وآمنة لكي أستمتع بطعام صحي وشهي.

Gluten-Free Meal Card   Chinese

To the chef:

I am on a medically required diet and need special assistance with my meal. I cannot eat wheat and gluten (gluten is found in wheat, rye and barley). Even the smallest amount of gluten can make me sick and therefore I must avoid any food, sauce or garnish containing gluten and any of its byproducts including wheat flour, oats, breadcrumbs, soy sauce, bouillon cubes and purchased stocks, teriyaki sauce, commercial seasoning blends, marinades and sauces (unless they are labeled gluten free).

I can safely eat fruits, vegetables, rice, quinoa, buckwheat, amaranth, corn, potatoes, peas, legumes, millet, sorghum and nuts, chicken, red meats, fish, eggs, dairy products, fats and oils, distilled vinegars, and homemade stocks and gravies, as long as they are not cooked with wheat flour, breadcrumbs or sauce.

Please prepare my food in a way that avoids cross contamination with wheat. Use fresh water, separate oil, pots, pans and utensils. If you are not sure about an ingredient that the food contains, please let me know and I may be able to give you more information.

Thank you for helping me to have a safe and pleasant dining experience.

Traditional Chinese

致廚師：

　　在醫學上，我被指定遵循特殊的飲食需要和幫助。我不能食用麥類和麩類的食物(小麥，黑麥和大麥含有麩類)。既使是最小量的麩類也會使我惡心，因此我不得不避免任何含有麩類的食品，湯及配料，任何可能含有麩類的副產品包括麥粉，燕麥，面包屑，醬油，牛肉和雞肉湯，及各种湯料，腌和醬食品(除非他們是標明不含麩類食品)。

對我安全的食物有：水果，蔬菜，大米，黎，喬麥，莧菜，玉米，馬鈴薯，豌豆，豆類，小米，高粱和堅果，雞肉，紅肉類，魚，蛋，乳制品，脂肪和油類，蒸餾水，自制湯料和鹵汁。只要上述食物不与小麥面粉，面包屑，湯汁同煮即可。

在准備我的食物時，請避免与小麥產品及副產品接觸。請用淡水，單獨的烹調油，平底鍋，盤及餐具。如果你對任何食物的所含原料不确定，請告訴我。我可以提供更多的信息給你。

感謝你為我提供一個既安全又愉快的用餐經歷。

Gluten Free Meal Card   Traditional Chinese

To the Chef:

I am on a medically required diet and need to know how my food is prepared. I cannot eat wheat and gluten (gluten is found in wheat, rye and barley). Even the smallest amount of gluten can make me sick, and therefore I must avoid any food, sauce, or garnish containing gluten, and any of its byproducts. If you are not sure if a menu item, recipe or ingredient contains gluten, please let me know and I may be able to give you more information.

Foods that I can safely eat include:
- Beef, fish, lamb, pork, duck, goose and other poultry, rabbit, seafood, tofu, and most soy products (except soy sauce made with wheat)
- Eggs
- Dairy products
- Fruits and juice, vegetables, coconut, bean sprouts
- All legumes, beans, nuts, peanut butter
- Rice, rice noodles, spring roll wrappers that are 100% rice
- Homemade stocks and broths (that do not contain wheat)
- Pure spices and herbs, distilled vinegars that do not contain malt, wheat free soy sauce, fish sauce
- Oils
- Distilled alcohol, wine

Foods that I cannot safely eat (unless they have been checked to be gluten free) include:
- Imitation crab meat, seitan and artificial meat substitutes
- Chinese crispy noodles, egg roll wrappers, egg or wheat based noodles or dishes that contain these noodles such as lo mein and chow mein, fortune cookies, pancakes, spring roll wrappers that are not 100% rice, wonton wrappers
- Any foods with a flour based coating or breadcrumbs or pastry coating such as sesame chicken or sweet and sour chicken
- Any foods containing a sauce that has been thickened with wheat flour
- Seasoning blends (that have not been checked for gluten), Chinese five spice seasoning mixes, hoisin sauce, plum sauce, some barbecue sauces, soy sauce, tamari sauce, teriyaki sauce
- Bouillon cubes, canned stocks and broths, packaged soup bases, some marinades, rice and malt vinegar, beer, food additives, hydrolyzed vegetable protein

If a label says that a food product was made on equipment that processes wheat, rye or barley, I cannot eat it. If the label says malt or barley, I cannot eat it.

In the Preparation of my Food:

Please prepare my food in a safe way to avoid cross contamination with wheat, rye, and barley. Use fresh water, separate oil, pots, pans, colanders and utensils.

Thank you for preparing my meal in a creative way that includes safe foods so I can have a wonderful dining experience.

不含麩類食物卡 (中文) Traditional Chinese

致廚師：

在醫學上，我有特殊的飲食要求。我需要知道我的食物是如何制作的。我不能食用含有麥類和麩類的食物 (麥類存在于小麥，黑麥和大麥產品 中)。既使是最小量的麩類也會使我惡心，因此我不得不避免任何含有麩類及其副產品的食品，醬油和湯汁 。如果你對任何一個菜單，菜譜及原材 料是否含有麩類不确定，請告訴我，我或許能提供更多的信息給你。

對我安全的食物包括：

- 牛肉，魚，羊肉，豬肉，鴨子，鵝及其他家禽，兔肉，海鮮，豆腐和大多數的豆制品 (除 外用小麥制作的醬油)．
- 雞蛋
- 乳制品
- 水果及水果汁，蔬菜，椰子，豆芽
- 所有豆類，各色堅果，花生醬
- 大米，米粉，用100%大米粉制作的春卷皮
- 自家制作的不含麩類的湯料
- 純香料和香草，不含有麥芽的蒸餾醋，不含麥粉的醬油，魚子醬
- 油類
- 蒸餾酒和葡萄酒

對我不安全的食物有(除非這些食物被證實是不含麩類的產品)：

- 人工蟹肉，seitan和人工肉類替代品
- 中國油炸面條，春卷皮，蛋或小麥面粉制作的面條及其含這類面條的食品，例如：撈面, chowmei, 簽語餅，烙餅，不是100%純米粉的春卷，及混沌皮
- 所有用小麥面粉包裹的食物，面包屑及糕點，例如：芝麻雞和甜酸雞
- 任何用小麥面粉做添稠劑的醬油
- 食品調味劑 (未經檢驗麩類含量的)，含5种香料的調味劑，hoisin 醬，李子醬，一些燒烤
- 醬汁，醬油，tamari 調味汁，teriyaki調味汁
- 罐裝湯汁，袋裝醬料，一些腌菜，米及麥芽醋，啤酒，食品添加劑，水解植物蛋白 如果商標證明此种食物曾經用處理過小麥，黑麥和大麥的器械，那么我不能食用。

如果商標上顯示該食品為麥芽或大麥，我也不能食用。

如何准備我的食物：

在准備我的食物時，請避免接觸任何含有小麥，黑麥和大麥的用俱。用淡水，單獨的油，鍋，盤，過濾用 品及餐具。

非常感激你能用具有創新性的途徑，為我准備安全的食品，讓我享受這美好的就餐体驗。

Gluten-Free Meal Card   French

To the Chef:

I am on a medically required diet and need special assistance with my meal. I cannot eat wheat and gluten (gluten is found in wheat, rye, and barley). Even the smallest amount of gluten can make me sick, and therefore I must avoid any food, sauce, or garnish containing gluten and any of its byproducts, including wheat flour, oats, breadcrumbs, soy sauce, bouillon cubes and purchased stocks, teriyaki sauce, commercial seasoning blends, marinades, and sauces (unless they are labeled gluten-free) .

I can safely eat fruits, vegetables, rice, quinoa, buckwheat, amaranth, corn, potatoes, peas, legumes, millet, chicken, red meats, fish, eggs, dairy products, fats and oils, distilled vinegars, and homemade stocks and gravies, as long as they are not cooked with wheat flour, breadcrumbs, or sauce.

Please prepare my food in a way that avoids cross-contamination with wheat. Use fresh water, separate oil, pots, pans, and utensils. If you are not sure about an ingredient that the food contains, please let me know and I may be able to give you more information.

Thank you for helping me to have a safe and pleasant dining experience.

French

Pour la Cuisine:

Je suis à un régime médicalement prié et ai besoin de l'aide spéciale avec mon repas. Je ne peux pas manger le blé et le gluten (du gluten est trouvé dans le blé, le seigle et l'orge) . Même un peu de gluten peut me faire le malade et donc je moût éviter n'importe quelle nourriture, sauce ou garnis contenant le gluten et n'importe lequel de ses sous-produits comprenant la farine de blé, l'avoine, la chapelure, la sauce de soja, les cubes en bouillon et les stocks achetés, la sauce à teriyaki, les mélanges commerciaux d'assaisonnement, les marinades et les sauces (à moins qu'ils sont marqués gluten libre).

Je peux sans risque manger des fruits, des légumes, riz, quinoa, sarrasin, amaranthe, maïs, des pommes de terre, des pois, des légumineuses, millet, sorgho et des écrous, poulet, des viandes rouges, des poissons, des oeufs, des produits laitiers, des graisses et des pétroles, des vinaigres distillés, et des stocks et des sauces au jus faits maison, tant que ils ne sont pas faits cuire avec la farine de blé, la chapelure ou la sauce.

Veuillez préparer ma nourriture d'une manière dont évite la contamination transversale avec du blé. Utilisez l'eau doux, le pétrole séparé, les pots, les casseroles et les ustensiles. Si vous n'êtes pas sûr au sujet d'un ingrédient que la nourriture contient, faites-le moi savoir et je peux pouvoir te fournir plus d'information.

Merci de m'aider à avoir une expérience dinante sûre et plaisante.

Gluten-Free Meal Card   French

To the Chef:

I am on a medically restricted diet and need to know how my food is prepared. I cannot eat wheat and gluten (gluten is found in wheat, rye, and barley) . Even the smallest amount of gluten can make me sick, and therefore I must avoid any food, sauce, or garnish containing gluten and any of its byproducts. If you are not sure if a menu item recipe or ingredient contains gluten, please let me know and I may be able to give you more information.

Foods that I can safely eat include:
- Beef, fish, pork, poultry, seafood, tofu, and most soy products
- Eggs
- Dairy products
- Fruits and juices, vegetables, including canned tomato products
- All beans, legumes, nuts, including peanut butter and nut butters
- Potatoes, rice
- Homemade stocks and broths (without added wheat)
- Butter, margarine, olives, olive and vegetable oils
- Pure spices and herbs, distilled vinegars that do not contain malt, wheat-free soy sauce
- Distilled alcohol, wine

Foods that I cannot safely eat (unless they have been checked to be gluten-free) include:
- Chicken, beef, pork, or seafood that has been dredged or dusted with wheat flour, breaded with breadcrumbs, or dipped in a wheat-flour batter such as chicken français, chicken cordon bleu, imitation crabmeat, artificial bacon bits, dried sausage
- Baguette, bread, croissants, crepes (made from wheat flour) , pasta and pastries
- Seasoning blends, modified wheat starch, soy sauce, teriyaki sauce, hydrolyzed vegetable protein, Worcestershire sauce
- Au gratin, bechamel, beurre marie, bouillon cubes, packaged stocks and broths, cream soups and sauces, some salad dressings, fondues thickened with wheat flour
- Beer

If a label says that a food product was made on equipment that processes wheat, rye, or barley, I cannot eat it. If the label says malt or barley, I cannot eat it.

In the preparation of my food:

Please prepare my food in a safe manner in order to avoid cross-contamination with wheat, rye, and barley. Use fresh water and separate oil, pots, pans, colanders, and utensils.

Thank you for preparing my meal in a creative way using safe foods so that I may have a wonderful dining experience.

Gluten-Free Meal Card   Français/French

Pour la Cuisine:

Je suis sur un régime alimentaire médicalement nécessaires et ont besoin de savoir comment ma nourriture est préparée. Je ne peux pas manger le blé et le gluten (le gluten est présent dans le blé, le seigle et l'orge) . Même la plus petite quantité de gluten peut me rendez malade, et donc je dois éviter toute nourriture, de sauce, garnir ou contenant du gluten, et l'un de ses sous-produits. Si vous n'êtes pas sûr si un élément de menu, la recette ou un ingrédient contenant du gluten, s'il vous plaît laissez-moi savoir et je mai être en mesure de vous donner de plus amples informations.

Les aliments que je peux manger les suivants:
- Bœuf, poisson, porc, volaille, fruits de mer, tofu et la plupart des produits à base de soja
- Oeufs
- Les produits laitiers
- Fruits et jus de fruits, légumes, y compris les produits à base de tomate en conserve
- Tous les haricots, les légumineuses, les noix, y compris: le beurre d'arachide et beurres de noix
- Pommes de terre, riz
- Stocks et bouillons maison (sans blé)
- Beurre, margarine, olives, huile d'olive et les huiles végétales
- Pure épices et des herbes, des vinaigres distillée ne contenant pas de malt, le blé libre de la sauce de soja
- De l'alcool distillé, de vin

Les aliments que je ne peux pas manger sans danger (sauf si elles ont été vérifiées pour être sans gluten) sont les suivants:
- Poulet, bœuf, porc ou fruits de mer qui a été dragué ou saupoudrée de farine de blé, pané avec des miettes, ou trempé dans une pâte de farine de blé francais comme le poulet, le poulet cordon bleu, crabe d'imitation, artificielles morceaux de bacon, saucisson
- Baguette, pain, croissants, des crêpes (à base de farine de blé) , les pâtes et les pâtisseries
- Mélanges assaisonnements, amidon de blé modifié, la sauce soya, sauce teriyaki, protéines végétales hydrolysées, la sauce Worcestershire
- Au gratin, sauce béchamel, beurre marie, cubes de bouillon, emballés stocks et bouillons, soupes et sauces crème, des sauces à salade, fondue épaissie avec de la farine de blé
- Bière

Si une étiquette d'un produit alimentaire a été faite sur le matériel que les processus de blé, le seigle ou l'orge, je ne peux pas manger. Si l'étiquette indique de malt ou d'orge, je ne peux pas manger.

Dans la préparation de mon alimentation:

S'il vous plaît préparer mes repas d'une manière sûre d'éviter la contamination croisée avec le blé, le seigle et l'orge. L'utilisation d'eau douce, de séparer l'huile, casseroles, ustensiles et colanders.

Merci pour la préparation de mon repas d'une manière créative de sécurité qui comprend des aliments de sorte que je puisse avoir une belle expérience culinaire.

Gluten-Free Meal Card   German

To the Chef:

I am on a medically required diet and need special assistance with my meal. I cannot eat wheat and gluten (gluten is found in wheat, rye, and barley). Even the smallest amount of gluten can make me sick, and therefore I must avoid any food, sauce, or garnish containing gluten and any of its byproducts, including wheat flour, oats, breadcrumbs, soy sauce, bouillon cubes and purchased stocks, teriyaki sauce, commercial seasoning blends, marinades, and sauces (unless they are labeled gluten-free).

I can safely eat fruits, vegetables, rice, quinoa, buckwheat, amaranth, corn, potatoes, peas, legumes, millet, sorghum, nuts, chicken, red meats, fish, eggs, dairy products, fats and oils, distilled vinegars, and homemade stocks and gravies, as long as they are not cooked with wheat flour, breadcrumbs, or sauce.

Please prepare my food in a way that avoids cross-contamination with wheat. Use fresh water and separate oil, pots, pans, and utensils. If you are not sure about an ingredient that the food contains, please let me know and I may be able to give you more information.

Thank you for helping me to have a safe and pleasant dining experience.

German

An den Kochlch ernähre mich nach einer medizinisch erforderlichen Diät und benötige spezielle Hilfe mit meiner Mahlzeit. Ich kann nicht Weizen und Gluten (Gluten wird im Weizen, im Roggen und in der Gerste gefunden) essen. Selbst eine kleine Menge an Gluten kann mich krank machen und folglich muß ich jede Nahrung, Soße oder Beilage die Gluten und ihre Nebenprodukte wie Weizenmehl, Hafer, Brotkrumen, Sojasoße, Brühwürfel und gekaufte Brühen, Teriyaki Soße, handelsübliche Gewürzmischungen, Marinaden und Soßen enthält, meiden (es sei denn sie sind als Gluten-frei beschriftet).

Ich kann Früchte, Gemüse, Reis, Reismelde, Buchweizen, Amarant, Mais, Kartoffeln, Erbsen, Hülsenfrüchte, Hirse, Sorghum und Nüsse, Huhn, rotes Fleisch, Fisch, Eier, Milchprodukte, Fette und Öle, destillierten Essig und selbstgemachte Brühen und Soßen sicher essen, solange sie nicht mit Weizenmehl, Brotkrumen oder Soße gekocht werden.

Bereiten Sie bitte meine Nahrung in einer Weise zu, die Querkontamination mit Weizen vermeidet. Benutzen Sie frisches Wasser und trennen Sie Öle, Töpfe, Pfannen und Küchenutensilien. Falls Sie sich nicht über eine Zutat sicher sind die in der Nahrung enthalten ist, fragen Sie mich bitte und ich kann Ihnen mehr Information geben.

Vielen Dank da_ sie mir dabei helfen, eine sichere und angenehme Mahlzeit zu geniessen.

Gluten-Free Meal Card   German

To the Chef:

I am on a medically restricted diet and need to know how my food is prepared. I cannot eat wheat and gluten (gluten is found in wheat, rye, and barley). Even the smallest amount of gluten can make me sick, so I must avoid any food, sauce, or garnish containing gluten or any of its byproducts. If you are not sure whether a menu item, recipe, or ingredient contains gluten, please let me know and I may be able to give you more information.

Foods that I can safely eat include:
- Beef, bratwurst (gluten-free), fish, kielbasa, pork, poultry such as chicken and turkey, seafood, and most soy products
- Eggs
- Dairy products
- Fruits and juice, vegetables, cabbage, canned tomato products
- All legumes, beans, nuts
- Rice, potatoes, potato salad (made with distilled vinegar)
- Homemade stocks and broths (that do not contain wheat)
- Pure spices and herbs, distilled vinegars that do not contain malt
- Butter, margarine, and vegetable oils
- Distilled alcohol, wine

Foods that I cannot safely eat (unless they have been checked to be gluten-free) include:
- Beer brats
- Meats that have been dusted or dredged in flour such as Weiner Schnitzel and Sauerbraten
- Blintzes, bread, kuchen (cake), kugel, potato dumplings, quark, spaetzle
- Any foods containing a sauce that has been thickened with wheat flour
- Seasoning blends, some barbecue sauces, gravies and sauces thickened with wheat flour
- Bouillon cubes, canned stocks and broths, packaged soup mixes, some marinades, rice and malt vinegar, food additives, salad dressing, some mustards
- Beer and lagers

If a label says that a food product was made on equipment that processes wheat, rye, or barley, I cannot eat it. If the label says malt or barley, I cannot eat it.

In the preparation of my food:

Please prepare my food in a safe way to avoid cross-contamination with wheat, rye, and barley. Use fresh water and separate oil, pots, pans, colanders, and utensils.

Thank you for preparing my meal in a creative way that includes safe foods so I can have a wonderful dining experience.

Gluten-Freie Mahlzeit Karte   Deutsch/German

An den Koch:

Ich ernähre mich nach einer medizinisch erforderlichen Diät und muß wissen, wie meine Nahrung zubereitet wird. Ich kann nicht Weizen und Gluten (Gluten wird im Weizen, im Roggen und in der Gerste gefunden) essen. Selbst eine kleine Menge an Gluten kann mich krank machen, und folglich muß ich jegliche Nahrung, Soße oder Beilage vermeiden die Gluten enthält oder eines ihrer Nebenprodukte. Sollten Sie sich nicht sicher sein, ob ein Gericht auf der Speisekarte, ein Rezept oder eine Zutat Gluten enthält, informieren Sie mich bitte und ich kann Ihnen mehr Auskunft geben.

Nahrungsmittel, die ich sicher essen kann, schließen ein:

Rindfleisch, Bratwurst (Gluten-frei) , Fisch, Polnische Wurst, Schweinefleisch, Geflügel wie Huhn und Truthahn, Meeresfrüchte und die meisten Sojaprodukte

*   Eier
*   Milchprodukte
*   Früchte und Saft, Gemüse, Kohl, Tomatenprodukte aus der Dose
*   Alle Hülsenfrüchte, Bohnen, Nüsse
*   Reis, Kartoffeln, Kartoffelsalat (mit destilliertem Essig angerührt)
*   Selbstgemachte Brühen und Suppen (die nicht Weizen enthalten)
*   Reine Gewürze und Kräuter, destillierter Essig, der nicht Malz enthält
*   Butter, Margarine und Pflanzenöle
*   Destillierter Alkohol, Wein

Nahrungsmittel, die ich nicht sicher essen kann (es sei denn es wurde geprüft, da_ sie kein Gluten beinhalten), schließen ein:

Bratwürste

*   Fleisch, das mit Mehl bestäubt oder im Mehl gewendet wurde wie Wiener Schnitzel und Sauerbraten
*   Pfannenkuchen, Brot, Kuchen, Kartoffelklöße, Quark, Spätzle
*   Alle Nahrungsmittel die eine Soße enthalten, die mit Weizenmehl verdickt worden ist
*   Gewürzmischungen, einige Grill-Soßen, Bratensoßen und Soßen die mit Weizenmehl verdickt wurden
*   Brühwürfel, Brühen und Suppen aus der Dose, handelsübliche Fertigsuppen, einige Marinaden, Reis- und Malzessig, Nahrungsmittelzusätze, Salatsoßen, einige Senfe
*   Bier und Lagerbier

Wenn ein Aufkleber sagt, daß ein Nahrungsmittel mit Geräten zubereitet wurde, die auch Weizen, Roggen oder Gerste verarbeiten, kann ich es nicht essen. Wenn der Aufkleber Malz oder Gerste sagt, kann ich es ebenfalls nicht essen.

Zur Zubereitung meiner Nahrung:

Bitte bereiten Sie meine Nahrung auf eine sichere Art und Weise zu, um Querkontamination mit Weizen, Roggen und Gerste zu vermeiden. Benutzen Sie frisches Wasser, trennen sie Öl, Töpfe, Pfannen, Siebe und Utensilien.

Vielen Dank dafür, da_ Sie mein Essen auf eine kreative Weise zubereiten die sichere Nahrungsmittel einschließt, so da_ ich eine wundervolle Mahlzeit genie_en kann.

Gluten-Free Meal Card   Greek

To the chef:

I am on a medically required diet and need special assistance with my meal. I cannot eat wheat and gluten (gluten is found in wheat, rye and barley). Even the smallest amount of gluten can make me sick and therefore I must avoid any food, sauce or garnish containing gluten and any of its byproducts including wheat flour, oats, breadcrumbs, soy sauce, bouillon cubes and purchased stocks, teriyaki sauce, commercial seasoning blends, marinades and sauces (unless they are labeled gluten free).

I can safely eat fruits, vegetables, rice, quinoa, buckwheat, amaranth, corn, potatoes, peas, legumes, millet, sorghum and nuts, chicken, red meats, fish, eggs, dairy products, fats and oils, distilled vinegars, and homemade stocks and gravies, as long as they are not cooked with wheat flour, breadcrumbs or sauce.

Please prepare my food in a way that avoids cross contamination with wheat. Use fresh water, separate oil, pots, pans and utensils. If you are not sure about an ingredient that the food contains, please let me know and I may be able to give you more information.

Thank you for helping me to have a safe and pleasant dining experience.

Greek

Προς τον μάγειρα / chef:

Βρίσκομαι σε μια αυστηρή ιατρική δίαιτα και χρειάζομαι ειδική βοήθεια όσον αφορά το γεύμα μου. Δεν μπορώ να φάω σιτάρι και γλουτένη (η γλουτένη βρίσκεται στο σιτάρι, στη σίκαλη και στο κριθάρι). Ακόμη και το μικρότερο ποσό γλουτένης μπορεί να με κάνει να αρρωστήσω και επομένως πρέπει να αποφύγω οποιαδήποτε φαγητό, σάλτσα ή γαρνίρισμα που περιέχει γλουτένη και οποιοδήποτε από τα υποπροϊόντα της, συμπεριλαμβανομένου του σιτάλευρου, της βρώμης, των τριμμένων φρυγανιών, της σάλτσας σόγιας, των κύβων σούπας και των αγορασμένων ζωμών, της σάλτσας τεριγιάκι, των εμπορικών μιγμάτων καρυκευμάτων, των μαρινάδων και των σαλτσών (εκτός κι αν αναγράφουν στην ετικέτα ότι δεν περιέχουν γλουτένη).

Μπορώ ακίνδυνα να φάω φρούτα, λαχανικά, ρύζι, κινόα, μπακγουήτ, αμάρανto, καλαμπόκι, πατάτες, μπιζέλια, όσπρια, κεχρί, σόργο και καρύδια, κοτόπουλο, κόκκινα κρέατα, ψάρια, αυγά, γαλακτοκομικά προϊόντα, λίπη και έλαια, αποσταγμένο ξίδι, και τα σπιτικούς ζωμούς και τους ζωμούς, εφ' όσον δεν μαγειρεύονται με αλεύρι σίτου, τριμμένες φρυγανιές ή σάλτσα.

Παρακαλώ προετοιμάστε το γεύμα μου με τέτοιο τρόπο ώστε να αποφευχθεί η μόλυνση από το σιτάρι. Χρησιμοποιήστε καθαρό νερό, λάδι, δοχεία, τηγάνια και εργαλεία. Εάν δεν είστε βέβαιοι για ένα συστατικό που τα τρόφιμα περιέχουν, παρακαλώ ενημερώστε με και μπορώ να είμαι σε θέση να σας δώσω περισσότερες πληροφορίες.

Gluten Free Meal Card   Greek

To the Chef:

I am on a medically required diet and need to know how my food is prepared. I cannot eat wheat and gluten (gluten is found in wheat, rye and barley). Even the smallest amount of gluten can make me sick, and therefore I must avoid any food, sauce, or garnish containing gluten, and any of its byproducts. If you are not sure if a menu item, recipe or ingredient contains gluten, please let me know and I may be able to give you more information.

Foods that I can safely eat include:
- Beef, fish, goat, lamb, pork, poultry, seafood, tofu and most soy products
- Eggs
- Dairy products, yogurt
- Fruits and juices, baba ganoush, all vegetables including cabbage, eggplant, grape leaves, zucchini, and canned tomato products
- All beans, fava beans, legumes, seeds and nuts including: peanut butter, nut butters, tahini
- Potatoes, rice
- Homemade stocks and broths (without added wheat)
- Butter, margarine, olives, olive and vegetable oil
- Pure spices and herbs, distilled vinegars that do not contain malt, wheat free soy sauce
- Distilled alcohol, wine

Foods that I cannot safely eat (unless they have been checked to be gluten free) include:
- Any meat or seafood that has been dusted or dredged in wheat flour or basted with wheat flour based marinades
- Bread, egg noodles, phyllo, pita, or any items made with these such as baklava, gyros, pastries, pies (cheese, meat or vegetable), souvlaki spanakopita
- Seasoning blends, modified wheat starch, soy sauce, teriyaki sauce, hydrolyzed vegetable protein, Worcestershire sauce
- Bechamel sauce, bouillon cubes, canned stocks and broth, packaged soup and soup bases, gravies, cream sauces and some marinades
- Salad dressings, and sauces that include malt or any gluten containing byproduct
- Beer

If a label says that a food product was made on equipment that processes wheat, rye or barley, I cannot eat it. If the label says malt or barley, I cannot eat it.

In the Preparation of my Food:

Please prepare my food in a safe way to avoid cross contamination with wheat, rye, and barley. Use fresh water, separate oil, pots, pans, colanders and utensils. Thank you for preparing my meal in a creative way that includes safe foods so I can have a wonderful dining experience

Κάρτα Γευμάτων Χωρίς Γλουτένη   **Greek**
Προς τον μάγειρα / Σεφ:
    Βρίσκομαι σε μια αυστηρή ιατρική δίαιτα και πρέπει να ξέρω πώς προετοιμάζεται το γεύμα μου. Δεν μπορώ να φάω το σιτάρι και τη γλουτένη (η γλουτένη βρίσκεται στο σιτάρι, τη σίκαλη και το κριθάρι). Ακόμη και το μικρότερο ποσό γλουτένης μπορεί να με κάνει να αρρωστήσω, και επομένως πρέπει να αποφύγω οποιαδήποτε τρόφιμα, σάλτσα, ή γαρνίρισμα που περιέχει γλουτένη και οποιωνδήποτε από τα υποπροϊόντα της. Εάν δεν είστε βέβαιοι για ένα συστατικό του μενού, μια συνταγή ή ένα τρόφιμο περιέχουν γλουτένη, παρακαλώ ενημερώστε με και μπορεί να είμαι σε θέση να σας δώσω περισσότερες πληροφορίες.

Τρόφιμα που μπορώ ακίνδυνα να φάω:
• Βοδινό κρέας, ψάρια, γίδα, αρνί, χοιρινό κρέας, πουλερικά, θαλασσινά, τοφού και τα περισσότερα προϊόντα σόγιας
• Αυγά
• Γαλακτοκομικά προϊόντα, γιαούρτι
• Φρούτα και χυμοί, τραχανάς, όλα τα λαχανικά συμπεριλαμβανομένου του λάχανου, μελιτζάνας, αμπελόφυλλων, κολοκυθιών, και των κονσερβοποιημένων προϊόντων ντομάτας
• Όλα τα φασόλια, φασόλια φάβας, όσπρια, σπόρους και καρύδια συμπεριλαμβανομένων των: φυστικοβούτυρο, βούτυρα καρυδιών, ταχίνι
• Πατάτες, ρύζι
• Σπιτικοί ζωμοί και ζωμοί (χωρίς προστιθέμενο σιτάρι)
• Βούτυρο, μαργαρίνη, ελιές, από ελιά και φυτικό έλαιο
• Καθαρά καρυκεύματα και χορταρικά, αποσταγμένο ξίδι που δεν περιέχει βύνη, σάλτσα σόγιας χωρίς σιτάρι
• Εμφιαλωμένα αλκοολούχα ποτά, κρασί

Τρόφιμα που δεν μπορώ να φάω ακίνδυνα (εκτός αν έχουν ελεγχθεί και είναι χωρίς γλουτένη):
• Οποιοδήποτε κρέας ή θαλασσινά που έχουν βουτηχτεί στο αλεύρι σιταριού ή έχουν ραντιστεί με μαρινάδα βασισμένη σε αλεύρι σιταριού
• Ψωμί, noodles αυγών, φύλλο, πίτα, ή οποιαδήποτε τρόφιμα που γίνονται από αυτά όπως ο μπακλαβάς, γύρος, ζυμαρικά, πίτες (με τυρί, κρέας ή λαχανικό), σπανακόπιτα ή σουβλάκι
• Μίγματα καρυκευμάτων, τροποποιημένο άμυλο σιταριού, σάλτσα σόγιας, σάλτσα τεριγιάκι, υδρολυμένη φυτική πρωτεΐνη, σάλτσα Γουορτσέστεσαηαρ.
• Σάλτσα Μπεσαμέλ, κύβοι σούπας, κονσερβοποιημένοι ζωμοί, συσκευασμένες σούπες και βάσεις σούπας, σάλτσες κρέμας και μερικές μαρινάδες
• Σάλτσες σαλάτας, και σάλτσες που περιλαμβάνουν τη βύνη ή οποιοδήποτε υποπροϊόν που περιέχει γλουτένη
• Μπύρα
    Εάν στην ετικέτα αναγράφει ότι κάποια τρόφιμα έγιναν σε μηχάνημα που επεξεργάζεται το σιτάρι, τη σίκαλη ή το κριθάρι, δεν μπορώ να τα φάω. Εάν η ετικέτα αναγράφει βύνη ή κριθάρι, δεν μπορώ να τα φάω.
Κατά την προετοιμασία των τροφίμων μου:
    Παρακαλώ προετοιμάστε το γεύμα μου με ασφαλή τρόπο ώστε να αποφευχθεί η μόλυνση από το σιτάρι, τη σίκαλη, και το κριθάρι. Χρησιμοποιήστε καθαρό νερό, λάδι, δοχεία, τα τηγάνια, τρυπητά και εργαλεία.
    Σας ευχαριστώ για την προετοιμασία του γεύματός μου με δημιουργικό τρόπο που περιλαμβάνει τα ασφαλή τρόφιμα έτσι ώστε εγώ να μπορώ να έχω μια θαυμάσια εμπειρία δείπνου.

Gluten-Free Meal Card   Hebrew

To the chef:

I am on a medically required diet and need special assistance with my meal. I cannot eat wheat and gluten (gluten is found in wheat, rye and barley). Even the smallest amount of gluten can make me sick and therefore I must avoid any food, sauce or garnish containing gluten and any of its byproducts including wheat flour, oats, breadcrumbs, soy sauce, bouillon cubes and purchased stocks, teriyaki sauce, commercial seasoning blends, marinades and sauces (unless they are labeled gluten free).

I can safely eat fruits, vegetables, rice, quinoa, buckwheat, amaranth, corn, potatoes, peas, legumes, millet, sorghum and nuts, chicken, red meats, fish, eggs, dairy products, fats and oils, distilled vinegars, and homemade stocks and gravies, as long as they are not cooked with wheat flour, breadcrumbs or sauce.

Please prepare my food in a way that avoids cross contamination with wheat. Use fresh water, separate oil, pots, pans and utensils. If you are not sure about an ingredient that the food contains, please let me know and I may be able to give you more information.

Thank you for helping me to have a safe and pleasant dining experience.

Hebrew

לכבוד השף

אני על דיאטה רפואת וצריכה עזרה בהכנת הארוחה. אין באפשרותי לאכל חיטה ועמילן (עמילן נימצא בחיטה, שיפון) גם הכמויות הקטנות הנימצאות בעמילן גורמות לי לחלות ולכן אנני יכולה לאכל עלי להימנע מכל מאכל המכיל עמילן וכל מוצרו כולל קמח לבן, שיבולת שועל, פרורי לחם, רוטב סוייה, קוביות מרק צח, קופסאות שימורים, רוטב טריאקי תארובת תבלינים (אלה עם כן התוית מראה שלא נימצא עמילן)

אני יכולה לאכל פירות, ירקות, אורז, קינואה, כוסמת, חידע, תירס, תפוח אדמה, אפונה, קטניות, דוחן, אגוזים, עוף, בשר אדום, דגים, ביצים, דיברי חלב, שמן ושומנים, חומץ, רוטב ביתי ורוטב בשר כל עוד לא נעשו ובשלו עם קמח או פרורי לחם.

בבקשה להכין עבורי את האוכל ללא תערובת של חיטה להישתמש במים נקיים להפריד שמן מהמחבטים, הסירים והמסננים. אם אתה לא בטוח בקשר למרכיב שהמזון מכיל תידע אותי ואני אוכל לתת לך יותר פרטים.

תודה רבה

Gluten Free Meal Card   Hebrew

To the Chef:

I am on a medically required diet and need to know how my food is prepared. I cannot eat wheat and gluten (gluten is found in wheat, rye and barley). Even the smallest amount of gluten can make me sick, and therefore I must avoid any food, sauce, or garnish containing gluten, and any of its byproducts. If you are not sure if a menu item, recipe or ingredient contains gluten, please let me know and I may be able to give you more information.

Foods that I can safely eat include:
Beef, fish, poultry such as chicken and turkey, seafood, and most soy products
Eggs
Dairy products
Fruits and juice, vegetables, cabbage, canned tomato products
All legumes, lentils, beans, hummus, nuts
Rice, potatoes,
Homemade stocks and broths (that do not contain wheat)
Pure spices and herbs, distilled vinegars that do not contain malt
Butter, margarine and vegetable oils
Distilled alcohol, wine

Foods that I cannot safely eat (unless they have been checked to be gluten free) include:
Meats that have been dusted or dredged in flour or cooked with matzoh meal such as gefilte fish and meatballs
Bagels, blintzes, bread, butter cakes, challah, cookies, couscous, falafel made with wheat flour, knishes, kugel, matzoh, matzoh balls, noodles, potato dumplings, spelt
Any foods containing a sauce that has been thickened with wheat flour
Seasoning blends, some barbecue sauces, gravies and sauces thickened with wheat flour
Bouillon cubes, canned stocks and broths, packaged soup mixes, some marinades, rice and malt vinegar, food additives, salad dressing, some mustards
Beer

If a label says that a food product was made on equipment that processes wheat, rye or barley, I cannot eat it. If the label says malt or barley, I cannot eat it.

In the Preparation of my Food:

Please prepare my food in a safe way to avoid cross contamination with wheat, rye, and barley. Use fresh water, separate oil, pots, pans, colanders and utensils.

Thank you for preparing my meal in a creative way that includes safe foods so I can have a wonderful dining experience.

Hebrew

כרטיס ארוחה ללא עמילן

לכבוד השף

אני בדיאטה רפואית וצריכה לדעת איך מכינים לי את המזון. אני יכולה לאכול מאכלים
העשוים מחיטה ועמילן (עמילן מצוי בחיטה ובגריסים) . אפילו כמות קטנה של עמילן
גורמת לי לחלות עלי להימנע מכל מאכל הכולל עמילן ומצרו. אם אינך בטוח שהתפריט
מכיל עמילן בבקשה לידע אותי בכדי שאוכל לתת לך יותר פרטים.

המאכלים שבאפשרותי לאכול כוללים :
-בשר בקר, דגים, עופות תרנגול והודו, מאכלי ים, ומאכלי סויה למיניהם
-ביצים
-מוצרי חלב
-פירות ומיצים, ירקות, כרוב, ושימורי עגבניות
-קטניות, עדשים שעועים, חומוס, אגוזים
-אורז, תפוח אדמה
-מרק בשר ביתי (שאין בו חיטה)
-תבלינים, עשבי תיבול וחומץ שאינו מכיל בירה שחורה
-חמאה מרגרינה ושמן ירקות
-אלכוהל יין וזוככים

המאכלים שאינם בריאים לי (אלה עם כן נבדקי ולא נמצא בהם עמילן) כולל :
-בשרים שתובלו או בושלו עם קמח או פרורי מצה כמו גפילטפיש וכדורי בשר
-כעכים בליינצ'ס, לחם, עוגת חמאה, חלה, עוגיות, קוס קוס, פלאפל שעשוי עם קמח,
  קוגל, כדורי מצה, איטריות או כל סוגי החיטה
-כל סוג של אוכל עם קמח לבן
-תבלינים מעורבבים חלק מסוגי רוטב ברבקיו ורוטבים שיש בהם קמח
-מרק צח קופסאות שימורים תערובת של אבקת מרק ורוטבים, אורז חומץ שעורה, צבעי
  מאכל ושימור, רוטבי סלט וחרדל למיניהם
-בירה

אם התוית מראה שהמאכל מכיל מוצרי קמח או גריסים אין באפשרותי לאכל .
אם התוית מראה על שעורה או גריסים אין באפשרותי לאכל .

הכנת האוכל
בבקשה להכין את האוכל ולהימנע ממוצרי חיטה שיפון וגריסים השתמשו במים נקיים
להפריד את השמן מהמחבטים והסירים מסננים וכלים .
תודה שהכנתם את הארוחה בצורה שאני יכול לאכול את האוכל בביטחון וללא חשש
ושאוכל להנות .

Gluten-Free Meal Card　Indian (Hindi)

To the chef:

I am on a medically required diet and need special assistance with my meal. I cannot eat wheat and gluten (gluten is found in wheat, rye and barley). Even the smallest amount of gluten can make me sick and therefore I must avoid any food, sauce or garnish containing gluten and any of its byproducts including wheat flour, oats, breadcrumbs, soy sauce, bouillon cubes and purchased stocks, teriyaki sauce, commercial seasoning blends, marinades and sauces (unless they are labeled gluten free).

I can safely eat fruits, vegetables, rice, quinoa, buckwheat, amaranth, corn, potatoes, peas, legumes, millet, sorghum and nuts, chicken, red meats, fish, eggs, dairy products, fats and oils, distilled vinegars, and homemade stocks and gravies, as long as they are not cooked with wheat flour, breadcrumbs or sauce.

Please prepare my food in a way that avoids cross contamination with wheat. Use fresh water, separate oil, pots, pans and utensils. If you are not sure about an ingredient that the food contains, please let me know and I may be able to give you more information.

Thank you for helping me to have a safe and pleasant dining experience.

Hindi

रसोइये के लिए:

मैं एक चिकित्सकीय आवश्यक आहार पर हूँ और मुझे अपने भोजन के साथ विशेष सहायता की जरूरत है. मैं गेहूं और ग्लूटेन (लस) नहीं खा सकता/सकती (ग्लूटेन गेहूं, रागी और जौ में पाया जाता है). ग्लूटेन की थोड़ी सी मात्रा भी मुझे बीमार कर सकती है और इसलिए मुझे ग्लूटेन युक्त कोई भी भोजन, सॉस या सजावट की सामग्री और गेहूं का आटा, ओट्स (जई), ब्रेड के टुकड़े, सोया सॉस, शोरबे के क्यूब्स और खरीदे गए व्यंजन, तेरियाकी सॉस, वाणिज्यिक मसालों के मिश्रण, सिरके और सॉस (जब तक कि उन पर ग्लूटेन मुक्त होने के लेबल ना लगे हों) सहित ग्लूटेन के कोई उप-उत्पाद खाने से बचना चाहिए.

मैं फल, सब्जियाँ, चावल, कीन्वा [quinoa], बकव्हीट (कुट्टू), चौली, मक्का, आलू, मटर, फलीदार सब्ज़ियाँ, बाजरा, ज्वार और मेवा, चिकन, लाल गोश्त, मछली, अंडे, डेयरी उत्पाद, वसा और तेल, आसुत सिरके, और घर के बने व्यंजन और शोरबे सुरक्षित रूप से खा सकता/सकती हूँ, जब तक कि वे गेहूं के आटे, ब्रेड के टुकड़ों या चटनी के साथ पकाए नहीं गए हों.

कृपया मेरा खाना इस प्रकार बनाएँ कि वह गेहूं से संदूषित होने से बचे. ताज़े पानी, अलग तेल, पतीलों, तवों और बर्तनों का इस्तेमाल करें. यदि आप भोजन में शामिल किसी भी सामग्री के बारें में निश्चित रूप से नहीं जानते हैं तो कृपया मुझे बताएँ, शायद मैं आपको और जानकारी दे सकूँ.

मुझे भोजन का एक सुरक्षित और सुखद अनुभव लेने में मदद करने के लिए धन्यवाद.

Gluten Free Meal Card   Indian (Hindi)

To the Chef:

I am on a medically required diet and need to know how my food is prepared. I cannot eat wheat, and gluten (gluten is found in wheat, rye and barley). Even the smallest amount of gluten can make me sick, and therefore I must avoid any food, sauce, or garnish containing gluten, and any of its byproducts. If you are not sure if a menu item, recipe or ingredient contains gluten, please let me know and I may be able to give you more information.

Foods that I can safely eat include:
- Beef, fish, pork, poultry, seafood, tofu and most soy products
- Eggs
- Dairy products, yogurt, coconut milk
- Fruits and juices, coconut, vegetables, including canned tomato products
- All beans, legumes, lentils, split peas, nuts including: peanut butter, and nut butters
- Bhajis (made with 100% chick pea flour), pakoras (made with 100% garbanzo flour), papadum (made with 100% lentil flour), potatoes, rice, sweet potatoes
- Butter, margarine and vegetable oils
- Pure spices and herbs, distilled vinegars that do not contain malt, wheat free soy sauce, homemade stocks and broths (without added wheat)
- Distilled alcohol, wine

Foods that I cannot safely eat (unless they have been checked to be gluten free) include:
- Skewered meat, vegetables and shrimp dusted with wheat flour or wheat flour based marinades
- Bread, chapattis, naan parathas, pooris, roti, samosas
- Hing and spice blends that contain hing, curry powder, curries and chutneys thickened with wheat flour, seasoning blends, modified wheat starch, soy sauce, teriyaki sauce, hydrolyzed vegetable protein
- Bouillon cubes, canned stocks and broth, packaged soup, and soup abd curry bases,
- Salad dressings, and sauces that include malt or any gluten containing byproduct
- Beer
- Food fried in the same oil as wheat and gluten products such as samosas and pooris.

If a label says that a food product was made on equipment that processes wheat, rye or barley, I cannot eat it. If the label says malt or barley, I cannot eat it.

In the Preparation of my Food:

Please prepare my food in a safe way to avoid cross contamination with wheat, rye, and barley. Use fresh water, separate oil, pots, pans, colanders and utensils.

Thank you for preparing my meal in a creative way that includes safe foods so I can have a wonderful dining experience.

Hindi

ग्लूटेन मुक्त भोजन कार्ड   भारतीय (हिंदी)

रसोइये के लिए:

मैं एक चिकित्सकीय आवश्यक आहार पर हूँ और मेरे लिए यह जानना ज़रूरी है कि मेरा खाना कैसे तैयार किया जाता है. मैं गेहूं और ग्लूटेन (लस) नहीं खा सकता/सकती हूँ (ग्लूटेन गेहूं, रागी और जौ में पाया जाता है). ग्लूटेन की थोड़ी सी मात्रा भी मुझे बीमार कर सकती है, और इसलिए मुझे ग्लूटेनयुक्त कोई भोजन, सॉस या सजावट की सामग्री, और उसके कोई भी उप-उत्पाद खाने से बचना चाहिए. यदि आपको निश्चित तौर पर नहीं पता कि मेनू आइटम, व्यंजन या सामग्री में ग्लूटेन है या नहीं, तो कृपया मुझे बताएँ, हो सकता है मैं आपको और जानकारी दे सकूँ.

ऐसे खाद्यपदार्थ जिन्हें मैं सुरक्षित रूप से खा सकता/सकती हूँ:

- बीफ (गाय का गोश्त), मछली, पोर्क (सूअर का गोश्त), पोल्ट्री (अंडे, मुर्गियाँ, बतखें इत्यादि), समुद्री भोजन, टोफू (सोयाबीन का दही) और अधिकतर सोया उत्पाद
- अंडे
- डेयरी उत्पाद, दही, नारियल का दूध
- फल और रस, नारियल, कैन्ड टमाटर उत्पाद सहित सब्ज़ियाँ
- सभी फलियाँ, फलीदार सब्ज़ियाँ, मसूर, मूँग, दालें, मेवे जिनमें: मूंगफली के मक्खन, और मेवे के मक्खन शामिल हैं
- भाजियाँ (100% बेसन से बनी), पकौड़े (100% बेसन से बने), पापड (100% दाल के आटे से बने), आलू, चावल, शकरकंद
- मक्खन, मार्जरीन और वनस्पति तेल
- शुद्ध मसाले और जड़ी बूटियाँ, आसुत सिरके जिनमें मॉल्ट न हो, सोया सॉस जिसमें गेहूँ न हो, घर के बने व्यंजन और शोरबे (जिनमें गेहूँ डाला न गया हो)
- आसुत आल्कोहॉल, वाइन

ऐसे खाद्यपदार्थ जिन्हें मैं सुरक्षित रूप से नहीं खा सकता/सकती (जब तक कि उनके ग्लूटेन मुक्त होने की जाँच ना कर ली गई हो):

- सीख गोश्त, गेहूँ का आटा छिड़की सब्ज़ियाँ और झींगी या गेहूँ के आटे आधारित सिरके
- ब्रेड, चपातियाँ, नान पराठे, पूरियाँ, रोटी, समोसे
- हींग और हींगयुक्त मसालों के मिश्रण, गरम मसाला, गेहूँ के आटे से गाढ़ी बनाई गई सब्ज़ियाँ और चटनियाँ, मसालों के मिश्रण, रूपान्तरित गेहूँ का स्टार्च, सोया सॉस, तेरियाकी सॉस, हाइड्रोलाइज्ड वनस्पति प्रोटीन
- शोरबे के क्यूब्स, कैन्ड व्यंजन और शोरबा, पैकेज्ड सूप और सूप व सब्ज़ी का गूदा
- सलाद ड्रेसिंग, और सॉस जिनमें मॉल्ट या कोई ग्लूटेनयुक्त उप-उत्पाद हो
- बीयर
- गेहूँ और ग्लूटेन के उत्पाद तले गए हों उस तेल में तले गए समोसे और पूरियों जैसे खाद्यपदार्थ.

यदि लेबल पर लिखा हो कि खाद्य पदार्थ ऐसे उपकरण पर बनाया गया है जो गेहूँ, रागी [rye] या बार्ली (जौ) को प्रोसेस (प्रसंस्कृत) करता है, तो मैं नहीं खा सकता/सकती. यदि लेबल पर मॉल्ट या बार्ली लिखा हो तो मैं नहीं खा सकता/सकती.

मेरा भोजन तैयार करने से संबंधित:

कृपया मेरा खाना सुरक्षित तरीके से बनाएँ ताकि वह गेहूं, रागी, और जौ से संदूषित होने से बचे. ताज़े पानी, अलग तेल, पतीलों, तवों, छलनियों और बर्तनों का इस्तेमाल करें.

मुझे खाने का एक अद्भुत अनुभव मिल सके इसके लिए सुरक्षित खाद्य पदार्थों का इस्तेमाल करके सृजनात्मक तरीके से मेरा खाना तैयार करने के लिए धन्यवाद.

Gluten-Free Meal Card   Italian

To the Chef:

I am on a medically required diet and need special assistance with my meal. I cannot eat wheat and gluten (gluten is found in wheat, rye, and barley) . Even the smallest amount of gluten can make me sick, and therefore I must avoid any food, sauce, or garnish containing gluten and any of its byproducts, including wheat flour, oats, breadcrumbs, soy sauce, bouillon cubes and purchased stocks, teriyaki sauce, commercial seasoning blends, marinades, and sauces (unless they are labeled gluten-free).

I can safely eat fruits, vegetables, rice, quinoa, buckwheat, amaranth, corn, potatoes, peas, legumes, millet, sorghum, nuts, chicken, red meats, fish, eggs, dairy products, fats and oils, distilled vinegars, and homemade stocks and gravies, as long as they are not cooked with wheat flour, breadcrumbs, or sauce.

Please prepare my food in a way that avoids cross-contamination with wheat. Use fresh water and separate oil, pots, pans, and utensils. If you are not sure about an ingredient that the food contains, please let me know and I may be able to give you more information.

Thank you for helping me to have a safe and pleasant dining experience.

Italian

Allo Chef:

Sono in una dieta medicamente richiesta e ho bisogno di una assistenza speciale per il mio pasto. Non posso mangiare il frumento ed il glutine (il glutine si trova nel frumento, nella segale e nell' orzo) . Anche la più piccola quantità di glutine può farmi male e quindi devo evitare tutto l'alimento, e qualsiasi condimento contenente glutine e ogni suo relativo sottoprodotto, compresi la farina di frumento, avena, pangrattato, salsa di soia, estratti di brodo comprati, salsa di teriyaki, miscele commerciali di condimento, marinate e salse (a meno che siano identificati libero da glutine) .

Posso mangiare con sicurezza gli ortofrutticoli, riso, quinoa, grano saraceno, amaranto, mais, patate, piselli, legumi, miglio, sorgo e nocciole, pollo, carni rosse, pesci, uova, latticini, grassi e olii, aceti distillati, brodi e sughi casalighi, purche non siano cucinati con la farina di frumento, il pangrattato o la salsa.

Per favore prepara il mio cibo in in modo da evitare la contaminazione trasversale con frumento. Utilizza acqua fresca, separare l'olio le pentole e gli utensili. Se non siete sicuri circa un ingrediente che l'alimento contiene, per favore fatemelo sapere cosi' posso darvi piu' informazioni.

Grazie per il vostro aiuto nel farmi avere una piacevole e sicura esperienza culinaria.

Gluten-Free Meal Card   Italian

To the Chef:

I am on a medically required diet and need to know how my food is prepared. I cannot eat wheat and gluten (gluten is found in wheat, rye, and barley) . Even the smallest amount of gluten can make me sick, and therefore I must avoid any food, sauce, or garnish containing gluten and any of its byproducts. If you are not sure if a menu item, recipe, or ingredient contains gluten, please let me know and I may be able to give you more information.

Foods that I can safely eat include:
- Beef, fish, goat, lamb, pork, poultry, seafood, wild boar, tofu, and most soy products
- Eggs
- Dairy products
- Fruits and juices, vegetables (including canned tomato products)
- All beans, legumes, and nuts, including peanut butter and other nut butters
- Polenta, potatoes, rice, risotto
- Homemade stocks and broths (without added wheat)
- Butter, margarine, olives, olive and vegetable oils
- Pure spices and herbs, distilled vinegars that do not contain malt, wheat-free soy sauce
- Distilled alcohol, wine

Foods that I cannot safely eat (unless they have been checked to be gluten-free) include:
- Any meat or seafood that has been dredged or dusted with wheat flour, breaded with breadcrumbs, or dipped in a wheat flour batter, such as piccata, scallopini, marsala, and parmesan, some processed meat, meatballs, imitation crabmeat, artificial bacon bits
- All breads, bulgur, cakes, pastas, and pastries made with wheat flour, durum, semolina, and spelt
- Seasoning blends, modified wheat starch, soy sauce, teriyaki sauce, hydrolyzed vegetable protein, Worcestershire sauce
- Alfredo sauce, cream sauces, gravies, some marinades, bouillon cubes, packaged stocks and broths, cream soups, some salad dressings
- Beer

If a label says that a food product was made on equipment that processes wheat, rye, or barley, I cannot eat it. If the label says malt or barley, I cannot eat it.

In the preparation of my food:

Please prepare my food in a safe way to avoid cross-contamination with wheat, rye, and barley. Use fresh water and separate oil, pots, pans, colanders, and utensils.

Thank you for preparing my meal in a creative way that includes safe foods so I can have a wonderful dining experience.

Scheda libera del pasto del glutine   Italiano/Italian

Allo Chef:

Sono in una dieta medicamente richiesta e devo sapere come il mio alimento è preparato. Non posso mangiare il frumento ed il glutine (glutine si trova nel frumento, nella segale e nell' orzo) . Anche la più piccola quantità di glutine può farmi male e quindi devo evitare tutto l'alimento, e qualsiasi condimento contenente il glutine e ogni suo sottoprodottoi. Se non siete sicuri circa una voce del menu', una ricetta o un ingrediente contiene glutine, per favore fatemelo sapere cosi posso darvi piu' informazioni.

Gli alimenti che posso mangiare sicuro includono:
- Manzo, pesce, capretto, agnello, maiale, pollame, frutti di mare, cinghiale, tofu e la maggior parte dei prodotti della soia
- Uova
- Latticini
- Frutte e spremute, verdure, compreso i prodotti inscatolati del pomodoro
- Tutti i fagioli, legumi, nocciole compreso: burro di arachidi e burro di nocciole
- Polenta, patate, riso, risotto
- Sughi e brodi casalinghi (senza frumento aggiunto)
- Burro, margarina, olive, olio vegetale e di olive
- Spezie ed erbe pure, aceti distillati che non contengono il malto, salsa di soya non contenente grano
- L'alcool distillato, vino

Alimenti che non posso mangiare con sicurezza (a meno che siano stati controllati e siano esenti da glutine) includono:
- Qualsiasi carne o frutti di mare che sono stati infarinati o impanati con la farina di frumento, con il pangrattato, o sono inzuppati in una pastella di farina di frumento, come per esempio la piccata, le scallopini al marsala ed alla parmigiana, carne preparata come le polpette, imitazione di carne di granchio, punte artificiali di pancetta affumicata
- Tutti i pani, bulgur, torte, paste e dolci fatti con la farina di frumento, grano duro, semolino ed ortografati
- Le miscele di condimento, amido di grano modificato, salsa di soia, salsa di teriyaki, proteine vegetali idrolizzate, salsa del worcestershire
- La salsa Alfredo, le salse cremose, i sughi, alcune marinate, dadi di brodo, brodi confezionatii, le minestre cremose, alcuni condimenti per 'insalata
- Birra

Se un'etichetta dice che un prodotto alimentare è stato fatto su apparecchiatura che trasforma il frumento, la segale o l'orzo, non posso mangiarlo. Se l'etichetta dice il malto o l'orzo, non posso mangiarlo.

Nella preparazione del mio alimento:

Per favore Prepari il mio alimento in un modo sicuro onde evitare la contaminazione trasversale con frumento, segale ed orzo. Utilizzi l'acqua fresca, separe l'olio le pentole i contenitori, gli scolini e gli utensili.

Grazie per la preparazione del mio pasto in un modocreativo e che includa alimenti sicuri per me, in modo tale che io possa avere una meravigliosa esperienza culinaria

Gluten-Free Meal Card   Japanese

To the chef:

I am on a medically required diet and need special assistance with my meal. I cannot eat wheat and gluten (gluten is found in wheat, rye and barley). Even the smallest amount of gluten can make me sick and therefore I must avoid any food, sauce or garnish containing gluten and any of its byproducts including wheat flour, oats, breadcrumbs, soy sauce, bouillon cubes and purchased stocks, teriyaki sauce, commercial seasoning blends, marinades and sauces (unless they are labeled gluten free).

I can safely eat fruits, vegetables, rice, quinoa, buckwheat, amaranth, corn, potatoes, peas, legumes, millet, sorghum and nuts, chicken, red meats, fish, eggs, dairy products, fats and oils, distilled vinegars, and homemade stocks and gravies, as long as they are not cooked with wheat flour, breadcrumbs or sauce.

Please prepare my food in a way that avoids cross contamination with wheat. Use fresh water, separate oil, pots, pans and utensils. If you are not sure about an ingredient that the food contains, please let me know and I may be able to give you more information.

Thank you for helping me to have a safe and pleasant dining experience.

Japanese

シェフの方へ **-Japanese**

私は治療に必要な食事をしているので、その食事に対して特別な助けが必要です。私は小麦とグルテンが摂取できません。（グルテンは小麦、ライ麦、大麦に含まれています。）ほんの少量のグルテンでさえ症状がでてしまうので、グルテンを含む食べ物、ソース、付け合わせを避けなければなりません。グルテンが含まれていないと表示されていない限り、小麦粉、オート麦、パン粉、醤油、ブイヨン、市販のだし、照り焼きソース、そしてさらに市販のブレンド済みの調味料やマリーネード、ソースを含みます。

私は小麦粉やパン粉、ソースを使って調理されてない限り、差し支えなくフルーツ、野菜類、米、キノア、蕎麦、アマランス、とうもろこし、ジャガイモ、豆、豆類、キビ、モロコシ、ナッツ、鶏肉、赤い肉、魚、卵、乳製品、油脂、蒸留酢、自家製のだしやグレービーソースは食べる事ができます。

どうか小麦を使わないで私の食事を作ってください。新鮮な水を使い、油や鍋、フライパンや調理器具も別にしてください。もし、材料の中身が確かでないときは、私にお知らせください。もう少し情報を提供できるかもしれません。
　安全で快適な食事の為にご協力いただきありがとうございます。

Gluten Free Meal Card   Japanese

To the Chef:

I am on a medically required diet and need to know how my food is prepared. I cannot eat wheat and gluten (gluten is found in wheat, rye and barley). Even the smallest amount of gluten can make me sick, and therefore I must avoid any food, sauce, or garnish containing gluten, and any of its byproducts. If you are not sure if a menu item, recipe or ingredient contains gluten, please let me know and I may be able to give you more information.

Foods that I can safely eat include:
- Beef, fish, lamb, pork, duck, goose and other poultry such as chicken and turkey, rabbit, seafood, sushi, sashimi, tofu, and most soy products (except soy sauce made with wheat)
- Eggs
- Dairy products
- Fruits and juice, vegetables, coconut, bean sprouts
- All legumes, beans, nuts, peanut butter
- Rice, rice noodles, soba noodles that are 100% buckwheat, spring roll wrappers that are 100% rice
- Homemade stocks and broths (that do not contain wheat)
- Pure spices and herbs, distilled vinegars that do not contain malt, wheat free soy sauce, fish sauce
- Oils
- Distilled alcohol, wine

Foods that I cannot safely eat (unless they have been checked to be gluten free) include:
- Imitation crab meat, fish cakes, packaged roe, seitan and artificial meat substitutes
- Bread, cookies, gyoza, panko bread crumbs, soba noodles that are not 100% buckwheat, udon
- Any foods with a flour based coating or breadcrumbs or pastry coating such as tempura (unless a 100% rice flour coating is used)
- Any foods containing a sauce that has been thickened with wheat flour
- Seasoning blends, hoisin sauce, plum sauce, some barbecue sauces, soy sauce, tamari sauce, teriyaki sauce

If a label says that a food product was made on equipment that processes wheat, rye or barley, I cannot eat it. If the label says malt or barley, I cannot eat it.

In the Preparation of my Food:

Please prepare my food in a safe way to avoid cross contamination with wheat, rye, and barley. Use fresh water, separate oil, pots, pans, colanders and utensils.

Thank you for preparing my meal in a creative way that includes safe foods so I can have a wonderful dining experience.

シェフの方へ　　**Japanese**

　　　私は、治療に必要な食事をとっています。そしてどのように私の食事が用意されるのかを知る必要がります。私は、小麦とグルテン（グルテンは小麦、ライ麦、大麦に含まれます）を食べる事ができません。ほんの少しの量でさえ症状がでてしまうので、私はグルテンやグルテンからできたものを含むすべての食品、ソース、デコレーションは避けなければなりません。もしあなたが、メニューやレシピ、材料にグルテンが含まれているか分らなければお知らせください。もう少し情報を伝えられるかもしれません。

私が安全に食べられる食品は、以下を含みます。

- 牛肉、魚、豚肉、ひな鳥や七面鳥などの鶏肉類、シーフード、寿司、刺身、豆腐、ほとんどの大豆製品（小麦からできた醤油を除く）
- 卵
- 乳製品
- 果物、ジュース、野菜、ココナッツ、もやし
- すべての豆類、ナッツ類、ピーナッツバター
- 米、ビーフン、そば粉を１００％使用したそば、米１００％で作られた春巻きの皮
- 自家製の出し汁やブイヨンスープ（小麦を含まない）
- 純スパイス、ハーブ、麦芽を含まない蒸留された酢、小麦を含まない醤油、魚のソース
- 油類
- 蒸留されたアルコール、ワイン

私が安全に食べられない食品（グルテンが含まれていないことをチェックされない限り）は以下を含みます。

- カニかまぼこ、つみれ、パッケージされた魚の卵、人工的に作られた肉や人工肉の代用品
- パン、クッキー、餃子、パン粉、１００％のそば粉からできていないそば、うどん
- 小麦粉や、パン粉、パイなどでコーティングしてある食品、例えば天ぷら（米粉１００％のコーティング使われていない限り）
- 小麦粉でとろみをつけたソースを含むすべての食品
- ブレンド調味料、海鮮醤（ハイシェンジャン）、プラムソース、一部のバーベキューソース、醤油、たまり醤油、照り焼きソース

もしラベルに食品が小麦やライ麦、大麦を加工処理する器具で作られていると書いてあれば、私はその食品を食べられません。もしラベルに麦芽や大麦と書いてあったら、私は食べる事ができません。

Gluten-Free Meal Card   Polish

To the Chef:

I am on a medically required diet and need special assistance with my meal. I cannot eat wheat and gluten (gluten is found in wheat, rye, and barley). Even the smallest amount of gluten can make me sick, and therefore I must avoid any food, sauce, or garnish containing gluten and any of its byproducts, including wheat flour, oats, breadcrumbs, soy sauce, bouillon cubes and purchased stocks, teriyaki sauce, commercial seasoning blends, marinades, and sauces (unless they are labeled gluten-free).

I can safely eat fruits, vegetables, rice, quinoa, buckwheat, amaranth, corn, potatoes, peas, legumes, millet, sorghum, nuts, chicken, red meats, fish, eggs, dairy products, fats and oils, distilled vinegars, and homemade stocks and gravies, as long as they are not cooked with wheat flour, breadcrumbs, or sauce.

Please prepare my food in a way that avoids cross-contamination with wheat. Use fresh water and separate oil, pots, pans, and utensils. If you are not sure about an ingredient that the food contains, please let me know and I may be able to give you more information.

Thank you for helping me to have a safe and pleasant dining experience.

Polish

Szef Kuchni:

Jestem na diecie i lekarskie potrzebuję szczególnej pomocy ze swoim posiłkiem. Nie mogę jeść glutenu (glutenu występuje w pszenicy, żyta i jęczmienia) . Nawet najmniejsze ilości glutenu może mnie zrobic chore i dlatego należy unikać wszelkich żywności, sos lub dekorować zawierające gluten i wszystkich jej byproducts w tym mąki pszennej, owsa, sos sojowy kostki i zakupionych zapasów, handlowych przypraw mieszanek, marynat i sosów (chyba że są one odpowiednio oznaczone bezglutenowy) .

Mogę bezpiecznie jeść owoce, warzywa, ryż, quinoa, gryki, amarant, kukurydza, ziemniaki, groch, rośliny strączkowe, proso, sorgo i orzechy, kurczak, czerwonych mięs, ryb, jaj, nabiału, tłuszczów i olejów, destylowanego octu i domowych zapasów i gravies, tak długo jak nie są one gotowane z mąki pszennej, lub sos.

Proszę przygotować moje żywności w taki sposób, aby uniknąć zanieczyszczeń krzyżowych z pszenicy. Używać świezą wodę, oddzielne olej, garnki, patelnie i naczyńia. Jeśli nie jesteś pewien jaki składnik, środek spożywczy zawiera, proszę dać mi znać i mogą być w stanie podać więcej informacji.

Dziękujemy za pomoc mi będę miał bezpieczne i przyjemne odżywianie.

Gluten-Free Meal Card   Polish

To the Chef:

I am on a medically required diet and need to know how my food is prepared. I cannot eat wheat and gluten (gluten is found in wheat, rye, and barley). Even the smallest amount of gluten can make me sick, and therefore I must avoid any food, sauce, or garnish containing gluten and any of its byproducts. If you are not sure if a menu item, recipe, or ingredient contains gluten, please let me know and I may be able to give you more information.

Foods that I can safely eat include:
- Beef, bratwurst (gluten-free), chicken livers, fish, kielbasa, lamb, pork, poultry such as chicken and turkey, seafood, steak tartar, and most soy products
- Eggs
- Dairy products
- Fruits and juice, vegetables, cabbage, canned tomato products
- All legumes, beans, and nuts
- Buckwheat groats, kasza, potatoes, potato salad (made with distilled vinegar) , rice
- Homemade stocks and broths (that do not contain wheat) , borscht (made with wheat-free stock)
- Pure spices and herbs, distilled vinegars that do not contain malt, oils
- Distilled alcohol, wine

Foods that I cannot safely eat (unless they have been checked to be gluten-free) include:
- Beer brats
- Meats that have been dusted or dredged in flour, breaded pork or chicken cutlets, meatloaf
- Blintzes, bread, cake, doughnuts, dumplings, egg noodles, pastry, pierogis, potato pancakes
- Any foods containing a sauce that has been thickened with wheat flour, barley soup, soups thickened with wheat starch or rye
- Beer sauce, seasoning blends, some barbecue sauces, gravies and cream sauces
- Bouillon cubes, canned stocks and broths, packaged soup mixes, some marinades, rice and malt vinegar, food additives, salad dressing, some mustards
- Beer and lagers

If a label says that a food product was made on equipment that processes wheat, rye, or barley, I cannot eat it. If the label says malt or barley, I cannot eat it.

In the preparation of my food:

Please prepare my food in a safe way to avoid cross-contamination with wheat, rye, and barley. Use fresh water and separate oil, pots, pans, colanders, and utensils.

Thank you for preparing my meal in a creative way that includes safe foods so I can have a wonderful dining experience.

Bezglutenowy Meal Card   Polski/Polish

Szef Kuchni:

Jestem na diecie i lekarskie wymagane muszą wiedzieć, w jaki sposób moje jedzenie jest przygotowywane. Nie mogę jeść glutenu (glutenu występuje w pszenicy, żyta i jęczmienia) . Nawet najmniejsze ilości glutenu może mnie zrobic chore, i dlatego należy unikać wszelkich żywność, sos lub dekorować zawierające gluten, a wszelkie jego produkty. Jeśli nie jesteś pewien, czy dieta zawiera glutenu, proszę dać mi znać i mogą być w stanie podać więcej informacji.

Żywność, że mogę bezpiecznie jeść obejmują:
- Wołowiny, Bratwurst (bezglutenowy) , wątróbek z kurczaka, ryby, Kiełbasa, wątröbzka, wieprzowina, drób, takich jak kurczak i indyk, ryba, steyk tatarski, większość produktów sojowych
- Jaja
- Nabiał
- Owoce i sok, warzyw, kapusty, pomidorów konserwowanych produktów Wszystkie rośliny strączkowe, fasola, orzechy
- Gryka kasz, kasza, ziemniaki, sałatka ziemniaczana (wykonane z destylowanego octu) , ryż
- Domowe buliony (które nie zawierają pszenicy) , barszcz (produkowany z pszenicy domowcj)
- Pure przyprawy i zioła, destylowanego octu, które nie zawierają słód, oleJe
- Destylowany alkohol, wino

Żywność, I ktore nie mogę bezpiecznie jeść (chyba że zostały one sprawdzone ze są bezglutenowy) :
- Piwo brats
- Mięso, które zostały posypane mąką, panierowane kotlety wieprzowe lub drobiowe, Meatloaf
- Blintzes, chleb, ciasta, pączki, dumplings jajka makaron, ciasta, pierogis, ziemniaków naleśników
- Wszystkie środki spożywcze zawierające sos, który został zagęszczony z mąki pszennej, jęczmiennej zupy, zupy zagęszczana skrobi z pszenicy lub żyta
- Piwo sos przyprawowy mieszanki, niektóre z grilla sosy, sosy gravies i śmietana
- Bouillon kostek, zapasy konserw i buliony, zupy pakowane mieszanki niektórych marynat, ryżu i słodu ocet, dodatków do żywności, sos sałatkowy, niektóre musztardy
- Piwo

Jeśli etykiety mówi, że product byt żrobiony pszenicy, żyta i jęczmienia, nie mogę go jeść.

W Przygotowanie moje Żywności
Proszę przygotować moje żywności w bezpieczny sposób, aby uniknąć zanieczyszczeń krzyżowych z pszenicy, żyta i jęczmienia. Wykorzystanie wody świeżej oddzielne olej, garnków, patelni i naczyń.

Dziękuje za moje przygotowanie posiłku w twórczy sposób, że obejmuje żywność bezpieczną, więc mogę mieć wspaniały obia

Gluten-Free Meal Card   Spanish

To the Chef:

I am on a medically required diet and need special assistance with my meal. I cannot eat wheat and gluten (gluten is found in wheat, rye, and barley) . Even the smallest amount of gluten can make me sick, and therefore I must avoid any food, sauce, or garnish containing gluten and any of its byproducts, including wheat flour, oats, breadcrumbs, soy sauce, bouillon cubes and purchased stocks, teriyaki sauce, commercial seasoning blends, marinades, and sauces (unless they are labeled gluten-free).

I can safely eat fruits, vegetables, rice, quinoa, buckwheat, amaranth, corn, potatoes, peas, legumes, millet, sorghum, nuts, chicken, red meats, fish, eggs, dairy products, fats and oils, distilled vinegars, and homemade stocks and gravies, as long as they are not cooked with wheat flour, breadcrumbs, or sauce.

Please prepare my food in a way that avoids cross-contamination with wheat. Use fresh water, separate oil, pots, pans, and utensils. If you are not sure about an ingredient that the food contains, please let me know and I may be able to give you more information.

Thank you for helping me to have a safe and pleasant dining experience.

Spanish

Al cocinero:

Estoy en una dieta medicamente requerida y necesito ayuda especial con mi comida. No Puedo comer trigo y/o gluten (el gluten se encuentra en el trigo, centeno y cebada) . Incluso la cantidad mas pequena de gluten puede hacer que me enferme y por lo tanto debo evitar cualquier alimento, salsa o adobo que contengan gluten y/o cualquiera de sus derivados, incluyendo harina de trigo, avena, migajas de pan, salsa de soya, cubos de caldo comprados almacenados, salsa teriyaki, mezclas de condimentos comerciales, adobos y las salsas (amenos que esten etiquetadas libres de gluten) .

Puedo comer con seguridad frutas, vegetales, arroz, quinoa, alforfon, amaranto, maiz, patatas, guisantes, legumbres, mijo, sorgo, nueces, pollo, carnes rojas, pescado, huevos, productos lacteos, grasas, aceites, vinagre destilado, productos almacenados y salsas hechas en casa mientras no se cocinen con harina de trigo, migajas de pan o salsa.

Por favor prepare mi comida de una manera que evite la contaminacion cruzada con trigo. Utilice agua fresca, aceites separados, los potes, las cacerolas, y los utencilios. Si usted no esta seguro de un alimento o ingrediente que este contenga dejeme saber para darle mas informacion.

Gracias por ayudarme a tener una experiencia de cena mas segura y agradable.

Gluten-Free Meal Card   Spanish

To the Chef:
   I am on a medically required diet and need to know how my food is prepared. I cannot eat wheat and gluten (gluten is found in wheat, rye, and barley) . Even the smallest amount of gluten can make me sick, and therefore I must avoid any food, sauce, or garnish containing gluten and any of its byproducts. If you are not sure if a menu item, recipe, or ingredient contains gluten, please let me know and I may be able to give you more information.

Foods that I can safely eat include:
*   Beef, fish, pork, poultry such as chicken and turkey, seafood, and most soy products
*   Eggs
*   Dairy products
*   Fruits and juice, vegetables, canned tomato products, plantains
*   All legumes, beans, nuts
*   Corn tortillas, rice, potatoes
*   Homemade stocks and broths (that do not contain wheat)
*   Pure spices and herbs, distilled vinegars that do not contain malt
*   Oils
*   Distilled alcohol, wine

Foods that I cannot safely eat (unless they have been checked to be gluten-free) include:
*   Any sauce that has been thickened with wheat flour such as mole, enchilada and salsa, and cheese dip
*   Bread, churros, empanadas, flour tortillas
*   Any soup or stew, including gazpacho that has been thickened with breadcrumbs or wheat flour
*   Tapas that contain bread or bread crumbs
*   Spice and seasoning blends, seasoned rice mixes
*   Bouillon cubes, canned stocks and broths, packaged soup mixes, some marinades, rice and malt vinegar, some barbecue sauces, food additives, salad dressing
*   Beer
*   Corn chips that have been fried in the same oil as flour tortillas or other gluten-containing products

If a label says that a food product was made on equipment that processes wheat, rye, or barley, I cannot eat it. If the label says malt or barley, I cannot eat it.

In the preparation of my food:
   Please prepare my food in a safe way to avoid cross-contamination with wheat, rye, and barley. Use fresh water separate oil, pots, pans, colanders, and utensils.
   Thank you for preparing my meal in a creative way that includes safe foods so I can have a wonderful dining experience.

Carta o Menu de comida libre de gluten   Español/Spanish

Al cocinero:
Estoy en una dieta medicamente requerida y necesito saber como esta preparada mi comida. No puedo comer trigo y/o gluten (el gluten se encuentra en el trigo, centeno y cebada) . Incluso la cantidad mas pequeña de gluten puede hacer que me enferme, y por lo tanto debo evitar cualquier comida, salsa o adobo que contengan gluten o cualquiera de sus derivados. Si usted no esta seguro si un articulo del menu, receta o ingrediente contiene gluten, por favor dejeme saberlo para darle mas informacion.

Los alimentos que puedo comer con seguridad son:
- Carne de vaca, pescado, cerdo, aves de corral tales como pollo, pavo, mariscos y la mayoria de los productos de la soya
- Huevos
- Productos lacteos
- Las frutas y jugos, vegetales, productos de tomate en lata, platanos
- Todos los legumbres, frijoles y nueces
- Tortillas de maiz, arroz y patatas
- Productos almacenados y caldos hechos en casa (que no contengan trigo)
- Especies puras y hierbas, vinagres destilados que no contienen malta
- Aceites
- Alcohol destilado y vino

Alimentos que no puedo comer con seguridad (amenos que sean comprobados libres de gluten)
- Cualquier salsa que se haya espesado con harina de trigo tal como topo, enchilada, salsa e inmersion de queso
- Pan, churros, empanadas y tortillas de harina
- Cualquier sopa o guisado, incluyendo el gazpacho que se ha espesado con las migajas de pan o la harina de trigo
- Tapas que contiene el pan o las migajas de pan
- Mezclas de especies y condimentos, mezclas de arroz sasonados
- Cubos de caldos, productos y caldos conservados, mezclas de sopas empaquetadas, algunos adobos de vinagre, del arroz y de la malta, algunas salsas de barbacoa, comidas aditivas y salsas para ensaladas
- Cervesa
- Las virutas de maiz que hayan sido fritas en el mismo aceite que las tortillas de harina u otros productos con gluten

Si una etiqueta dice que un producto alimenticio fue hecho con el mismo equipo que procesa trigo, centeno o cebada, no puedo comerlo. Si la etiqueta dice malta o cebada, no puedo comerlo.

En la preparacion de mi alimento:
Prepare por favor mi alimento de una manera segura y evite la contaminacion cruzada con trigo, centeno, y cebada. Utilice agua fresca, aceites separados, los potes, las cacerolas, los colanders y los utencilios.
Gracias por preparar mi comida de una manera creativa que incluya alimentos seguros para poder tener una experiencia maravillosa de cena.

Gluten-Free Meal Card   Thai

To the chef:

I am on a medically required diet and need special assistance with my meal. I cannot eat wheat and gluten (gluten is found in wheat, rye and barley). Even the smallest amount of gluten can make me sick and therefore I must avoid any food, sauce or garnish containing gluten and any of its byproducts including wheat flour, oats, breadcrumbs, soy sauce, bouillon cubes and purchased stocks, teriyaki sauce, commercial seasoning blends, marinades and sauces (unless they are labeled gluten free).

I can safely eat fruits, vegetables, rice, quinoa, buckwheat, amaranth, corn, potatoes, peas, legumes, millet, sorghum and nuts, chicken, red meats, fish, eggs, dairy products, fats and oils, distilled vinegars, and homemade stocks and gravies, as long as they are not cooked with wheat flour, breadcrumbs or sauce.

Please prepare my food in a way that avoids cross contamination with wheat. Use fresh water, separate oil, pots, pans and utensils. If you are not sure about an ingredient that the food contains, please let me know and I may be able to give you more information.

Thank you for helping me to have a safe and pleasant dining experience.

Thai

ถึง พ่อครัว/แม่ครัว: Thai

ฉันมีความจำเป็นทางการแพทย์ที่จะต้องควบคุมอาหารบางอย่าง และต้องการความช่วยเหลือเป็นพิเศษในการเตรียมอาหารของฉัน ฉันทานข้าวสาลีและกลูเท็นไม่ได้ (กลูเท็นเป็นโปรตีนที่อยู่ในข้าวสาลี ข้าวไรย์ และข้าวบาร์เลย์) ถ้าฉันทานกลูเท็นแม้แต่เพียงนิดเดียวก็ตาม จะทำให้ฉันป่วย ดังนั้นฉันจึงต้องหลีกเลี่ยงอาหาร ซอส หรือของแต่งหน้าทุกชนิดที่มีกลูเท็นเป็นส่วนประกอบ ตลอดจนผลผลิตพลอยได้ทั้งหมดของสิ่งเหล่านี้ ซึ่งได้แก่แป้งสาลี ข้าวโอ๊ต ขนมปังป่น ซอสถั่วเหลือง ซุปก้อน และน้ำซุปที่ซื้อมา ซอสเทอริยากิ ผงปรุงรสต่างๆ ที่จำหน่ายในท้องตลาด ซอสสำหรับหมัก และซอสต่างๆ (เว้นเสียแต่ว่าจะระบุบนฉลากสินค้าว่า "ปลอดกลูเท็น")

ฉันทานผลไม้ ผัก ข้าว ข้าวคีนัว บัควีท ผักโขม ข้าวโพด มันฝรั่ง พืชตระกูลถั่ว พืชฝักตระกูลถั่ว ข้าวเดือย ข้าวฟ่างและถั่วต่างๆ ไก่ เนื้อแดง ปลา ไข่ ผลิตภัณฑ์ที่ทำจากนม ไขมันและน้ำมัน น้ำส้มสายชูกลั่น และซุปและน้ำเกรวี่ที่ทำเองได้ ตราบเท่าที่ไม่ใช้แป้งสาลี ขนมปังป่น หรือซอสในการปรุงอาหารเหล่านี้

กรุณาเตรียมอาหารของฉันโดยไม่ให้มีการปนเปื้อนกับข้าวสาลีเลย ขอให้ใช้น้ำใหม่ และใช้น้ำมัน หม้อ กะทะ และเครื่องมือเครื่องใช้ในการปรุงอาหารแยกต่างหาก ถ้าคุณไม่แน่ใจเกี่ยวกับส่วนผสมในอาหารชนิดหนึ่งๆ กรุณาบอกให้ฉันรู้ เพราะฉันอาจให้ข้อมูลเพิ่มเติมแก่คุณได้

ขอบคุณมากที่ช่วยให้ฉันเพลิดเพลินกับการรับประทานอาหารที่ปลอดภัย

Gluten Free Meal Card   Thai

To the Chef:
    I am on a medically required diet and need to know how my food is prepared. I cannot eat wheat and gluten (gluten is found in wheat, rye and barley). Even the smallest amount of gluten can make me sick, and therefore I must avoid any food, sauce, or garnish containing gluten, and any of its byproducts. If you are not sure if a menu item, recipe or ingredient contains gluten, please let me know and I may be able to give you more information.

Foods that I can safely eat include:
- Beef, lamb, pork, duck, goose and other poultry such as chicken and turkey, fish, rabbit, tofu, and most soy products (except soy sauce made with wheat)
- Eggs
- Dairy products
- Fruits and juice, vegetables, bean sprouts, canned tomato products, coconut
- All beans, legumes, nuts, and peanut butter
- Rice, rice noodles, spring roll wrappers that are 100% rice
- Homemade stocks and broths (that do not contain wheat)
- Pure spices and herbs, distilled vinegars that do not contain malt, wheat free soy sauce, and fish sauce
- Oils
- Distilled alcohol, wine

Foods that I cannot safely eat (unless they have been checked to be gluten free) include:
- Imitation crab meat, seitan and artificial meat substitutes
- Chinese noodles, egg noodles, egg roll wrappers, wonton wrappers,
- Fish or oyster sauce thickened with wheat flour
- Seasoning blends (that have not been checked for gluten), soy sauce, tamari sauce, teriyaki sauce, hydrolyzed vegetable protein
- Bouillon cubes, canned stocks and broths, packaged soup and curry bases, some marinades, rice and malt vinegar
- Beer

If a label says that a food product was made on equipment that processes wheat, rye or barley, I cannot eat it. If the label says malt or barley, I cannot eat it.

In the Preparation of my Food:
    Please prepare my food in a safe way to avoid cross contamination with wheat, rye, and barley. Use fresh water, separate oil, pots, pans, colanders and utensils.
    Thank you for preparing my meal in a creative way that includes safe foods so I can have a wonderful dining experience.

บัตรมื้ออาหารที่ปลอดกลูเท็น ภาษาไทย Thai

ถึง พ่อครัว/แม่ครัว:

ฉันมีความจำเป็นทางการแพทย์ที่จะต้องควบคุมอาหารบางอย่าง และจำเป็นต้องทราบว่าอาหารของ
ฉันได้รับการเตรียมอย่างไร ฉันทานข้าวสาลีและกลูเท็นไม่ได้ (กลูเท็นเป็นโปรตีนที่อยู่ในข้าวสาลี ข้าวไรย์
และข้าวบาร์เลย์) ถ้าฉันทานกลูเท็นแม้แต่เพียงนิดเดียวก็ตาม จะทำให้ฉันป่วย ดังนั้น ฉันจึงต้องหลีกเลี่ยง
อาหาร ซอส หรือของแต่งหน้าทุกชนิดที่มีกลูเท็นเป็นส่วนประกอบ และผลผลิตพลอยได้ทั้งหมดของสิ่ง
เหล่านี้ ถ้าคุณไม่แน่ใจว่ารายการในเมนู สูตรอาหาร หรือส่วนผสมใดมีกลูเท็นเป็นส่วนประกอบหรือไม่ กรุณา
บอกให้ฉันรู้ เพราะฉันอาจให้ข้อมูลเพิ่มเติมแก่คุณได้

อาหารที่ฉันทานได้อย่างปลอดภัย ได้แก่
- เนื้อวัว เนื้อลูกแกะ เนื้อหมู เป็ด ห่าน และสัตว์ปีกอื่นๆ เช่น ไก่ ไก่งวง ปลา กระต่าย เต้าหู้ และ
  ผลิตภัณฑ์จากถั่วเหลืองส่วนใหญ่ (ยกเว้นซอสถั่วเหลืองที่ทำจากข้าวสาลี)
- ไข่
- ผลิตภัณฑ์ที่ทำจากนม
- ผลไม้และน้ำผลไม้ ผัก ถั่วงอก ผลิตภัณฑ์มะเขือเทศบรรจุกระป๋อง มะพร้าว
- พืชตระกูลถั่วทั้งหมด พืชฝักตระกูลถั่ว ถั่ว และเนยถั่ว
- ข้าว ก๋วยเตี๋ยวที่ทำจากข้าว แผ่นแป้งห่อเปาะเปี๊ยะที่ทำจากข้าว 100%
- น้ำซุปและน้ำซุปเนื้อที่ทำเอง (ที่ไม่มีข้าวสาลีเป็นส่วนประกอบ)
- เครื่องเทศและสมุนไพรบริสุทธิ์ที่ไม่มีสิ่งเจือปนใดๆ น้ำส้มสายชูกลั่นที่ไม่มีส่วนผสมของข้าวมอลต์
  ซอสถั่วเหลืองที่ไม่มีข้าวสาลีผสม และน้ำปลา
- น้ำมันต่างๆ
- แอลกอฮอล์กลั่น ไวน์

อาหารที่อาจไม่ปลอดภัยสำหรับฉัน (เว้นเสียแต่ว่าจะได้รับการตรวจแล้วว่าปลอดกลูเท็น) ได้แก่
- ปูอัด หมี่กึง และผลิตภัณฑ์เนื้อสัตว์เทียม
- ก๋วยเตี๋ยวจีน บะหมี่ แผ่นแป้งห่อเปาะเปี๊ยะทอด แผ่นแป้งห่อเกี๊ยว
- น้ำปลาหรือน้ำมันหอยที่ทำให้ข้นด้วยแป้งสาลี
- ผงปรุงรส (ที่ยังไม่ได้รับการตรวจว่ามีกลูเท็นหรือไม่) ซอสถั่วเหลือง ซอสทามาริ ซอสเทอริยากิ
  โปรตีนไฮโดรไลซ์จากพืช
- ซุปก้อน น้ำซุปและน้ำซุปเนื้อบรรจุกระป๋อง ซุปและเครื่องแกงบรรจุห่อ ซอสสำหรับหมักบางชนิด
  และน้ำส้มสายชูที่ทำจากข้าวและข้าวมอลต์
- เบียร์

ถ้าฉลากกำกับเขียนว่า ใช้เครื่องแปรรูปอาหารจำพวกข้าวสาลี ข้าวไรย์ หรือข้าวบาร์เลย์ในการทำ
ผลิตภัณฑ์อาหารนั้น ฉันก็ทานผลิตภัณฑ์นั้นไม่ได้ ถ้าฉลากเขียนว่า ข้าวมอลต์หรือข้าวบาร์เลย์ ฉันก็ทาน
ไม่ได้เช่นกัน

ในการเตรียมอาหารให้แก่ฉัน:

กรุณาเตรียมอาหารของฉันโดยไม่ให้มีการปนเปื้อนกับข้าวสาลี ข้าวไรย์ และข้าวบาร์เลย์เลย ขอให้
ใช้น้ำใหม่ และใช้น้ำมัน หม้อ กะทะ กระชอน และเครื่องมือเครื่องใช้ในการปรุงอาหารแยกต่างหาก

ขอบคุณมากที่เตรียมอาหารของฉันอย่างสร้างสรรค์และปลอดภัยแก่ฉัน เพื่อให้ฉันได้รับ
ประสบการณ์การทานอาหารที่ดี

Gluten-Free Meal Card   Vietnamese

To the chef:

I am on a medically required diet and need special assistance with my meal. I cannot eat wheat and gluten (gluten is found in wheat, rye and barley). Even the smallest amount of gluten can make me sick and therefore I must avoid any food, sauce or garnish containing gluten and any of its byproducts including wheat flour, oats, breadcrumbs, soy sauce, bouillon cubes and purchased stocks, teriyaki sauce, commercial seasoning blends, marinades and sauces (unless they are labeled gluten free).

I can safely eat fruits, vegetables, rice, quinoa, buckwheat, amaranth, corn, potatoes, peas, legumes, millet, sorghum and nuts, chicken, red meats, fish, eggs, dairy products, fats and oils, distilled vinegars, and homemade stocks and gravies, as long as they are not cooked with wheat flour, breadcrumbs or sauce.

Please prepare my food in a way that avoids cross contamination with wheat. Use fresh water, separate oil, pots, pans and utensils. If you are not sure about an ingredient that the food contains, please let me know and I may be able to give you more information.

Thank you for helping me to have a safe and pleasant dining experience.

Vietnamese

Kính gỵi quí vỹ ỵ̈yu bỵp: **Vietnamese**

Do nhu cỵu sỵc khỵe, tôi ỵ̈yỵc yêu cỵu ỵn uỵng theo mỵt chỵ ỵ̈y ỵ̈yc biỵt và cỵn sỵ giúp ỵ̈y cỵa bỵn ỵ̈yi vỵi thỵc ỵ̈yn cỵa tôi. Tôi không thỵ ỵn lúa mì và gluten* (có trong lúa mì, lúa mỵch ỵen và lúa mỵch). Ngay cỵ vỵi mỵt lỵỵng gluten nhỵ nhỵt cỵng có thỵ làm cho tôi bỵ bỵnh và vì vỵy tôi phỵi tránh bỵt kỵ thỵc ỵn, xỵt, hay các lỵai thỵo mỵc dùng ỵ̈y trang trí trên thỵc ỵn có chỵa gluten và các sỵn phỵm phỵ cỵa nó bao gỵm bỵt mì, ỵ̈yn mỵch, ruỵt bánh mì, tỵ̈yng, bỵt nêm súp cô ỵ̈yc và nỵỵc súp hỵp, xỵt teriyaki, bỵt nêm tỵng hỵp, xỵt ỵ̈yp gia vỵ và các lỵai xỵt khác (ngỵ̈ai trỵ sỵn phỵm có nhãn không chỵa chỵt gluten)

Tôi có thỵ ỵn trái cây, rau cỵi, gỵo, quinoa, bỵt kiỵu mỵch, giỵng rau dỵn, bỵp, khoai tây, ỵ̈yu, các lỵai rau ỵ̈yu, hỵt kê, cây và hỵt bo bo, gà, các lỵai thỵt ỵ̈y, cá, trỵng, bỵ sỵa, chỵt béo và dỵu ỵn, dỵm cỵt, nỵỵc súp nỵu, và nỵỵc cỵt thỵt làm xỵt, nỵu nhỵ các thỵc ỵn này không nỵu chung vỵi bỵt mì, ruỵt bánh mì hoỵc các lỵai xỵt.

Xin vui lòng chuỵn bỵ thỵc ỵn cỵa tôi theo phỵỵng thỵc tránh liên hỵ vỵi lúa mì. Sỵ dỵng nỵỵc sỵch, dỵu, nỵi, chỵo và muỵng nỵa riêng biỵt. Nỵu nhỵ bỵn không chỵc chỵn vỵ các chỵt chỵa trong thỵc phỵm, xin vui lòng cho tôi biỵt, tôi có thỵ cung cỵp thêm vỵ thông tin này. Xin cỵm ỵn bỵn giúp tôi thỵỵng thỵc mỵt bỵa ỵn ngon miỵng và an tòan cho sỵc khỵe.

(*Gluten la hon hop dam co tinh dinh (nhu nhua), con lai sau khi loc tinh bot. Chat nay co chua trong lua mi va lua mach den, giu mot vai tro quan trong trong viec lam banh mi. Khi nhoi voi nuoc, gluten tro nen dinh va giu duoc khong khi de tao thanh bot nhoi. Tre em nhay cam voi chat nay se bi benh tang phu.)

Gluten Free Meal Card   Vietnamese

To the Chef:

I am on a medically required diet and need to know how my food is prepared. I cannot eat wheat and gluten (gluten is found in wheat, rye and barley). Even the smallest amount of gluten can make me sick, and therefore I must avoid any food, sauce, or garnish containing gluten, and any of its byproducts. If you are not sure if a menu item, recipe or ingredient contains gluten, please let me know and I may be able to give you more information.

Foods that I can safely eat include:
- Beef, fish, lamb, pork, duck, goose and other poultry such as chicken and turkey, rabbit, seafood, tofu, and most soy products (except soy sauce made with wheat)
- Eggs
- Dairy products
- Fruits and juice, vegetables, coconut, bean sprouts
- All beans, legumes, nuts, peanut butter
- Bean threads, cellophane noodles, congee, crepes (banh xeo) made with 100% rice flour, dumplings made with 100% rice flour, glass noodles, rice, rice noodles, rice sticks, rice vermicelli, spring roll wrappers that are 100% rice
- Homemade stocks and broths (that do not contain wheat)
- Pure spices and herbs, distilled vinegars that do not contain malt, wheat free soy sauce, fish sauce (nuoc mam, nuoc cham)
- Oils
- Distilled alcohol, wine

Foods that I cannot safely eat (unless they have been checked to be gluten free) include:
- Imitation crab meat, seitan and artificial meat substitutes
- Chinese noodles, dumplings made with wheat flour, egg noodles, egg roll wrappers, French bread, wonton wrappers
- Puddings, nems (fried pastry)
- Fish or oyster sauce thickened with wheat flour
- Seasoning blends (that have not been checked for gluten), soy sauce, tamari sauce, teriyaki sauce, hoisin sauce, hydrolyzed vegetable protein
- Bouillon cubes, canned stocks and broths, packaged soup bases, some marinades, rice and malt vinegar
- Beer

If a label says that a food product was made on equipment that processes wheat, rye or barley, I cannot eat it. If the label says malt or barley, I cannot eat it.

In the Preparation of my Food:

Please prepare my food in a safe way to avoid cross contamination with wheat, rye, and barley. Use fresh water, separate oil, pots, pans, colanders and utensils.

Thank you for preparing my meal in a creative way that includes safe foods so I can have a wonderful dining experience.

Thÿc ÿÿn không chÿa gluten Vietnamese
Do nhu cÿu sÿc khÿe,
tôi ÿÿÿc yêu cÿu ÿn uÿng theo mÿt chÿ ÿÿ ÿÿc biÿt và cÿn biÿt thÿc ÿÿn cÿa tôi ÿÿÿc chuÿn bÿ nhÿ thÿ nào. Tôi không thÿ ÿn lúa mì và gluten (có trong lúa mì, lúa mÿch ÿen và lúa mÿch). Ngay cÿ vÿi mÿt lÿÿng gluten nhÿ nhÿt cÿng có thÿ làm cho tôi bÿ bÿnh và vì vÿy tôi phÿi tránh bÿt kÿ thÿc ÿn, xÿt, hay các lÿai thÿo mÿc dùng ÿÿ trang trí trên thÿc ÿn có chÿa gluten và các sÿn phÿm phÿ cÿa nó. Nÿu nhÿ bÿn không rõ là trong các món trong thÿc ÿÿn, công thÿc pha chÿ hay nguyên vÿt liÿu có chÿa chÿt gluten hay không, xin vui lòng cho tôi biÿt, tôi có thÿ cung cÿp thêm vÿ thông tin này.

Các thÿc ÿn tôi có thÿ dùng an tòan gÿm có:
- Thÿt bò, cá, thÿt cÿu, heo, vÿt, ngÿng và các lÿai gia cÿm nhÿ gà thÿÿng và gà tây, thÿ, ÿÿ biÿn, ÿÿu hÿ, và hÿu hÿt các sÿn phÿm ÿÿu nành (ngÿai trÿ tÿÿng làm vÿi lúa mì)
- Trÿng
- Bÿ sÿa
- Trái cây và nÿÿc trái cây, rau cÿi, dÿa, giá.
- Tÿt cá các lÿai ÿÿu, rau ÿÿu, hÿt, bÿ ÿÿu phÿng
- Bean threads, bún sÿi, congee, bánh xèo làm bÿng 100% bÿt gÿo, bánh bao làm bÿng 100% bÿt gÿo, bún trong, gÿo, bún gÿo, miÿn, bánh tráng gói gÿi cuÿn làm bÿng 100% gÿo.
- Nÿÿc súp thÿt và gà nÿu (không chÿ a lúa mì)
- Các lÿai thÿo mÿc và gia vÿ nguyên chÿt, dÿm cÿt không chÿa mÿch nha, tÿÿng không chÿa gluten, nÿÿc mÿm
- Dÿu ÿn
- Cÿn và rÿÿu chÿng cÿt

Các thÿc ÿn không an tòan cho sÿc khÿe mà tôi không thÿ dung (trÿ khi ÿÿÿc kiÿm tra là không chÿa chÿt gluten) gÿm có:
- Thÿt cua giÿ, seitan và thÿc phÿm thÿt nhân tÿo
- Mì, bánh bao bÿt làm bÿng bÿt mì, mì trÿng, vÿ bánh gói chÿ giò, bánh mì Pháp, vÿ bánh gói hòanh thánh
- Bánh pudding, chÿ giò chiên
- Nÿÿc mÿm hoÿc dÿu hào ÿÿc làm vÿi bÿt mì
- Bÿt nêm tÿng hÿp (không ÿÿÿc kiÿm tra chÿt gluten), tÿÿng ÿÿu nành, tÿÿng me, tÿÿng teriyaki, tÿÿng hoisin, rau ÿÿm ÿÿÿc thÿy phân
- Bÿt nêm súp cô ÿÿc, nÿÿc súp thÿt và gà lon, nÿÿc cÿt súp ÿóng gói, mÿt sÿ nÿÿc sÿt ÿÿp thÿt, gÿo và dÿm mÿch nha
- Bia

- Nÿu trên nhãn cho biÿt thÿc phÿm ÿã ÿÿÿc sÿn xuÿt bÿng các thiÿt bÿ chÿ biÿn lúa mì, lúa mÿch ÿen hay lúa mÿch, tôi không thÿ ÿn ÿÿÿc. Nÿu trên nhãn cho biÿt có lúa mÿch hay mÿch nha, tôi cÿng không thÿ ÿn ÿÿÿc.

Chuÿn bÿ cho thÿc ÿn cÿa tôi:
Xin vui lòng chuÿn bÿ thÿc ÿn cÿa tôi theo phÿÿng thÿc an tòan, tránh liên hÿ vÿi lúa mì, lúa mÿch ÿen và lúa mÿch. Sÿ dÿng nÿÿc sÿch, dÿu, nÿi, cháo, rÿ và muÿng nÿa riêng biÿt.
Xin cám ÿn ÿã chuÿn bÿ cho tôi mÿt thÿc ÿÿn ÿÿy sáng tÿo cùng vÿi các thÿc ÿn tÿt cho sÿc khÿe ÿÿ tôi có thÿ thÿÿng thÿc mÿt bÿa ÿn tuyÿt vÿi.

PART III: MAKING YOUR LIFE HEALTHY, HAPPY, AND UNCOMPLICATED

Making It Easy for Family and Friends

Telling Others about Your Gluten Sensitivity

Most people who change their diet for medical reasons are able to vary their food choices during special events such as a birthday, wedding, or vacation. However, with celiac disease this is not the case. Cheating is never allowed—this is the most difficult thing to get others to understand. After all, "a little taste can't hurt once in a while, can it?" And you will have to explain to them that it will.

You are following a gluten-free diet because you are ill, and as long as you follow this diet strictly, you won't get sick. It is important to convey to them what gluten is, how it is added to many foods, and that even the smallest amount can hurt you.

Encourage them to read about it, and explain to them that this is not your choice, but something which is medically required. Most importantly, stress the difficulties of cross-contamination. Be understanding. It is a hard concept to grasp. After all, they have seen you eating gluten in the past; how could it be such a big problem all of a sudden? Remember how difficult and confusing it was for you, too, when you first heard about it.

It will be hard for them to learn what is safe to eat when they are not living with it every day. They will be as shocked as you were that soups, salad dressings, and seasonings may have gluten added to them. They will try to prepare special meals for you only to find out you can't have the salad because of the croutons, or the turkey because it is self-basting. In an effort to make things easier for you, they may even search out gluten-free restaurants. These are the acts of a caring, supportive friend or relative.

Of course, some individuals are more supportive than others. There are those who just don't get it, and don't want to get it. These people won't even try to understand. They may think that you are just being picky and are making a big deal out of nothing. This is especially true when you have not been officially labeled or diagnosed with celiac disease and are saying that you have a non-celiac gluten sensitivity. In these situations, expect little support: you are on your own, and they may not go out of their way to accommodate you.

Most of us know both types of people, so instead of trying to explain why you are following a gluten-free diet, start out by giving them a copy of "*Getting Started Living GlutenFree,*" or print a copy of the chart at www.glutenfreehasslefree.com/facts/living/living.asp. In addition, print them out a copy of the English dining-out sheets found in Chapter 12 or at www.glutenfreeeasy.com/facts/living/cards.asp to make it easier for them to understand what foods are gluten-free.

Getting Started Living Gluten-Free

Living with someone who has celiac disease or non-celiac gluten sensitivity can be hard. But as hard as it is for you, it is ten times harder for them, because they have to deal with it every single time they eat.

Celiac disease and non-celiac gluten sensitivity are conditions in which a person can't eat gluten without getting sick. Gluten is a protein found in wheat, rye, and barley. The biggest difficulty in avoiding gluten is that it is often added to foods where you wouldn't expect to find it. It can turn up in seasonings, sauces, dressings, and condiments, and it can be used in fillers, thickeners, and binders. That's why people who have to live gluten-free have to question every single food that they put into their mouths.

Celiac disease and non-celiac gluten sensitivity is permanent; it never goes away. Even eating the smallest amount of gluten will start a whole array of negative reactions within their body. Crazy as it sounds, if a crouton gets put on their salad and they remove it, those few crouton crumbs may contain enough gluten to make them ill.

When someone is unable to eat gluten, they can't even use a toaster that has previously toasted wheat bread—or mayonnaise when someone might have spread some on a piece of bread and then put the knife back into the jar.

Unlike other health problems that let you make exceptions from your eating regimen once in a while, people who have celiac disease never can. Each exposure to gluten may cause an attack. That's why they may seem absurdly careful—and why they'll be so adamant about never eating the slightest bit of gluten, even on a special occasion like their birthday. (For someone with celiac disease, it can take up to three years of being completely gluten-free to recover from any damage that eating gluten may do to their body.)

When the gluten sensitivity is due to celiac disease, there is a risk of developing other health problems if a gluten-free diet is not followed strictly, such as

- Thyroid disease
- Cancer
- Type 1 diabetes
- Anemia
- Osteoporosis
- Autoimmune liver failure
- Lupus
- Rheumatoid arthritis
- Severe gastrointestinal problems
- Frequent infections
- Skin problems

So when someone in your life suffers from any gluten sensitivity, take seriously what they say and do—and what they ask of you—because it may make the difference between sickness and health for them.

Make It Easier for Children

As difficult as it is for adults to follow a gluten-free diet, it is so much harder for children. Sometimes children are so young you can't even explain to them why they can't eat like everybody else. Many times, others looking after them, such as babysitters or daycare or preschool workers, may not understand the diet. Another issue is that people with good intentions frequently offer food to children as a treat. Even if you have made every effort to inform others about your child's dietary needs, there is always a possibility that someone doesn't really understand the instructions you have provided. Also let's not forget that children often share their food with friends, so the source of the gluten-containing food could be another child.

Make sure you take extra steps as needed to ensure safety. Write a note to the school and the teachers explaining the seriousness of your child's dietary needs. Keep a quick list of safe and unsafe foods to give to every caregiver. Bring in an assortment of safe snacks that are similar to those the school will be giving out to make sure your child doesn't feel left out. Make it clear that you do not want your child sitting there watching other children having cupcakes while they can't have anything. You need to be informed ahead of time about parties so you can arrange for special treats. It is always a good idea to make delicious frosted gluten-free cupcakes in batches and freeze them so all you need to do is take them out of the freezer whenever a quick gluten-free treat is needed.

Make sure you pack fun lunches, and get your child involved with label-reading and meal planning so he or she can better understand what is safe to eat. Make sure holidays and special occasions are just as special for your child. Make most holiday choices gluten-free so everyone can have the same meal with less chance of cross-contamination.

When it comes to parties, it is absolutely necessary to call the host ahead of time and find out about the menu. Prepare choices that are similar to those that the other children will be having. The last thing you want is for your child to feel like he or she is missing something. Try to bring foods that will be appealing to everyone so that the gluten-free food seems like a special treat, not a penalty. When it comes to camps and activities, look into gluten-free camps so kids can feel part of a group instead of feeling singled out.

In your house, keep gluten-free food within reach for your children and unsafe foods out of sight. Help teenagers discover safe choices that are available at fast food restaurants and on the go so that they can hang out with their friends without feeling like they don't fit in. The easier and more enjoyable you can make it, the better it will be for both you and your children.

How Not to Be a Party Pooper

Going to a party is all about having fun, seeing family and friends, mingling, and catching up. The last thing you want to have happen is to have a bad reaction to the gluten in the food and have to leave early. But going around and asking a million questions about the food, or telling everyone that you cannot eat anything, is bound to make you and others feel bad. So what to do?

Call the host ahead and find out about the menu. Offer to bring a dish and a dessert—this way, you'll know there will be some safe choices for you. If it is a set menu, explain that you are on a medically required diet and ask if it is okay to just bring a separate dish of food for you. This will be especially helpful when it is a large party and the host is already overwhelmed. In many cases, the host will ask what you can have and offer to prepare items in a way that will be safe for you. Each situation is unique and should be handled as you think will work best.

Sometimes you may not know the host well enough to call ahead about the menu. In this case, find out what you can, have a little something before you go to the party, and always bring something with you to complement any meal, such as an appetizer or dessert. If you are not a great cook, prepare one of the simple recipes in this book, pick up something at a gluten-free restaurant, or make up a cold antipasta platter—always a great option. Don't make the party just about the food. It's about having a good time!

Making Social Events Easier for Everyone

If you are following a gluten-free diet, being prepared will make social events easier for everyone. Always carry snacks with you so that when everyone stops to grab something at the local hot dog/pretzel stand, you can have something, too. Look up lists of gluten-free restaurants, or call other restaurants ahead of time so you can evaluate what will be available for you. When you are confident about what you can have, it is much more enjoyable. Planning ahead makes it better for everyone. The trick is to find ways to enjoy every situation. Bring gluten-free candy or popcorn to the movie theater, bring your favorite gluten-free cookies to a birthday party, and bring a show-stopping appetizer to a barbecue.

You should never have to feel deprived—social events are made to be social, and they should always be enjoyed.

Making It Easy for Yourself

Tips for Everyday Gluten-Free Eating

There are many foods that are naturally gluten-free; it is only when we start combining and mixing foods that gluten secretly creeps in. Although wheat has been used as the base of many recipes, it does not have to be. When it comes to our foods, we really shouldn't have to refer to our gluten-free foods as gluten-free—they are just foods. But since gluten is added to so many food choices, for now we will have to identify which foods are safe for us to eat, and which are unsafe.

Today, the world is starting to discover the importance of having gluten-free selections, and in the future it will be increasingly easier to live gluten-free. For now, in order for us to find safe food choices, stick with these simple tips:

1. Pick foods that are naturally gluten-free.

2. Learn how to read labels to identify gluten-free products.

3. Call manufactures when you are in doubt.

It is important to stay on track with gluten-free eating. Even if you don't feel ill when you eat gluten, many people have silent celiac disease. Having even the smallest amounts of gluten can cause silent damage to your health. Knowing how to deal with a gluten-contaminated world is essential to protecting your health. Here are some easy tips: (1) carry toaster-safe bags to make it possible to toast up your gluten-free breads when using shared toasters; (2) look up gluten-free restaurants for safe selections; (3) carry safe foods and seasoning agents with you; (4) join local celiac organizations to benefit from the research that other people have done; (5) when in doubt, reach for one of your safe snack options.

Easy-to-Carry Gluten-Free Snacks

Snacks are an important part of everybody's day. Most people don't plan ahead, they just grab snacks while they are on the run. Since gluten-free snacks may not be available everywhere you go, it is important to know what to pack so that you will always be prepared. The following are some gluten-free snacks:

- Dried fruits (double-check to make sure your dried fruit isn't dusted with wheat or oat flour)

- Dried vegetables

- Fresh fruit or fruit cups

- Gluten-free crackers or cheese puffs or crisps or chips

- To the gluten-free crackers add dried fruit or any of the following; unseasoned nuts, cheese sticks, and peanut butter (available in individual single servings)

- Individual gluten-free puddings, canned fruit, and Jell-O

- Gluten-free yogurt or yogurt shakes

- Gluten-free pretzels

- Gluten-free popcorn, potato chips, apple chips, or corn chips

- Gluten-free fruit rollups

- Gluten-free cereal blends

- Gluten-free rice cakes

- Gluten-free energy bars and cookies

- Gluten-free shakes such as Boost, Ensure, Glucerna, Pediasure, Nutrashake, Nutren, and Nutren Jr.

- Fruit juices

Gluten-Free Eating in Unexpected Situations

No matter how carefully you try to plan, there will inevitably be situations when you will need to just wing it. Imagine that

- You are on a cruise to an exotic island, it is 100 degrees, and the buffet meal is being served by individuals who don't speak English.

- You are on a three-day scuba diving and boating trip.

- You are at a ski resort, and all your gluten-free supplies are back at the cabin.

- You have gotten last-minute tickets to a baseball game and didn't have time to pick up your supplies.

- You are in a business meeting where you are the low man on the chain of command, and it is a three-day meeting, 9 a.m. to 9 p.m., with all meals being catered in.

We live in the real world, and we can't account for everything. It is important to try to make the most appropriate choices whenever possible. There will be times when you just have to do what you can, so learning as much as you can about gluten-free living and cooking techniques makes you better prepared to deal with each situation as it comes up. Although it may not be easy to carry snacks with you everywhere, or to call ahead to evaluate menus for every restaurant, following these guidelines makes it possible for you to have the best experience you can.

Can Just a Little Gluten Hurt?

It is usually the consumption of small amounts of gluten that keeps a person with celiac disease from getting well. Most people who are trying to follow a gluten-free diet do so with a majority of their food choices. They stock up on gluten-free breads and snacks, watch what they order when they go out, they generally feel that they are making the best possible choices. It is the things they forget to check, such as medications, vitamins, mouthwash, and toothpaste (check out www.glutenfreedrugs.com for the gluten-free status of many medications).

Today, many scientists are working on methods to reduce gluten sensitivity for those with celiac disease. The future seems promising, and it may provide a way to consume gluten again, at least in small amounts. But for now, even the smallest amount of gluten can cause a reaction, and so it should always be avoided. Knowing what questions to ask can make things so much easier.

D's Dieting Dilemmas

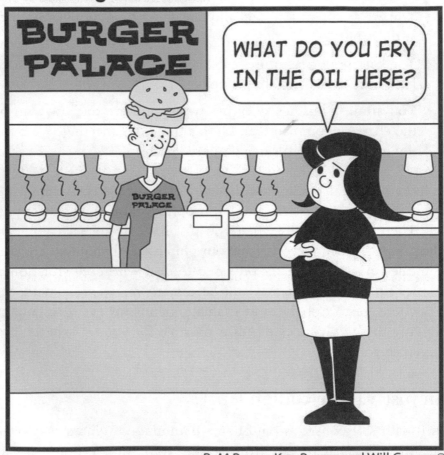

ByM Brown Ken Brown and Will Cypser ©

Learning More about Gluten and Your Health

The Hidden Faces of Celiac Disease

The dangers of untreated or undiagnosed celiac disease may have many consequences. In this section, we will explore the dangers we commonly see when gluten is not eliminated from the diet.

Vitamin and Mineral Deficiencies

Untreated celiac disease often leads to vitamin and mineral deficiencies, which may lead to conditions such as anemia and osteoporosis. The deficiencies might not be obvious, as is the case with calcium and vitamin D (causing osteoporosis). It is a cycle where continued consumption of gluten will continue to negatively affect the absorption of these key vitamins and minerals.

Neurological Disorders

Another common problem found with untreated celiac disease is neurological disorders. These nervous system disorders can lead to problems such as ataxia, seizures, and neuropathy. Ataxia is a lack of coordination. It can occur in your muscles or in your ability to speak. It can be also effect the inner ear. This means that you can suffer from vertigo and dizziness. If it affects your eyes, you might have poor hand–eye coordination.

Seizures are changes in behavior that occur from abnormal electrical activity in the brain. Seizures can be very mild or severe. The mild forms could lead to simple changes in feelings, such as a sudden feeling of fear or changes in vision. The most severe types will cause unconsciousness and terrible body twitching. Neuropathy is a broad term that means problems with your nerves. It can present as pain, numbness, weakness, or tingling. Some people may even feel an extreme sensitivity to touch.

The Dangers of Untreated Celiac Disease

Some other complications that occur from untreated celiac disease can range from things as simple as lactose intolerance to things as dangerous as primary biliary cirrhosis (which in severe cases may require a liver transplant). In some cases, illnesses may be reversed from switching to a gluten-free diet; in other cases, the damage is irreversible. The list of health issues that may be related to celiac disease is so extensive that it is hard to believe; many of them are listed in Chapter 1. Some of the more common problems include infertility, osteoporosis, gastrointestinal problems, anemia, and thyroid disease.

It is important to understand that even though the treatment for celiac disease is only a change in diet, not changing your diet could be life-threatening.

Cancers

Cancer is one of the more serious risks of untreated celiac disease. Most frequently, such cancer is located in the intestinal tract, which includes the esophagus (the tube that brings food from your mouth to your stomach), stomach, and small intestine. Other cancers that might occur include thyroid or lymphoma (specifically, non-Hodgkin's lymphoma).

Autoimmune Diseases

When celiac disease goes undiagnosed, there is an increased risk of other autoimmune diseases. Autoimmune diseases occur when our immune system attacks our own body. The following diseases that have been associated with celiac disease.

Type 1 diabetes, an autoimmune disease, causes your body to stop making the hormone insulin by damaging the cells of the pancreas that make the hormone. The insulin is needed to move the sugar from your blood into your cells. Without it, your body cells cannot get the energy from the foods you eat, and the amount of sugar in your blood becomes very high, causing damage to the eyes, kidneys, nerves, and blood vessels.

The thyroid is the organ that regulates your metabolism. It also determines how many calories a day you need to live. There are two autoimmune diseases of the thyroid: Grave's disease and Hashimoto's thyroiditis. In Grave's disease, the metabolism runs too quickly. Someone with Grave's disease loses weight, has frequent bowel movements, feels irritable, loses sleep, and has bulging eyes. Palpitations, increased blood pressure, and tremor may also occur. The thyroid grows and may need to be removed. In Hashimoto's thyroiditis, conversely, the metabolism runs too slowly. Those with this disease gain weight, are sensitive to cold, and have constipation, depression, migraines, muscle cramps, and infertility. If left untreated, it can cause failure of the muscles to work—including failure of the heart, which may lead to death. The disease is treated with thyroid hormone taken in a pill.

Connective tissue is a tissue in the body that is fibrous. It is what holds our organs in place, makes up the ligaments and tendons surrounding our joints, and forms the lymphoid tissues in our body, the fatty tissue, and the elastic tissue. The connective tissue diseases we often see in untreated celiac disease include systemic lupus erythematosus (SLE), rheumatoid arthritis, scleroderma, and Sjögren's syndrome. Let's look at each of these.

SLE is a disease that leads to an inflammation of the connective tissue in your body; thus, it can affect many areas in the body. The name comes from the typical appearance of a red rash on the face. The rash looks like a butterfly as it spreads over nose from one cheek to the other. People with the disease will have times of remission (no inflammation) and other times with flares (times with inflammation). It is a difficult disease to diagnose because of its complexity.

Rheumatoid arthritis is different from regular arthritis—which is really called osteoarthritis. Osteoarthritis is caused by damage to the joint, leading to inflammation. However, in rheumatoid arthritis, your immune system attacks the membrane surrounding the joints. It causes severe pain in the joints, as well as deformity. Rheumatoid arthritis can affect many organs, including the heart, lungs, and eyes.

Scleroderma is a disease that causes the development of scar tissue in the skin, internal organs, and small blood vessels. It causes these tissues to harden. There are two kinds: a localized kind known as morphea and a generalized kind known as systemic sclerosis. The localized disorder causes hardening of tissues that leads to disability. The systemic type can damage the heart, lungs, kidneys, and intestine, any of which may be fatal.

Sjögren's disease is also called Sjögren's syndrome. It causes damage to the exocrine glands. Exocrine glands are the glands that secrete products into ducts (versus endocrine glands, which secrete products into the bloodstream). The exocrine glands in our body are the ones that produce sweat, tears, breast milk, digestive enzymes (the proteins we need to break down food), and hormones. The symptoms, as you may have already guessed, are dry mouth and eyes. Besides the dryness of these areas, often there is dry skin, nose, and, in women, vagina. This disorder very often occurs with other autoimmune disorders like rheumatoid arthritis and scleroderma.

Infertility is defined as an inability to have a baby either through not getting pregnant or because of miscarriages. When celiac disease is untreated, there is a higher rate of infertility, something that is not very well understood at this time. Some suggest that it is related to the nutritional deficiencies seen with the illness. However, other possibilities include a problem with the reproductive cycle in women (shorter periods and earlier menopause) and gonadal dysfunction in men (problems making sperm).

Non-celiac Gluten Sensitivities and Autism

Autism

Autism spectrum disorders are a set of conditions that affect the brain and development. People with this disorder have a difficult time with social interaction and communication. They often have symptoms that include sensory integration problems, repetitive behaviors, and muscle weakness. Many people with autism are unable to make eye contact. They can have restrictive interests—for instance, focusing only on trains.

Little is known about what causes this disorder. However, some believe that it occurs after the start of vaccinations. Other causes could be heavy metal toxins, disruptions to immune development, and inborn errors of metabolism. There is definitely a genetic link. Most likely, someone is genetically predisposed to the disorder but does not develop it unless it is triggered by something else.

Some people with autism have gastrointestinal problems. These problems cause constipation, diarrhea, and vomiting. There is also a greater incidence of allergies in a person with autism. Food allergies and intolerances are more common. Some get relief from the stomach problems by eliminating gluten, casein (a protein found in milk), and, less frequently, soy protein.

However, there are some who do not have clear stomach problems or a clear intolerance to gluten who still do better when they stop consuming it. The theory as to why this happens, which is still unproven, is called leaky gut syndrome. It is speculated that in leaky gut syndrome, the gluten and casein proteins cannot be broken down. These larger proteins should not get into the body without being broken down, but the gut can be permeable, letting things in (see our discussion of probiotics in Chapter 9). The gluten and casein get into the body and act like opiates, similar to drugs like morphine, codeine, and opium. The opiatelike protein, like these drugs, causes neurological disturbances. Another theory is that these proteins cause an unusual immune reaction in the body.

By removing the gluten and casein from the diet, these proteins cannot get into the body and cause their damage or the immune response. Some parents of children with autism have found improvements in many areas when they remove gluten and casein (dairy) from the diet. The improvements vary from decreases in sensory-seeking behavior (like handflapping and toewalking) to improvement in eye contact and verbal communication. Not all children on this diet see improvement; its success varies from one case to the next.

It is suggested that the diet be tried for six months. If behavior changes are noted, continue for another six. At the one-year mark, it is a good idea to challenge the child to see if it was really the proteins, not some other therapy, that made the difference. Reintroduce each of the proteins. If the behaviors do not return, you can leave them in the diet. If they do return, eliminate them for good. Some people can have casein and not gluten, others gluten and not casein. Some can have neither gluten, casein, nor soy.

Best Resources for Gluten-Free Living

Celiac Organizations and Research Centers

American Celiac Disease Alliance (ACDA)
Alexandria, VA
1 (703) 622-3331
info@americanceliac.org

American Dietetic Association Nutrition Evidence Analysis Project
"Gluten Intolerance/Celiac Disease"
http://www.adaevidencelibrary.com/topic.cfm?cat=1403

Canadian Celiac Association (CCA)
Mississauga, ON
1 (800) 363-7296
http://www.celiac.ca

Children's Digestive Health and Wellness Foundation
http://www.celiachealth.org

Celiac Disease Foundation (CDF)
Studio City, CA
1 (818) 990-2354
1 (818) 990-2379 (fax)
http://www.celiac.org
cdf@celiac.org

Celiac Disease Clinic, Department of Internal Medicine, Gastroenterology,
University of Iowa
Iowa City, IA
1 (319) 356-4060
http://www.uihealthcare.com

Celiac Disease Program at Boston Children's Hospital, Gastroenterology
and Nutrition Division
Boston, MA
1 (617) 355-2127

Celiac Forums
http://www.celiacforums.com

Celiac Sprue Association (CSA)
Omaha, NE
1 (877) 272-4272
1 (402) 558-0600
1 (402) 558-1347 (fax)
http://www.csaceliacs.org
celiac@csaceliacs.org

Children's Digestive Health and Nutrition Foundation: Celiac (CDHNF)
http://www.cdhnf.org
http://www.celiachealth.org

Gluten-Free Certification Organization (GFCO)
Auburn, WA
1 (253) 218-2956
http://www.gfco.org

Gluten Intolerance Group (GIG): SE
Seattle, WA
1 (206) 246-6652
1 (206) 246-6531 (fax)
http://www.gluten.net
info@gluten.net

National Institutes of Health (NIH) Celiac Disease Awareness Campaign:
Bethesda, MD
1 (800) 891-5389
http://www.celiac.nih.gov

National Institute of Digestive Diseases Information Clearinghouse:
Celiac Disease
http://www.digestive.niddk.nih.gov/ddiseases/pubs/celiac/

National Foundation for Celiac Awareness (NFCA)
1 (215) 325-1306
1 (215) 283-2335

http://www.celiacawareness.org
info@celiacawareness.org

North American Society for Pediatric Gastroenterology, Hepatology and Nutrition
http://www.naspghan.org/sub/celiac disease.asp

U.S. Department of Health and Human Services/National Institutes of Health
http://www.nih.gov

Educational Institutions

American College of Gastroenterology: Digestive Health SmartBrief
http://www.smartbrief.com/dhsb/?campaign=acg
Celiac Disease Clinic at Mayo Clinic
http://www.mayoclinic.org/celiac-disease
1 (507) 284-5255 (patients)
1 (507) 284-2631 (medical professionals)

William K. Warren Medical Research Center for Celiac Disease and the Clinical Center for Celiac Disease at the University of California
San Diego, CA
1 (858) 534-4622
http://celiaccenter.ucsd.edu/

Celiac Disease Center at Columbia University
http://www.celiacdiseasecenter.columbia.edu
1 (212) 305-5590

Celiac Center at Beth Israel Deaconess Medical Center, Harvard Medical School
http://www.bidmc.harvard.edu/celiaccenter
1(617) 667-1272

Celiac Group at University of Virginia Health System, Digestive Health Center of Excellence

http://www.healthsystem.virginia.edu/internet/digestive-health/
patientcare.cfm
1 (434) 243-9309

The Culinary Institute of America (culinary school offering gluten-free
cooking classes)
http://www.ciachef.edu/enthusiasts/programs
1 (800) 888-7850

The Natural Gourmet Cooking School, Natural Food Cooking School
http://www.naturalgourmetschool.com
1 (212) 645-5170

Mayo Clinic
http://www.mayoclinic.com
1 (480) 301-8000

Simon Fraser University
http://www.sfu.cal~jfremont/celiac.htlm

Stanford Celiac Sprue Management Clinic, Stanford Medical Center
Stanford, CA
1 (650) 723-6961
http://www.stanfordhospital.com/clincsmedservices/clincs/
gastroenterology/celiacsprue

St. Johns University, NY (brings together gluten-intolerant people from
around the world)
listserv@maelstrom.stjhns.edu

University of Chicago Celiac: Disease Program
1 (773) 702-7593
http://www.celiacdisease.net

University of Maryland Center for Celiac Research
http://www.celiaccenter.org
1 (410) 328-6749

University of Virgina: Celiac Support Group
http://www.healthsystem.virginia.edu/internet/digestive-health/
nutrition/celiacsupport.cfm

Autistic Sites

Autism Research Institute
http://www.autism.com/ari/

Autism Society of America
http://www.autism-society.org/site/PageServer

Autism Speaks
http://www.autismspeaks.org

National Institute of Child Health and Human Development
http://nichd.nih.gov/autism/

General Gluten Free Information

CarolFenster
http://www.Glutenfree101.com

Celiac.com
http://www.Celiac.com

Celiacs, Inc.
http://www.e-celiacs.org

The Celiac Site
http://www.TheCeliacSite.com

Celiac Frequently Asked Questions (FAQ)
http://www.enabling.org/ia/celiac/faq.html

Clan Thompson Celiac Page
http://www.celiacsite.com/index.php3

Finer Health & Nutrition
http://www.finerhealth.com

Gfree Cuisine (GF recipes & menus)
http://www.GfreeCuisine.com

Gluten-Free Easy
http://www.glutenfreeeasy.com

Glutenfreeda Online Cooking Magazine
http://www.glutenfreeda.com

Gluten-Free-Online.com
http://www.gluten-free-online.com

Karina's Kitchen (gluten-free recipes)
http://www.Glutenfreegoddess.blogspot.com

Marlisa Brown's Web site and blog
Web site: http://www.glutenfreeeasy.com
Blog: http://www.glutenfreeguru.com

Shelly Case's Gluten-Free Web site
http://glutenfreediet.ca

The Gluten-Free Kitchen (GF recipes)
http://gfkitchen.server101.com

The Gluten-Free Page: Celiac Disease/Gluten Intolerance Web sites
http://gflinks.com

Tricia Thompson's Web site
http://www.glutenfreedietitian.com

Meijer Stores (posts gluten-free products available at their locations)
http://www.meijerhealthyliving.com

Food Labeling Resources

United States

Information regarding the food allergen labeling and consumer protection act of 2004: http://www.cfsan.fda.gov/~dms/alrgqa.html

Questions and answers on the gluten-free labeling proposed rule: http://www.cfsan.fda.gov/~dms/glutqa.html

Keep an eye on gluten-free labeling in the United States: http://www.cfsan.fda.gov/~dms/lab-cat.html#gluten

U.S. Department of Health and Human Services Dietary Guidelines: http://www.health.gov/DietaryGuidelines

U.S. Department of Agriculture Food Safety and Inspection Service: http://www.fsis.usda.gov/regulations_&policies/FAQs_forNotice_45-05/index.asp

Canada

Information regarding the food allergen labeling amendments: http://www.hc-sc.gc.ca/fn-an/label-etiquet/allergen/guide_ligne_direct_indust-eng.php

Questions and answers on the labeling of food allergens: http://www.inspection.gc.ca/english/fssa/labeti/allerg/allergee.shtml

Europe

European Starch Association, allergen labeling: www.aaf-eu.org/PDF/Statement_on_permanent_obtained_for_allergen_labelling_11-2007.pdf

Labs

Kimball Genetics (DNA testing)
1 (800) 320-1807
http://www.kimballgenetics.com

Prometheus Labs (celiac diagnostic testing)
1 (888) 423-5227 Opt. #3
http://www.prometheuslabs.com

Medications and Supplements

Gluten-Free Drugs
http://www.glutenfreedrugs.com

Other

Alternative Cook (gluten-free cooking DVDs)
http://www.alternativecook.com

Dietary Guidelines
http://www.healthierus.gov/dietaryguidelines

Toaster bags
http://www.toastibags.com

Whole Grains Council (information on whole grains)
http://www.wholegrainscouncil.org

To find a registered dietitian in your area: http://www.glutenfreedietitian
.com/newsletter/?page_id=14

Allergy-Friendly Foods

Allergaroo
6614 Clayton Road
#226
Saint Louis, MO 63117
1 (314) 256-1433
1 (314) 667-3370 (fax)
info@allergaroo.com
http://www.allergaroo.com

Allergyfree Foods
310 West Hightower Drive
Dawsonville, GA 30534
1 (706) 265-1317
1 (706) 265-1281
info@allergyfreefoods.com
http://www.allergyfreefoods.com

Dining Out and Travel

AIC (Italian Celiac Association) Eating Out Project for Italy
http://www.celiachia.it/ristoratori/default_eng.asp

Bob and Ruth's Gluten-Free Dining and Travel Club (traveling gluten-free)
http://www.bobandruths.com

Celiac Travel
http://www.celiactravel.com/index.html

Dining Info Service from Coeliac UK (gluten-free travel information)
http://www.gluten-free-onthego.com

GIG Gluten Intolerance Group (restaurants with gluten-free restaurants)
http://www.gluten.net

Gluten-Free Culinary Summit (gluten-free annual culinary program)
http://www.theglutenfreelifestyle.com

Gluten-Free Delights (lists of gluten-free restaurants)
http://www.GFDelights.com

The Gluten-Free Guide to Italy, by Maria Ann Roglieri, PhD
http://www.gfguideitaly.com

The Gluten-Free Guide to New York
http://www.gfguideny.com

Gluten-Free Passport (booklets on gluten-free travel)
http://www.glutenfreepassport.com

Gluten-Free on the Go (Lists of gluten-free restaurants)
http://www.Glutenfreeonthego.com

Gluten-Free Restaurant Awareness Program (GFRAP) (lists of gluten-free restaurants) http://www.glutenfreerestaurants.org

Gluten-Free Travel Site (gluten-free travel information)
http://www.glutenfreetravelsite.com

Living with Cards
http://www.livingwithout.com/diningcards.html

Triumph Dining Cards (dining-out cards)
http://www.triumphdining.com/diningcards.aspx

Gluten-Free Books

American Dietetic Association's Celiac Disease Nutrition Guide, www.eatright.org

Canadian Celiac Association Pocket Dictionary: Ingredients for the Gluten-Free Diet

Celiac Disease: A Hidden Epidemic, Dr. Peter Green and Rory Jones

Celiac Disease: A Guide to Living with Gluten Intolerance, Sylvia Llewelyn Bower, Mary Kay Sharrett, and Steve Plogsted

Cooking Free, Carol Fenster

Gluten-Free Baking with the Culinary Institute of America, Richard J. Coppedge, Jr., and George Chookazian.

Gluten-Free Cooking for Dummies, Dana Korn and Connie Sarros

Gluten-Free Diet: A Comprehensive Resource Guide, Shelley Case

Gluten-Free Girl: How I Found the Food That Loves Me Back and How You Can, Too, Shauna James Ahern

Gluten-Free Everyday Cookbook, Robert M. Landolphi

Gluten-Free Grocery Shopping Guide (lists gluten-free foods), Matison and Matison

Gluten-Free 101, Carol Fenster

Going Gluten-Free: How to Get Started, Chris Ford and Rodney Ford

Guidelines for a Gluten-Free Lifestyle, Celiac Disease Foundation, www.celiac.org

Living with Celiac Disease: Abundance beyond Wheat and Gluten, Claudine Crangle

Living Gluten-Free for Dummies, Danna Korn

Living Gluten-Free Answer Book, Suzanne Bowland

Tell Me What to Eat If I Have Celiac Disease, Kimberly A. Tessmer

The Gluten-Free Nutrition Guide, Tricia Thompson

The Gluten-Free Gourmet Bakes Bread, Bette Hagman

The Gluten-Free Gourmet Cooks Comfort Foods: Creating Old Favorites with New Favorites, Bette Hagman

The Gluten-Free Gourmet Cooks Fast and Healthy: Wheat-Free and Gluten-Free with Less Fuss and Less Fat, Bette Hagman

1000 Gluten-Free Recipes, Carol Fenster

The Complete Idiot's Guide to Gluten-Free Eating, Eve Adamson and Tricia Thompson

The Essential Gluten-Free Restaurant Guide, Triumphdining

The Gluten-Free Bible, Jax Peters Lowell

The Gluten-Free Vegan, Susan O'Brien

The Gluten-Free Vegetarian Kitchen, Donna Klein

Wheat-Free Gluten-Free Cookbook for Kids and Busy Adults, Connie Sarros

Wheat-Free Gluten-Free Dessert Cookbook, Connie Sarros

The Wheat-Free Cook Gluten-Free Recipes for Everyone, Jacqueline Mallorca

Wheat-Free Recipes and Menus, Carol Fenster

Gluten-Free Publications

Living *Without* magazine
1 (847) 480-8810
http://www.livingwithout.com

The Gluten-Free Baker Newsletter
Sandra Leonard
1 (513) 878-3221
Thebakers@Cris.com

Gluten-Free Living
http://www.glutenfreeliving.com
Info@glutenfreeliving.com

Glutenfreeda (online cooking magazine)
http://www.glutenfreeda.com
Scott Free Newsletter
Scott Adams
http://www.celiac.com

Shopping Guides

Gluten-Free Grocery Shopping Guide, Matison & Matison
http://www.ceceliasmarketplace.com

Shopping Guide Data Base for PC and Palm OS, Pocket Shopping Guide
http://www.clanthompson.com

Tri-County Celiac Support Group Shopping Guide and Newsletter
http://www.tccg.com

Restaurants with Gluten-Free Menus

The following is a listing of restaurants that either have a gluten-free menu or have identified gluten-free menu choices:

Blooms Deli
http://www.bloomsnewyorkdeli.com

Bonefish Grill
http://www.bonefishgrill.com

Boston Market
http://www.bostonmarket.com

Buca di Beppo
http://www.bucadibeppo.com

Bugaboo Creek Steakhouse
http://www.bugaboocreeksteakhouse.com

Canyons Restaurant
http://www.canyonsrestaurant.com

Carrabba's Italian Grill
http://www.carrabbas.com

Cheeseburger in Paradise
http://www.cheeseburgerinparadise.com

Chevy's Fresh Mex
http://www.chevys.com

Don Pablo's
http://www.donpablos.com

El Chico
http://www.elchico.com

Legal Sea Foods
http://www.legalseafoods.com

Lilis 57
http://www.lilis57.com

Mamas
1352 Montauk Hwy
Oakdale, NY 11769
1 (631) 567-0909

Mitchell's Fish Market
http://www.mitchellsfishmarket.com

Naked Fish
http://www.nakedfish.com

Nizzo
http://www.nizzanyc.com

O'Naturals
http://www.onnaturals.com

Outback Steakhouse
http://www.outbacksteakhouse.com

P. F. Chang's China Bistro
http://www.pfchangs.com

Rice
http://www.riceny.com

Risotteria
http://www.risotteria.com

Sambuca
http://www.sambucanyc.com

Taco Del Mar
http://www.tacodelmar.com

Texas Roadhouse
http://www.texasroadhouse.com

Thaifoon
http://www.thaifoon.com

Uno's Chicago Pizeria
http://www.unos.com

Z'Tejas
http://www.ztejas.com

Marlisa Brown, MS, RD, CDE, CDN, is a registered dietitian, certified diabetes educator, chef, author, and international speaker. As president of Total Wellness Inc., for over 15 years Marlisa has worked as a nutritional consultant specializing in diabetes education, celiac disease, gastrointestinal disorders, cardiovascular disease, sports nutrition, culinary programs, and corporate wellness.

She is the author of *Gluten-Free, Hassle Free* and *Meal Plan Trios* and has contributed to many dietary programs and books, including Richard Simmons's *The Food Mover* program and cookbooks, Jorge Cruise's *The 3 Hour Diet*, Leslie Sansone's *Walk away the Pounds*, Kathy Smith's *Project: You! DM 2*, and Aspen's *Women's Sports Medicine and Rehabilitation*. Marlisa is also the creator of http://www.glutenfreeeasy.com, a comprehensive celiac Web site.

With over 30 years' culinary experience, she has been featured in over 50 cooking shows for the American Heart Association on International Cooking. Marlisa has also served as the past president of the New York State Dietetic Association and has been the recipient of the American Dietetic Association's "Emerging Dietetic Leader" award, the Long Island Dietetic Association's "Dietitian of the Year" award, LI Press's "2008/2009 Best of Long Island" award, and CW Post Long Island University's "Community Service Award."

Marlisa has a BS and MS from CW Post Long Island University and is currently listed on the university's Web site as an outstanding alumna. She has also studied at the Culinary Institute of America.

Index